# Left Brain, Right Brain

# Left Brain, Right Brain

## THIRD EDITION

### Sally P. Springer
University of California—Davis

### Georg Deutsch
University of Alabama—Birmingham

W. H. Freeman and Company
New York

bb:12135　　　# 18560131

Library of Congress Cataloging-in-Publication Data

Springer, Sally P.
　Left brain, right brain.

　Bibliography: p.
　Includes index.
　1. Cerebral dominance.　2. Brain—Localization of
functions.　3. Left and right (Psychology)　I. Deutsch,
Georg.　II. Title.
QP385.5.S67　1989　612′.825　88-30097
ISBN 0-7167-1999-1
ISBN 9-7167-2000-0 (pbk.)

Printed in the United States of America

3 4 5 6 7 8 9 0　VB　9 9 8 7 6 5 4 3 2 1

*To the memory of
Fanny Margulies and Peter Deutsch*

# Contents

# *Preface to the Third Edition*

Assigning functions to specific regions of the brain is a recurring theme in the relatively brief history of human brain research. Nowhere has this been more evident than in the attempt to divide human mental functions along the most obvious physical division of the brain—its separation into a left half and a right half. Asymmetries in hemispheric function were first discovered in the nineteenth century by observers who noted the differing effects of injury to the left and right halves of the brain. In the ensuing years, clinical investigators documented additional consistent differences in the behavioral consequences of such injuries.

Interest in hemispheric specialization dramatically increased after the split-brain operations of the 1960s and led to an explosion of research designed to characterize hemispheric differences and to explore their implications for human behavior. Considerable attention has been directed to seeing whether these differences may be related to such diverse phenomena as learning disabilities, psychiatric illness, and variations in cognitive styles among cultures. Although many advances in understanding have been made, the topic of functional asymmetry remains a controversial one, for at least two reasons. First, findings have not always been consistent; investigations designed to answer the same question have sometimes produced conflicting results. Second, the temptation to speculate and draw conclusions well beyond those justified by the data has been great.

This book is an attempt to bring together the major findings of research into the nature of hemispheric asymmetries. We first present basic findings on asymmetry in brain-damaged, split-brain, and normal subjects, and then we consider special topics such as left-handedness, sex differences in brain asymmetry, and the development of asymmetry. In providing an overview of the left brain and right brain, we have tried to separate what is reasonably established as fact from what is purely speculative without sacrificing the intrigue of either. In addition, we have sought wherever possible to identify potential explanations for inconsistent findings. We have also tried to show how the investigation of hemispheric asymmetry has yielded important insights about brain function in general. Studying the left brain and right brain is but one approach to brain research. We hope that this book conveys the sense in which it is a fruitful one.

For this, the third edition of *Left Brain, Right Brain*, we have not only updated the text with new information and discussions but we have also expanded the scope of the book. We have substantially expanded our coverage of the biological foundations of hemispheric asymmetry, reflecting the considerable progress that has been made in brain imaging techniques as well as the renewed theoretical interest in the biological bases of asymmetry. We believe that many of the discoveries to be made in the next decade will come from a biological orientation, and we wish to provide our readers with a state-of-the-art overview of the field as it is today. This new edition contains expanded theoretical discussions on a number of topics, including specific models of the nature of hemispheric differences and the function of the corpus callosum. The study of hemispheric asymmetry has matured over the last decade, and although much more remains to be learned, it has reached the stage where sophisticated theorizing is appropriate. We share some of that theorizing with our readers in this new edition.

As in the past, we have written with a relatively broad audience in mind. Our intention was to be as clear as possible without compromising accuracy or the complexity of the issues. We were pleased to see this book adopted in a variety of courses, including general studies in psychology and neuroscience, where cerebral laterality would be one aspect of a larger field. We also hope that this book will continue to interest general readers who would like to learn more about brain asymmetries and wish to go beyond oversimplified or exaggerated popular accounts.

We wish to thank several colleagues and friends for their contributions to *Left Brain, Right Brain* over the years. Bob Liebert got us started back in 1978 by asking for a reference reviewing the nature of hemispheric differences. When he was told that nothing appropriate was available, he suggested that perhaps it was time to write a book. Alan Rubens, Chuck Hamilton, Phil Bryden, Morris Moscovitch, Barry Lorinstein, Nick Goldberg, and Andy Papanicolaou each made valuable comments and suggestions on various aspects of the text. Our original, cumbersome title was shortened by Peter Schulman. At W. H. Freeman and Company, Judith Wilson and Jim Maurer provided us with the help needed to turn the manuscript of the first and the second editions, respectively, into books; Jonathan Cobb and Diane Maass have done the same for this new edition. In many ways we also owe a great debt to the readers of the previous editions of our book, especially those who took the trouble to tell us the ways in which they found the book useful and the topics they would like to see expanded or included. A very special note of thanks goes to our original editor, W. Hayward Rogers, who has now retired, for contributing unfailing enthusiasm for our efforts from the beginning.

Preparation of this new edition was complicated by the simultaneous start of new positions for both of us—the University of California, Davis for Sally P. Springer, and the University of Alabama, Birmingham for Georg Deutsch. Both institutions were very supportive of our efforts and made it possible for us to finish in a reasonable time frame. We would also like to thank our spouses, Håkon Hope and Martha Pezrow, for putting up with us during both the change in address and change in *Left Brain, Right Brain.*

Sally P. Springer<br>Georg Deutsch

August 1988

# Left Brain, Right Brain

# 1

# A Historical Overview of Clinical Evidence for Brain Asymmetries

In 1836, Marc Dax, an obscure country doctor, read a short paper at a medical society meeting in Montpellier, France. Dax had not been a frequent contributor to medical conferences. In fact, this paper was to be his first and only scientific presentation.

During his long career as a general practitioner, Dax had seen many patients suffering from loss of speech, known technically as *aphasia*, following damage to the brain. This observation in itself was not new. Cases of sudden, permanent disruption in the ability to speak coherently had been reported by the ancient Greeks. Dax, however, was struck by what appeared to be an association between the loss of speech and the side of the brain where the damage had occurred. In more than 40 patients with aphasia, Dax noticed signs of damage to the left half, or *hemisphere*, of the brain. He was unable to find a single case that involved damage to the right hemisphere alone. In his paper to the medical society, he summarized these observations and presented his conclusions: each half of the brain controls different functions; speech is controlled by the left half.

The paper was an unqualified flop. It aroused virtually no interest among those who heard it and was soon forgotten. Dax died the following year, unaware that he had anticipated one of the most exciting and active areas of scientific inquiry of the second half of the twentieth century: the investigation of the differences between the left brain and the right brain.

Although most of us think of the brain as a single structure, it is actually divided into halves. These two parts, or hemispheres, are tightly packed together inside the skull and are linked by several distinct bundles of nerve fibers that serve as channels of communication between them.

Each hemisphere appears to be approximately a mirror image of the other, very much in keeping with the general left–right symmetry of the human body. In fact, control of the body's basic movements and sensations is evenly divided between the two cerebral hemispheres. This occurs in a crossed fashion: the left hemisphere controls the right side of the body (right hand, right leg, and so on), and the right hemisphere controls the left side. Figure 1.1 shows this arrangement.*

The left–right physical symmetry of the brain and body does not imply, though, that the right and left sides are equivalent in all respects. We have only to examine the abilities of our two hands to see the beginnings of *asymmetry of function*. Few people are truly ambidextrous; most have a dominant hand. In many instances a person's handedness can be used to predict a great deal about the organization of higher mental functions in her or his brain. In right-handers, for example, it is almost always the case that the hemisphere that controls the dominant hand is also the hemisphere that controls speech.

Differences in the abilities of the two hands are but one reflection of basic asymmetries in the functions of the two cerebral hemispheres. A great deal of evidence has accumulated in recent years

*A brief overview of neuroanatomy may be found in the Appendix.

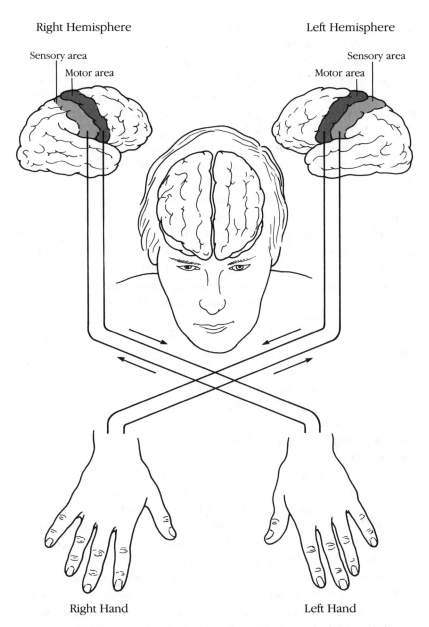

**Figure 1.1** Motor control and sensory pathways between the brain and the rest of the body are almost completely crossed. Each hand is served primarily by the cerebral hemisphere on the opposite side.

showing that the left brain and the right brain are not identical in their capabilities or organizations.

The earliest and most dramatic evidence of functional asymmetries comes from observations of the behavior of individuals with brain damage. Data of this type are known as clinical data because they are based on the study of patients with brain damage. Marc Dax's insight about the link between damage to the left hemisphere and loss of speech is an example of the use of clinical data. Later observations in the clinic led to the discovery of still other asymmetries.

In contrast to people who experience speech problems because of damage to the left hemisphere, patients with certain kinds of right-hemisphere damage are much more likely to have perceptual and attentional problems. These include serious difficulties in spatial orientation and memory for spatial relationships. For example, a patient may have great difficulty learning his or her way around a new building or may even be disoriented in familiar surroundings. Some right-hemisphere patients have difficulty recognizing familiar faces. Damage to the right hemisphere can also result in a problem called *neglect*. A patient experiencing the neglect syndrome pays no attention to the left side of space and sometimes pays no attention to the left side of the body. In many cases the patient will not eat food on the left side of the dinner plate and may refuse to acknowledge a paralyzed left arm as being his or her own. Surprisingly, similar damage to the left hemisphere usually does not produce such severe and long-lasting neglect of the right side of space.

Although clinical data pointing to brain asymmetries have been available for over 100 years, current interest in the left brain and right brain is traceable to recent work involving so-called split-brain patients. For medical reasons, these patients have undergone surgery to cut the cortical pathways that normally connect the cerebral hemispheres. Figure 1.2 shows the *corpus callosum*, the major pathway involved. To the untrained observer, this radical surgery seems to do little to interfere with the patient's normal functioning. To the inquisitive scientist, however, it affords an unparalleled opportunity to study the abilities of each hemisphere separately within the same head.

Special techniques make it possible to confine detailed sensory information to just one hemisphere. The limiting of stimuli to one hemisphere is often called *lateralization*. One way to accomplish lateralization is to let a blindfolded patient feel an object with only

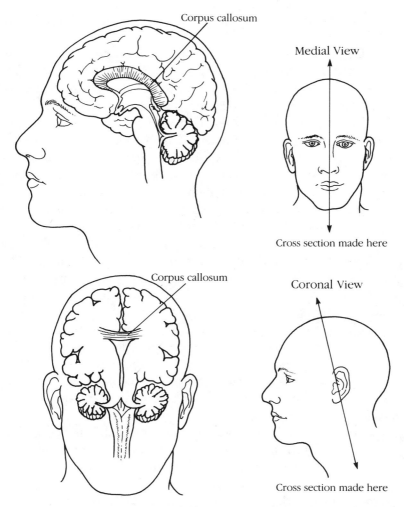

**Figure 1.2** Two views of the cerebral hemispheres and the corpus callosum, the major nerve-fiber tract connecting them.

one hand. A split-brain patient who does this with the right hand (which is controlled principally by the left hemisphere) will have no difficulty naming the object. But if the procedure is repeated using the left hand, the patient will be unable to name the object. Apparently, information about the object does not get through to the speech centers located in the left hemisphere. Nevertheless, the patient can easily use his or her left hand to retrieve the object from a number of other objects hidden from sight. A casual onlooker might conclude that the left hand knew and remembered what it held even though the patient did not.

Taking advantage of other techniques that confine visual and auditory information to one hemisphere at a time, researchers have demonstrated significant differences in the capabilities of the two hemispheres in split-brain patients. The left hemisphere has been found to be predominantly involved with analytic processes, especially the production and understanding of language, and it appears to process input in a sequential manner. The right hemisphere appears to be responsible for certain spatial skills and musical abilities and to process information simultaneously and holistically.

Encouraged by dramatic discoveries with brain-damaged and split-brain patients, investigators have sought ways to study hemispheric differences in neurologically normal subjects. Ideally, one would like to know if the differences between the left brain and the right brain found in brain-damaged patients have any consequences for the function of the normal brain. Techniques developed to answer this question have shown that they do.

Taken all together, this research has generated a great deal of excitement. It is now clear that there are differences in function between the two sides of the brain and that the differences are found in normal subjects as well as in patients. One consequence of these discoveries has been a wealth of speculation about what the asymmetries mean for behavior.

Results of the split-brain studies show that each half of the brain is capable of perceiving, learning, remembering, and feeling independently of the other, but that some differences exist in the way in which each hemisphere deals with incoming information. Roger Sperry, winner of the 1981 Nobel Prize in Physiology or Medicine for his pioneering work with split-brain patients, believes that an independent stream of consciousness resides in each of the separate hemispheres.[1] He has suggested that the surgical division of the brain divides the mind into two distinct realms of consciousness. Such speculation naturally leads to the possibility of dual consciousness in the intact, normal brain under certain conditions.

Other investigators have emphasized the significance of the differences between the hemispheres. It has been claimed that these differences clearly reflect the traditional dualisms of intellect versus intuition, science versus art, and the logical versus the mysterious. Psychologist Robert Ornstein believes brain research shows that these distinctions are not simply a reflection of culture or philosophy.[2] What used to be a belief in an Eastern versus a Western form of consciousness, he argues, now has a physiological basis in the differences between the two hemispheres.

It has also been suggested that lawyers and artists use different halves of the brain in their work and that the differences between the halves show up in activities not related to their work.[3] Others have extended this idea further and have claimed that everyone may be classified as a right-hemisphere person or a left-hemisphere person, depending on which hemisphere guides the bulk of an individual's behavior.[4]

Recent interest in brain asymmetries has sparked concern with the general issue of handedness. Studies have shown differences between left-handers and right-handers in the way the brain is organized. What are the consequences, if any, of these differences for intelligence and creativity? What factors produce left-handedness in the first place? Genes? Experience? Minor brain damage? These and other questions related to handedness have been the subject of intensive study in the last 15 years.

Various other issues have been related to research in hemispheric asymmetry. Diverse problems such as learning disabilities, stuttering, and schizophrenia have been associated with speculation about abnormalities in the division of labor between the two hemispheres. Joseph Bogen, a neurosurgeon involved in split-brain research, believes that research on hemispheric differences has important implications for education.[5] He argues that the current emphasis on the acquisition of verbal skills and the development of analytic thought processes neglects the development of important nonverbal abilities. As a result, he claims, "we are starving" one half of the brain and ignoring its potential contribution to the whole person.

From its modest beginnings in 1836, research on the left brain and right brain has gone on to capture the imaginations of scientists and laypersons alike. Few areas of scientific inquiry have generated so much interest from so diverse an audience. This has had both good and bad effects. On the positive side, vast quantities of new data have been collected in a short period of time, and investigators are hard at work considering the implications of their findings for important questions about human behavior.

On the negative side, there is a tendency to interpret every behavioral dichotomy, such as rational versus intuitive and deductive versus imaginative, in terms of left brain and right brain. This occupational hazard has been named "dichotomania" by some. In addition, the dividing line between fact and fantasy has often been blurred, making it difficult for nonspecialists to know what is speculation and what has been established firmly as fact.

Undoubtedly, however, important insights into brain function and its relation to behavior have resulted from the study of the left brain and right brain and many more important discoveries remain to be made. The goals of this book are to survey the current state of knowledge, to draw conclusions where possible, and to point out the gaps in knowledge that still exist.

We begin with an account of some of the clinical data that have given rise to current ideas concerning the left brain and right brain.

## LOSS OF SPEECH AND RIGHT-SIDED WEAKNESS: LONG-OVERLOOKED EVIDENCE OF ASYMMETRY

Anyone who walks through a stroke ward in a hospital cannot help but notice the fairly even distribution of patients into those with paralyzed left sides and those with paralyzed right sides. A stroke generally involves a stoppage of the blood supply to part of the brain and results in damage to the affected region. Because blood is supplied to each hemisphere separately, strokes usually affect only one half of the brain. Because each half controls the opposite side of the body, paralysis of the right side indicates a stroke in the left hemisphere, and left-sided paralysis indicates a stroke in the right hemisphere.

Throughout the long history of aphasia, the clinical combination of speech disturbances with weakness or paralysis of the right half of the body has been reported again and again. This amounted to a link between loss of speech and damage to the left hemisphere of the brain. The significance of the relationship, however, was not appreciated by the medical community as a whole until the second half of the nineteenth century.

It is perhaps not surprising that this evidence of hemispheric asymmetry was overlooked for so long. Early anatomical studies had shown that the halves of the brain are mirror images of each other, roughly equal in size and weight. Also, most scientists firmly believed that the brain functioned as a whole unit and, thus, the scientists were not predisposed to "see" evidence that suggested otherwise.

By the first decades of the nineteenth century, however, serious attention was being given to the idea that particular functions could be assigned to specific regions of the brain. The notion that one could study the role of specific regions became known as the doctrine of *cerebral localization.*

## The Concept of Cerebral Localization

Franz Gall, a German anatomist, was the first to propose that the brain is not a uniform mass and that various mental faculties could be localized to different parts of the brain. The faculty of speech, he believed, is located in the frontal lobes, the part of each hemisphere closest to the front of the head. Unfortunately, Gall also claimed that the shape of the skull reflects the underlying brain tissue and that an individual's mental and emotional characteristics could be determined through a careful study of bumps on the head.

In many scientific circles, Gall was dismissed as a quack on the grounds that no good evidence existed that skull shape could be used reliably to predict anything about the person whose head was being measured. The basic idea that different functions are controlled by different regions within the brain, however, did attract many followers. Among them was Jean Baptiste Bouillaud, a French professor of medicine. Bouillaud was so certain Gall had been correct in localizing speech to the frontal lobes that he offered 500 francs (a considerable sum at the time) to anyone who could produce a patient with damage to the frontal lobes that was unaccompanied by loss of speech.[6]

For many years, most scientists quietly aligned themselves with one of the two sides of this issue. One group firmly believed that speech was controlled by the frontal lobes; the other side argued that particular functions could not be localized to specific regions of the brain. At that time, there was little in the way of new data to change anyone's mind, and each group held firmly to its position in the absence of compelling evidence to the contrary. It was in this scientific climate that Marc Dax presented his work to the medical community in Montpellier in 1836. As we have seen, his observations pointing to a special role for the left hemisphere in speech were essentially ignored.

## A Turning Point: The Findings of Paul Broca

The stalemate was to end in 1861. At a meeting of the Society of Anthropology in Paris, Bouillaud's son-in-law, Ernest Auburtin, repeated Bouillaud's claim that the center controlling speech is to be found in the frontal lobes. His remarks impressed Paul Broca, a young surgeon who was present at the meeting. Just a few days before, an old man suffering from a serious leg infection had been admitted to Broca's service at a local hospital. Although the infection was recent, for many years the patient had suffered from loss of speech as well as from paralysis of one side of his body (*hemiplegia*).

After the Society of Anthropology meeting, Broca approached Auburtin and suggested it might be useful for them to examine this patient together. A day or so after they saw him, the man died, and Broca was able to perform a postmortem examination. It showed quite clearly a region of damaged tissue, or *lesion*, in part of the left frontal lobe. Broca brought the brain to the next meeting of the anthropological society and told the group of his findings. At first no one seemed to pay much attention.

A few months later, Broca again reported to the society that he had observed a similar lesion at autopsy in a second patient suffering from loss of speech. What changes had taken place in the minds of the Society of Anthropology members in the intervening months are not clear, but this time Broca's report was received with great excitement and touched off heated debate and controversy. Broca soon found himself viewed as the chief proponent of cerebral localization of function.

His new evidence did not convince everyone, however. Die-hard critics of the concept of localization directed their attacks at him. If speech is localized in the frontal lobes, he was challenged, why is it that monkeys with large frontal-brain areas do not possess the ability to speak? Similarly, how can one account for cases of extensive frontal-lobe damage that does not produce loss of speech?

Even Broca's terminology came under fire. He had been careful to differentiate between (1) loss of speech due to simple paralysis of the muscles used to produce speech and (2) the true loss of speech that he had seen in his patients (he called the latter *aphemia*). One critic, M. Trousseau, claimed that the word *aphemia* was derived from a Greek root meaning "infamous" and was not appropriate in this context. He suggested that *aphasia* was a better term to refer to the loss of speech. Although Broca ably defended his choice of words, investigators had already begun to use Trousseau's terminology, which has survived to the present day.

Broca was an unwilling participant in the controversy generated by his work. He later stated that his two reports to the Society of Anthropology were simply an attempt to bring to the attention of others a curious fact that he had observed by chance and that he did not desire to be involved in debates about the localization of speech

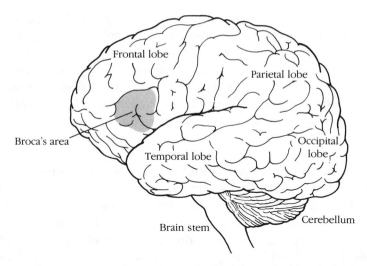

**Figure 1.3** The location of Broca's area in the left cerebral hemisphere.

centers. Despite his protests, Broca continued to figure centrally in the controversy. He went on to collect data from additional cases and was able to pinpoint more precisely the area of the brain involved in instances of speech loss. Figure 1.3 shows the location of this region, which has since become known as *Broca's area*. This figure also illustrates the division of a hemisphere into four lobes: frontal, parietal, occipital, and temporal.

### *Recognizing the Role of the Left Hemisphere.*

Although his two earliest cases had involved lesions of the frontal lobe of the left hemisphere, Broca did not immediately see the link between speech loss and the *side* of the lesion. For two years, he made no attempt to explain this coincidence. In commenting on other cases showing the same relationship, he noted: "Here are eight cases where the lesion is situated in the posterior portion of the third frontal convolution and a thing most remarkable in all of these patients (is that) the lesion is on the left side. I do not attempt to draw a conclusion and I await new findings."[7]

By 1864, however, Broca had become convinced of the importance of the left hemisphere in speech:

I have been struck with the fact that in my first aphemics the lesion always lay not only in the same part of the brain but always the same side—the left. Since then, from many postmortems, the lesion was always left sided. One has also seen many aphemics alive, most of them hemiplegic, and always hemiplegic on the right side. Furthermore, one has seen at autopsy lesions on the right side in patients who had shown no aphemia. It seems from all this that the faculty of articulate language is localized in the left hemisphere, or at least that it depends chiefly upon that hemisphere.[8]

This important insight embroiled Broca in yet another controversy, this time over who had priority in the discovery of this fundamental brain asymmetry. Shortly after learning of Broca's work, Gustav Dax, a physician and the son of Marc Dax, wrote a letter to the medical press claiming that Broca had willfully ignored his father's earlier paper showing that lesions affecting speech always occur in the left half of the brain. Broca replied, protesting that he had never heard of Dax or his work and could find no record of a paper by Dax having been delivered in 1836. Meanwhile, Gustav Dax located and proceeded to publish the text of his father's original talk in order to establish the elder Dax's priority.

Historians have disagreed about whether Broca was aware of Marc Dax's work at the time he published his own, and they will probably never resolve this question. Eventually, Broca presented a considerably more impressive argument for the association between aphasia and damage to the left hemisphere than had Dax. Dax's cases lacked verification of the location of damage as well as complete clinical histories. Broca's work, in contrast, contained extensive anatomical findings and information about the nature of the speech problems present.

Broca also went on to consider the relationship between handedness and speech. He suggested that both speech and manual dexterity are attributable to the inborn superiority of the left hemisphere in righthanders. "One can conceive," he speculated, "that there may be a certain number of individuals in whom the natural pre-eminence of the convolutions of the right hemisphere reverses the order of the phenomenon which I have just described."[9] These individuals, of course, are lefthanders. Broca's "rule" that the hemisphere controlling speech is on the side opposite to the preferred hand was influential well into the twentieth century.

Broca may be properly credited with being the first person to bring to the attention of the medical community the asymmetry of the human brain with regard to speech. He was also the first to link that asymmetry with hand preference.

## THE CONCEPT OF CEREBRAL DOMINANCE

Within ten years of the publication of Broca's initial observations, the concept now known as *cerebral dominance* began to emerge as the major view of the relationship between the two hemispheres of the brain. In 1864, the great British neurologist John Hughlings Jackson wrote, "Not long ago, few doubted the brain to be double in function as well as physically bilateral; but now that it is certain from the researches of Dax, Broca, and others, that damage to one lateral half can make a man entirely speechless, the former view is disrupted."[10]

Later, in 1868, Jackson proposed his idea of the "leading" hemisphere—a notion that may be viewed as precursor to the idea of cerebral dominance. "The two brains cannot be mere duplicates," he wrote, "if damage to one alone can make a man speechless. For these processes (of speech), of which there are none higher, there must surely be one side which is leading." Jackson further concluded "that in most people the left side of the brain is the leading side— the side of the so-called will, and that the right is the automatic side."[11]

By 1870, other investigators began to realize that many types of language disorders could result from damage to the left hemisphere. Early work concentrating on problems in *producing* speech that resulted from injury to the left hemisphere had overlooked the fact that patients frequently had difficulty *understanding* the speech of others. Karl Wernicke, a German neurologist, is credited with showing that damage to the back part of the temporal lobe of the left hemisphere could produce difficulties in understanding speech.

Similarly, problems in reading and writing were identified in some patients and were shown to result from damage to the left hemisphere, not from damage to the right. Clearly, the picture emerging by the end of the nineteenth century was one in which the left hemisphere played a role of great importance in language functions in general and not just in speech per se. It had also become apparent that different kinds of language problems resulted from damage to different areas within the left hemisphere.

Contributing still further evidence to the notion that the left hemisphere possesses functions not shared by the right was the work of Hugo Liepmann on a disorder known as *apraxia*. Apraxia is generally defined as the inability to perform purposeful movements on command.* An apraxic patient might have no difficulty brushing his or her teeth in the context of a normal bedtime routine, but he or she would be unable to reproduce the same movements when instructed to pretend to brush in an unrelated context.

Liepmann had shown that although such deficits are not due to a general inability to understand speech, they are associated with injury to the left hemisphere. He concluded that the left hemisphere controls "purposeful" movements as well as language, but that the specific areas of the left hemisphere involved are different in the two cases.

Taken together, these findings formed the basis of a widely held view of the relationship between the two hemispheres. One hemisphere, usually the left in right-handers, was seen as the director of speech and other higher functions; the right, or "minor," hemisphere, was without special functions and subordinate to control by the "dominant" left. Although the origin of the term is obscure, *cerebral dominance* nicely captures the idea of one half of the brain directing behavior. Although this notion underestimates the role of the right hemisphere, the term *cerebral dominance* is still widely used today.

## THE RIGHT BRAIN: THE NEGLECTED HEMISPHERE

Almost as soon as the concept of cerebral dominance became popular, evidence began to appear suggesting that the right, or minor, hemisphere also possesses specialized abilities. John Hughlings Jackson's notion of the left hemisphere as "leading" was the intellectual grandparent of the idea of dominance. Interestingly, Jackson was also one of the first to consider that an extreme, one-sided view of the way mental functions are localized in the brain was wrong. "If then," he wrote in 1865, "it should be proven by wider experience that the faculty of expression resides in one hemisphere, there is no absurdity in raising the question as to whether perception—its corresponding opposite—may be seated in the other."[12]

---

*Apraxia and other clinical disorders considered in this chapter are discussed in more detail in Chapter 6.

This speculation took more concrete form 11 years later when Jackson argued that the lobes at the rear of the brain are the seat of visual ideation or thought and that "the right posterior lobe is the leading side, the left the more automatic."[13] Jackson based this proposal on his observation of a patient with a tumor in the right hemisphere who experienced difficulty recognizing objects, persons, and places. But, like Dax's important insight 40 years earlier, Jackson's idea was way ahead of its time. Although other reports of a similar nature occasionally appeared, for the most part little attention was paid to this evidence. Investigators concerned themselves with localizing various functions within the left hemisphere and essentially ignored the right.

By the 1930s, however, enough data pointing to specialized roles for the right hemisphere had been collected to cause scientists to reconsider the functions of the minor half of the brain.

### Visuo-Spatial Abilities in the Right Hemisphere

One important development was the discovery of significant and fairly consistent differences in the way subjects with left-hemisphere damage and those with right-hemisphere damage performed on standard psychological tests. The tests were originally developed to study and compare normal subjects along such dimensions as verbal ability, appreciation of spatial relationships, and ability to manipulate forms.

The first large-scale effort using these tests to study the effects of brain damage involved over 200 patients and more than 40 different tests—an average of 19 hours of testing per patient.[14] The results of this and subsequent studies were impressive. It was found, as a general rule, that damage to the left, or dominant, hemisphere resulted in poor performance on the tests that emphasized verbal ability. Although this was not too surprising, it was also found that patients with damage to the right hemisphere did consistently more poorly on nonverbal tests involving the manipulation of geometric figures, puzzle assembly, completion of missing parts of patterns and figures, and other tasks involving form, distance, and space relationships. Two visuo-spatial tests are shown in Figure 1.4.

The most striking evidence for specialized right-hemisphere function came from direct observation of the patients themselves. Profound disturbances in orientation and awareness were seen in pa-

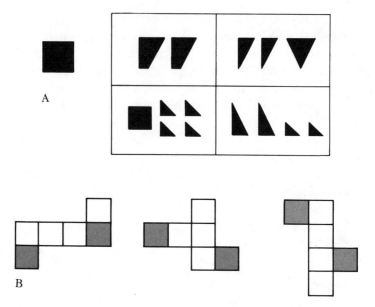

**Figure 1.4** Visuo-spatial tasks. A. Which boxed set(s) can form the square on the outside? B. If you fold these patterns into cubes, in which cube(s) will the dark sides meet at one edge?

tients with right-hemisphere damage. Such patients could be so disoriented in space that they were unable to find their way around a house in which they had lived for many years. Some showed neglect, or "hemispatial inattention": they consistently missed objects or events on their left.

Certain *agnosias*, or disturbances in the recognition or perception of familiar information, were also associated with damage to the right hemisphere. Spatial agnosia is a disorientation with respect to locations and spatial relationships. Some right-hemisphere patients have deficits in their ability to comprehend depth and distance relationships or to deal with mental images of maps and forms.

One of the most interesting forms of agnosia is *facial agnosia*. A patient with this condition is unable to recognize familiar faces and sometimes cannot discriminate between people in general. The deficit is quite specific. Recognition of scenes and objects, for example, may not be impaired. This problem has been found in cases where there was damage to both halves of the brain, although several investigators have argued for the importance of right-hemisphere lesions in this disorder.[15]

## The Role of the Right Hemisphere in Music

Additional evidence pointing to the specialization of the right hemisphere came from the observation that the ability to sing is frequently unaffected in patients suffering from severe speech disturbances. One of the earliest recorded cases of this type was described in 1745:

> . . . he had an attack of a violent illness which resulted in a paralysis of the entire right side of the body and complete loss of speech. He can sing certain hymns, which he had learned before he became ill, as clearly and distinctly as any healthy person. . . . Yet this man is dumb, cannot say a single word except "yes" and has to communicate by making signs with his hand.[16]

Similar cases were reported to the early 1900s, suggesting that the right hemisphere controls singing.

Other evidence consistant with this idea came from clinical reports that damage to the right half of the brain may result in the loss of musical ability, leaving speech unimpaired. This disorder, known as *amusia*, was most frequently reported in professional musicians who suffered from stroke or other brain damage. By the 1930s, the medical literature contained many case histories of people who suffered impairments in various aspects of musical ability after damage to the right hemisphere. Similar reports following damage to the left hemisphere were rarer, again suggesting that the right hemisphere is in some way critically involved in music.[17]

## Why "Discovery" of the Right Brain Took So Long

All this evidence shows that the view of the right hemisphere as the minor or passive hemisphere was inappropriate. Why did it take most scientists 70 years after Broca's findings concerning the left hemisphere to recognize that the right hemisphere controls important functions? There may be several reasons for this time lag.

First, it seemed that the right hemisphere was able to withstand greater damage without producing any obvious impairments. Small lesions in particular areas of the left hemisphere drastically affected speech abilities, but comparable damage in the right hemisphere did not appear to cause any serious dysfunction. This disparity was originally interpreted as a sign of the less important role played by the right hemisphere in human behavior. It has been suggested more recently, though, that this difference simply reflects the way processes are organized in the right hemisphere: specific processes are distributed over larger regions of brain tissue in the right half of the brain than in the left half.[18]

The most likely reason for the slow recognition of the importance of the right hemisphere, however, is that disabilities caused by lesions in the right hemisphere were not so easy to analyze and fit into the traditional ideas about brain function. Most damage to the right hemisphere does not abolish any obvious human abilities in an all-or-none fashion; instead, it disturbs behavior in fairly subtle ways. Some of the problems occurring with right-brain damage are not so easy to label as the problems associated with left-hemisphere injury. They often went unnoticed or were masked by more obvious physical disabilities, such as those found in most stroke victims.

It is important to keep in mind that the most debilitating effect of a stroke is the paralysis it often causes. The paralysis tends to be the patient's chief complaint or problem. Brain damage that arises from traumas such as accidents or gunshot wounds is also accompanied by complications that make it difficult to weed out subtle intellectual impairments from a host of other problems.

Despite its camouflaged role, the right hemisphere does play a vital part in human behavior. It is now clear that both hemispheres contribute in important ways to complex mental activity while differing in certain ways in their function and organization.

## HANDEDNESS AND THE HEMISPHERES

It is frequently the case in science that ideas are challenged by new evidence just as they have gained widespread acceptance. We have already seen how an extreme view of cerebral dominance was called into question by new findings dealing with the role of the right hemisphere. In the same way, Broca's "rule" linking aphasia with damage to the hemisphere opposite to the preferred hand was shown to be an oversimplification soon after Broca proposed it.

The rule accounted nicely for the relationship between damage to the left hemisphere and aphasia in right-handers. But left-handers appeared to come in two varieties—those with speech in the hemisphere opposite to their preferred hand (as predicted by Broca) and those with speech in the left hemisphere. The existence of the latter group was discovered through observations of left-handed patients who become aphasic following damage to the left hemisphere. These cases, known as instances of *crossed aphasia*, show rather dramatically that left-handedness is not necessarily the simple converse of right-handedness.[19]

The relationship of handedness to hemispheric asymmetry of function remains one of the most important questions to be resolved in the study of brain organization, and we shall return to it at various points throughout this book.

## FURTHER INSIGHTS FROM THE CLINIC

To complete our brief account of the contributions of clinical data to the understanding of hemispheric asymmetry of function, two highly specialized neurosurgical procedures developed in the 1930s and 1940s should be mentioned. Both were designed to help the neurosurgeon determine which hemisphere was controlling speech and language function in an individual about to undergo brain surgery for epilepsy. These procedures have also contributed significantly to our knowledge of hemispheric asymmetry of function in general.

### Direct Electrical Stimulation of the Hemisphere

Epilepsy, a disorder involving abnormal electrical activity generated within the brain, produces reactions that may range from short blackouts lasting a second or two to full-blown grand mal seizures. During an epileptic attack, the abnormal electrical activity often originates from a specific part of the brain and then spreads to other regions.

In the early 1930s, Wilder Penfield and his associates at the Montreal Neurological Institute pioneered the use of surgery to remove the area of the brain where the abnormal activity begins, as a treatment for epilepsy in patients who did not respond well to drug therapy. Although the procedure proved to be successful in many instances, surgeons were reluctant to undertake cases requiring the removal of tissue that was close to the parts of the brain controlling speech and language. They wished to avoid these regions to reduce the likelihood that the surgery would merely substitute one debilitating disorder (aphasia) for another (epilepsy). Penfield's own words aptly describe the situation facing him and his colleagues:

Twenty-five years ago we were embarking on the treatment of focal epilepsy by radical surgical excision of abnormal areas of brain. In the beginning it was our practice to refuse radical operation upon the dominant hemisphere unless a lesion lay anteriorly in the frontal lobe or posteriorly in the occipital lobe. Like other neurosurgeons, we feared that removal of cortex in other parts of this hemisphere would produce aphasia. (The) aphasia literature gave no clear guide as to just what might and what might not be removed with impunity.[20]

Clearly, what was required was a method for determining with precision the location of the centers controlling speech and language in a given patient. To meet this need, Penfield and his colleagues developed a procedure that involved mapping these areas by using direct electrical stimulation of the brain at the time of surgery.

Direct electrical stimulation of exposed brain tissue was not in itself a new procedure. Preliminary work in the early 1900s had shown that because the brain itself does not contain pain receptors, it is possible for a patient to remain fully conscious while a neurosurgeon removes a flap of skull under local anesthesia and applies small electrical currents directly to the brain surface. The electrode used for the procedure could be moved to stimulate different regions of the brain. Findings had shown that electrical stimulation of specific parts of the brain would cause patients to see, hear, smell, or feel in an elementary way. Stimulation of other regions caused involuntary motor responses, such as the movement of an arm or leg. The major contribution made by the Montreal group was the use of direct electrical stimulation as a tool for determining the location of the centers controlling speech and language in a given individual.*

During a typical procedure using direct electrical stimulation to map speech areas, the patient and surgeon are separated by a tent constructed of surgical drapes. A third person, acting as an observer, sits with the patient under the tent. While an electrical current is applied to the regions of the brain normally employed for speech, the patient is unable to speak. The interference is known as *aphasic arrest*.

These areas may be determined by having the observer show the patient a series of pictures and asking the patient to identify each

---

*Their work also had important implications for the way in which memories are stored in the brain, a topic that we discuss briefly in Chapter 6. The interested reader is directed to *Speech and Brain Mechanisms*, by W. Penfield and L. Roberts, a fascinating, well-written account of three decades of research on brain stimulation at the Montreal Neurological Institute.

one. The neurosurgeon moves the stimulating electrode over the surface of the brain to locate areas that produce interference with naming. Small, sterile squares of paper are dropped on the brain at the point of application of an electrode to provide a record of the areas stimulated and the patient's response. Throughout the procedure, the patient is fully conscious but unaware of when and where the electrode will be placed. The mapping takes about 15 minutes, a small amount of time compared with the duration of the surgery itself, which may last several hours. Figure 1.5 maps the points on the left hemisphere where stimulation has resulted in speech disturbance.

Aphasic arrest following the stimulation of a particular part of the brain is a sure sign that the region is part of the speech area of the language-specialized hemisphere. Penfield notes that aphasic arrest never follows from the stimulation of sites within the non-language-specialized half of the brain.

Several hundred patients have undergone direct electrical stimulation of the brain at the Montreal Neurological Institute and other institutions. The data obtained have proved to be of great theoretical as well as clinical value in localizing functions within a hemisphere. Another test, known as the Wada test after its inventor, Juhn Wada, has been very valuable in localizing functions *across* hemispheres.

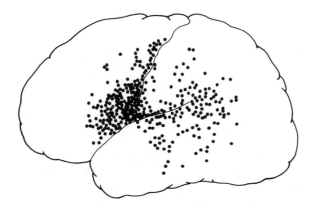

**Figure 1.5** Points along the surface of the left hemisphere where electrical stimulation resulted in interference with speech. The interference included total speech arrest, hesitation, slurring, repetition of words, and inability to name. [From Penfield and Roberts, *Speech and Brain Mechanisms*, Fig. VII-3, p. 122. (Princeton, N.J.: Princeton University Press, 1959). Reprinted by permission of Princeton University Press.]

## The Wada Test: Anesthetizing a Hemisphere

The Wada test temporarily anesthetizes one hemisphere at a time on separate days before surgery so that the neurosurgeon can see which side of the brain normally controls the ability to speak.[21] The first step in the Wada test is the insertion of a small tube into the carotid artery on one side of the patient's neck. The tube permits the neurosurgeon to inject the drug sodium amobarbital into that artery at a later time. The carotid artery on each side brings blood to the hemisphere on the same side as the artery. Thus, sodium amobarbital injected into the right artery is carried to the right hemisphere. The drug is a barbiturate, chemically similar to the ingredients used in sleeping pills. However, because of the way it is administered in the Wada test, it puts only one half of the brain to sleep at a time.

Moments before the drug is injected, the fully conscious patient lies flat on his or her back and is asked to count backward from 100 by threes. The patient is also asked to keep both arms raised in the air while counting. The drug is then slowly injected through the tube into the carotid artery. Within seconds of the injection, dramatic results occur.

First, the arm opposite to the side of the injection falls limp. Because each half of the brain controls the opposite side of the body, the falling arm tells the neurosurgeon that the drug has reached the proper hemisphere and has taken effect. Second, the patient generally stops counting, either for a few seconds or for the duration of the drug's effect, depending on which hemisphere is affected. If the drug is injected on the same side as the hemisphere controlling speech, the patient remains speechless for 2 to 5 minutes, depending on the dose administered. If it is injected on the other side, the patient generally resumes counting within a few seconds and can answer questions with little difficulty while the drug is still inactivating the other half of the brain.

The Wada test, like direct electrical stimulation, has been very useful in determining which hemisphere controls speech and language in patients about to undergo surgery involving areas of the brain that might control speech. Both procedures have also given investigators valuable information about the relationship of handedness to hemispheric asymmetry and the effects of early damage on asymmetry.

For example, from this work it has been determined that over 95 percent of all right-handers without any history of early brain damage have speech and language controlled by the left hemisphere; the remainder have speech controlled by the right hemisphere. Contrary to Broca's rule, a majority of left-handers also show left-hemisphere speech; the percentage (about 70 percent) is smaller, though, in left-handers than in right-handers. Roughly 15 percent of left-handers have speech in the right hemisphere, and 15 percent or so show evidence of speech control in both hemispheres (bilateral speech control).[22]

Data have also been collected using the Wada technique in patients who were known to have had some damage to the left hemisphere early in life. These patients show a much higher incidence of right-hemisphere or bilateral speech: 70 percent of the left-handers and 19 percent of the right-handers fall into one or the other of these categories. This evidence points to the adaptability of the brain and to the limited value of handedness per se as an index of brain organization, particularly in left-handers.

## THE LIMITATIONS OF CLINICAL DATA

We conclude this chapter with some remarks about the old and still controversial issue of localizing function to particular areas of the brain. Clinical observations of brain-damaged patients have formed the foundation of most of our ideas relating human behavior to brain function. The interpretation of these observations, however, has always been fraught with difficulty and subject to a great deal of criticism. The basic problem is that there is no simple way to relate the function of a piece of destroyed brain tissue to the disabilities a patient seems to incur as a result of the damage.

The oldest idea was to say simply that whatever a patient could not do was normally controlled by the area of the brain that was damaged. If a person had a lesion and could not see, for example, then the damaged area was said to control vision. If someone had a lesion in a different region and could not understand spoken language, then the area involved was said to be responsible for speech comprehension.

That approach has turned out to be much too simplistic. For one thing, most of the processes neatly labeled as visual perception, speech production, voluntary movement, or memory are really the result of many complex cerebral interactions. Whether they are diffusely spread over large areas of the brain or are limited to particular regions appears to be determined by which function we are studying, how precisely we are defining it, and how successfully we are able to limit our tests to what we assume they are testing. Just about any fairly limited damage to the brain is likely to interfere with a step or phase of some larger process (although not the entire process). It is also likely to interfere with a step or phase of more than one process. It is not unusual to see damage to a small area of the brain result in deficits in a number of different functions.

A rough analogy may be useful here. Imagine trying to figure out the function of different components in a radio by removing them and seeing how their removal affects the performance of the radio. The task would be a very difficult one, indeed. Similarly, the knowledge we gain about the role of particular brain regions from the effects of brain damage is tentative and most useful in combination with knowledge of brain function obtained in other ways.

Another major problem in deducing brain function from clinical data is the fact that the brain tends to adjust its operations as best it can in the presence of damage. We cannot assume that the remaining intact areas of a damaged brain are operating as they would in a normal brain. It is not as though a piece is missing but everything else is working as it was before. In most cases of brain damage there is some recovery of function over time—sometimes fairly dramatic recovery. The recovery can involve changes in the undamaged areas and is a tribute to the adaptability of the brain. This plasticity is a fascinating and obviously very useful feature, but it complicates the efforts of those who are trying to deduce brain function from clinical data.

For these reasons, other ways to study the functions of the left brain and the right brain have been sought. Other approaches are necessary both to corroborate brain-damage data and to add whatever knowledge can be gleaned from techniques that do not depend on great intrusions into normal functioning. We shall examine some of these approaches in the following chapters, and will review findings from clinical studies in more detail.

## IN SUMMARY

Notions about the role of the two cerebral hemispheres have ranged from the idea that the whole brain is involved in every function, to the belief that the left half is the dominant part, to the current idea that both hemispheres contribute to behavior in important ways through their specialized capabilities. Clinical evidence, despite its limitations, has yielded a sizable body of information about the left brain and right brain. Damage to one hemisphere leads to disabilities different from those arising from damage to the other hemisphere.

These differences strongly suggest that each hemisphere contributes certain specialized functions to overall human behavior. Moreover, within each hemisphere there is some specialization, because damage in certain locations can be quite selective in the way it affects behavior.

The clinical data form just part of the picture that has emerged about specialization within the brain. We will now consider how other approaches have led and are leading to additional insights into the workings of the left brain, the right brain, and the two together.

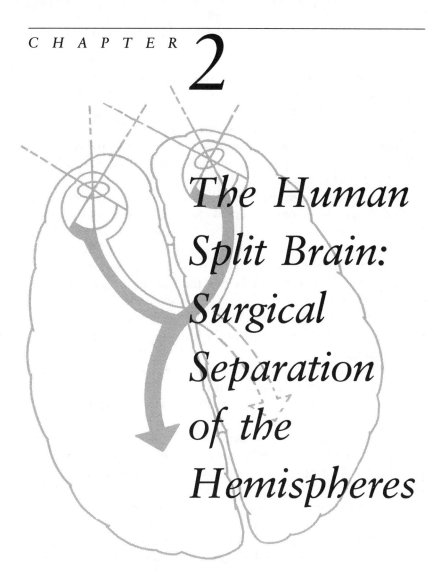

CHAPTER 2

# The Human Split Brain: Surgical Separation of the Hemispheres

In 1940, an article appeared in a scientific journal describing experiments on the spread of epileptic discharge from one hemisphere to the other in the brains of monkeys.[1] The author concluded that the spread occurred largely or entirely by way of the corpus callosum, the largest of several *commissures*, or bands of nerve fiber connecting regions of the left brain with similar areas of the right brain. Earlier, other investigators had observed that damage to the corpus callosum from a tumor or other problem sometimes reduced the incidence of seizures in human epileptics.[2] Together, these findings paved the way for a new treatment for patients with epilepsy that could not be controlled in other ways: the split-brain operation.

Split-brain surgery, or *commissurotomy*, involves surgically cutting some of the fibers that connect the two cerebral hemispheres. The first such operations to relieve epilepsy were performed in the early 1940s on approximately two dozen patients. The patients subsequently gave scientists their first opportunity to study systematically the role of the corpus callosum in humans, a role that had been speculated on for decades.

The corpus callosum was a puzzle for researchers who expected to find functions commensurate with its large size and strategic location within the brain. Animal research had shown the consequences of split-brain surgery on a healthy organism to be minimal. The behavior of split-brain monkeys, for example, appeared indistinguishable from what it was before the operation. The apparent absence of any noticeable changes following commissurotomy led some scientists to suggest facetiously that the corpus callosum's only function was to hold the halves of the brain together and keep them from sagging.

Speculations on the philosophical implications of split-brain surgery go back to the nineteenth century and the writings of Gustav Fechner, considered by many to be the father of experimental psychology. Fechner considered consciousness to be an attribute of the cerebral hemispheres, and he believed that continuity of the brain was an essential condition for unity of consciousness. If it were possible to divide the brain through the middle, he speculated, something like the duplication of a human being would result. "The two cerebral hemispheres," he wrote, "while beginning with the same moods, predispositions, knowledge, and memories, indeed the same consciousness generally, will thereafter develop differently according to the external relations into which each will enter."[3] Fechner considered this "thought experiment" involving separation of the hemispheres impossible to achieve in reality.

Fechner's views concerning the nature of consciousness did not go unchallenged. William McDougall, a founder of the British Psychological Society, argued strongly against the position that unity of consciousness depends on the continuity of the nervous system. To make his point, McDougall volunteered to have his corpus callosum cut if he ever got an incurable disease. He apparently wanted to show that his personality would not be split and that his consciousness would remain unitary.

McDougall never got the opportunity to put his ideas to the test, but the surgery Fechner thought an impossibility took place for the first time almost a century later. The issues these men raised have been among those explored by scientists seeking a fuller understanding of the corpus callosum through the study of split-brain patients.

## CUTTING 200 MILLION NERVE FIBERS: A SEARCH FOR CONSEQUENCES

### The First Split-Brain Operations on Humans

William Van Wagenen, a neurosurgeon from Rochester, New York, performed the first split-brain operations on humans in the early 1940s. Postsurgical testing by an investigator named Andrew Akelaitis showed surprisingly little in the way of deficits in perceptual and motor abilities.[4] The operation seemed to have had no effect on everyday behavior. Unfortunately, for some patients the surgery also seemed to do little to alleviate the condition responsible for the surgery in the first place. Success in relieving seizures seemed to vary greatly from patient to patient.

In retrospect, this variability seems attributable to two causes: (1) individual differences in the nature of the epilepsy in the patients and (2) variations in the actual surgical procedures used with each patient. Figure 2.1 shows the corpus callosum and the adjacent smaller commissures. Van Wagenen's operations varied considerably but usually included sectioning of the forward (anterior) half of the corpus callosum. In two patients, he also sectioned a separate fiber band known as the anterior commissure.

At the time, the importance of these factors was not known, and Van Wagenen soon discontinued the commissurotomy procedure in cases of intractable epilepsy. Clearly, it was not producing the dramatic results he had hoped for. Despite these discouraging findings, other investigators continued to study the functions of the corpus callosum in animals. A decade later, in the early 1950s, Ronald Myers and Roger Sperry made some remarkable discoveries that marked a turning point in efforts to study this enigmatic structure.

Myers and Sperry showed that visual information presented to one hemisphere in a cat with its corpus callosum cut would not be available to the other hemisphere.[5] In most higher animals, the visual system is arranged so that each eye normally projects to both hemispheres. But by cutting into the optic-nerve crossing, the *chiasm*, experimenters can limit where each eye sends its information. When this cut is made, the remaining fibers in the optic nerve transmit information to the hemisphere on the same side. Visual input to the

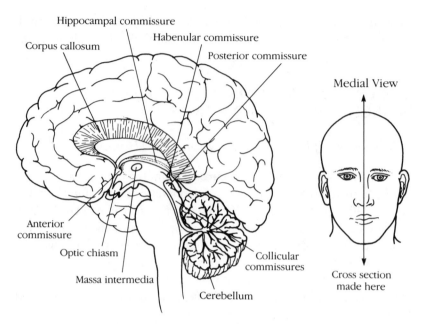

**Figure 2.**1 The major interhemispheric commissures. This is a sectional view of the right half of the brain as seen from the midline. [From Sperry, *The Great Cerebral Commissure*, Scientific American, 1964. All rights reserved.]

left eye is sent only to the left hemisphere, and input to the right eye projects only to the right hemisphere.

Myers performed this operation on cats and subsequently taught each animal a visual-discrimination task with one of its eyes patched. A discrimination task involves, for example, an animal's pressing a lever when it sees a circle but not pressing it when it sees a square. Even if this training is done with one eye covered, a normal cat can later perform the task using either eye. Myers found that cats with the optic chiasm cut were also able to perform the task using either eye when tested after the one-eyed training. However, when he cut the corpus callosum in addition to the optic chiasm, the results were dramatically different.

The cat trained with one eye open and one eye patched would learn to do a task well; but when the patch was switched to the other eye, the cat was unable to do the task at all. In fact, it had to be taught the same task over again, taking just as long to learn it as it had the first time. Myers and Sperry concluded that cutting the corpus callosum had kept information going into one hemisphere isolated from the other hemisphere. They had, in effect, trained only half of a brain. Figure 2.2 schematically illustrates the different conditions of their experiment.

These findings, as well as some further studies, led two neurosurgeons working near the California Institute of Technology, in Pasadena, to reconsider the use of split-brain surgery as a treatment for intractable epilepsy in human beings. The surgeons, Philip Vogel and Joseph Bogen, reasoned that some of the earlier work with human patients had failed because the disconnection between the cerebral hemispheres was not complete. As we have mentioned, Van Wagenen's operations varied considerably from patient to patient. Some parts of the corpus callosum as well as several smaller commissures were usually not included in his operations, and these remaining fibers may have connected the hemispheres sufficiently to mask the

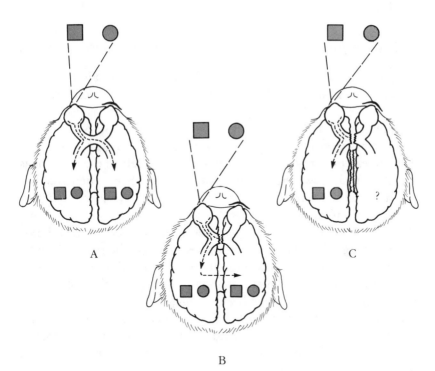

Figure 2.2 Split-brain experiment with animals. In a control situation, both eyes and both hemispheres see the stimuli. Experimental conditions alter this in the following ways: A. When one eye is patched, the other eye continues to send information to both hemispheres. B. When one eye is patched and the optic chiasm is cut, the visual information is transmitted to both hemispheres by way of the corpus callosum. C. When one eye is patched and both the optic chiasm and corpus callosum are cut, only one hemisphere receives visual information.

effects of the fibers that were cut. On the basis of this logic, coupled with new animal data showing no ill effects from the surgery, Bogen and Vogel performed a complete commissurotomy on the first of what was to be a new series of two dozen patients suffering from intractable epilepsy.

Bogen and Vogel's reasoning proved to be correct. In some of the cases, the medical benefits of the surgery even appeared to exceed expectations. In striking contrast to its consequences for seizure activity, the operation appeared to leave patients unchanged in personality, intelligence, and behavior in general, just as had been the case with Van Wagenen's patients. More extensive and ingenious testing conducted in Roger Sperry's California Institute of Technology laboratory, however, soon revealed a more complex story, for which Sperry was awarded the 1981 Nobel Prize in Physiology or Medicine.

## Testing for the Effects of Disconnecting Left from Right

Split-brain patient N.G., a California housewife, sits in front of a screen with a small black dot in the center. She is asked to look directly at the dot. When the experimenter is sure she is doing so, a picture of a cup is flashed briefly to the right of the dot. N.G. reports that she has seen a cup. Again, she is asked to fix her gaze on the dot. This time, a picture of a spoon is flashed to the left of the dot. She is asked what she saw. She replies, "No, nothing." She is then asked to reach under the screen with her left hand and to select, by touch only, from among several items the one that is the same as the one she has just seen. Her left hand palpates each object and then holds up the spoon. When asked what she is holding, she says, "Pencil."

Once again the patient is asked to fixate on the dot on the screen. A picture of a nude woman is flashed to the left of the dot. N.G.'s face blushes a little, and she begins to giggle. She is asked what she saw. She says, "Nothing, just a flash of light," and giggles again, covering her mouth with her hand. "Why are you laughing, then?" the investigator inquires. "Oh, doctor, you have some machine!" she replies.

The procedure just described is frequently used in studies with split-brain patients and is illustrated in Figure 2.3. The patient sits in front of a tachistoscope, a device that allows the investigator to control precisely the duration for which a picture or pattern is presented on a screen. The presentations are kept brief, about one- or two-tenths of a second (100 to 200 milliseconds), so that the

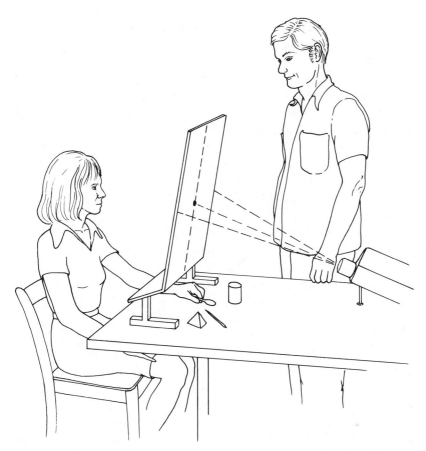

**Figure 2.3** The basic testing arrangement used to lateralize visual and tactile information and allow tactile responses.

patient does not have time to move his or her eyes away from the fixation point while the picture is still on the screen.* This procedure is necessary to ensure that visual information is presented initially to only one hemisphere. Stimuli presented to only one hemisphere are said to be *lateralized*.

The design of the human nervous system is such that each cerebral hemisphere receives information primarily from the opposite half of

---

*The rapid eye movements that occur when gaze is shifted from one point to another are known as *saccadic eye movements* or *saccades*. Although, once started, saccades are extremely rapid, they take about 200 milliseconds to initiate with the eye at rest. If a stimulus is presented for less than 200 milliseconds, the stimulus is no longer present by the time an eye movement can occur.

the body. This contralateral rule applies to vision and hearing as well as to body movement and touch (somatosensory) sensation, although the situation in vision and hearing is more complex.

In vision, the contralateral rule applies to the right and left sides of one's field of view (visual field), rather than to the right and left eyes per se. When both eyes are fixating on a single point, stimuli to the right of fixation are registered in the left half of the brain, while the right half of the brain processes everything occurring to the left of fixation. This split and crossover of visual information results from the manner in which the nerve fibers from corresponding regions of both eyes are divided between the cerebral hemispheres. Figure 2.4 shows both the optics and the neural wiring involved.

In animal studies, as we have seen, visual information can be directed to one hemisphere by cutting the optic chiasm so that the remaining fibers in the optic nerve are those transmitting information to the hemisphere on the same side as the eye. This allows experimenters to present a stimulus easily to either hemisphere alone by simply presenting the stimulus to the appropriate eye. The procedure is used only with animals, however, because cutting the chiasm substantially reduces peripheral vision, eliminates binocular depth perception, and plays no part in the rationale for the split-brain operation on humans. For these reasons, investigators wishing to transmit visual information to one hemisphere at a time in a human split-brain patient must do so through a combination of controlling the patient's fixation and presenting information to one side of space.

With this as background, let's return to an analysis of the tests administered to patient N.G. In those tests, the patient saw the left half of the screen (everything to the left of the fixation point) with the right side of her brain and everything to the right with her left hemisphere. The split in her brain prevented the normal interchange of information between the two sides that would have occurred before her surgery. In effect, each side of her brain was blind to what the other side was seeing, a state of affairs dramatically brought out by the knowledge that only one hemisphere controls speech.

As a consequence, the patient reported perfectly well any stimuli falling in the right visual field (projecting to the verbal left hemisphere), although she was unable to tell anything about what was flashed in her left visual field (sent to the mute right hemisphere). The fact that she "saw" stimuli in the left visual field is amply demonstrated by the ability of her left hand (basically controlled by the right brain) to select the spoon from among several objects

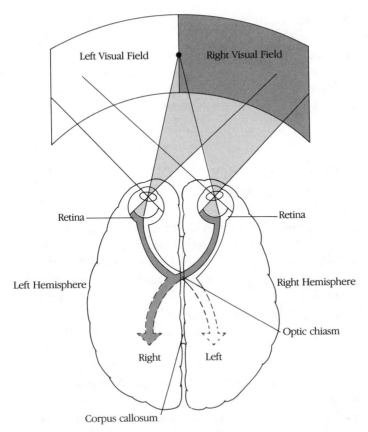

**Figure 2.4** Visual pathways to the hemispheres. When fixating on a point, each eye sees both visual fields but sends information about the right visual field only to the left hemisphere and information about the left visual field only to the right hemisphere. This crossover and split is a result of the manner in which the nerve fibers leading from the retina divide at the back of each eye. The visual areas of the left and right hemisphere normally communicate through the corpus callosum. If the callosum is cut and the eyes and head are kept from moving, each hemisphere can see only half of the visual world.

hidden from view. It is also demonstrated by her emotional reaction to the nude picture, despite her claim not to have seen anything.[6]

The patient's response to the nude picture is particularly interesting. She seemed puzzled by her own reactions to what had appeared. Her right hemisphere saw the picture and processed it sufficiently to evoke a general, nonverbal reaction—the giggling and the blushing. The left hemisphere, meanwhile, did not "know" what the right had seen, although its comment about "some machine" seems to be a sign that it was aware of the bodily reactions induced by the right hemisphere. It is very common for the verbal left hemisphere to try to make sense of what has occurred in testing situations where information is presented to the right hemisphere. As a result, the left brain sometimes comes out with erroneous and often elaborate rationalizations based on partial cues.


## EVERYDAY BEHAVIOR AFTER
## SPLIT-BRAIN SURGERY

It is natural to wonder what evidence of disconnection effects there is in the everyday behavior of split-brain patients. Some instances of bizarre behavior have been described by both patients and onlookers and are frequently mentioned in popular articles on split-brain research. One patient, for example, described the time he found his left hand struggling against his right when he tried to put his pants on in the morning: one hand was pulling them up while the other hand was pulling them down. In another incident, the same patient was angry and forcibly reached for his wife with his left hand while his right hand grabbed the left in an attempt to stop it.[7]

The frequency with which such stories are mentioned would lead one to believe that they are commonplace events. In fact, the frequency of such events is low in most patients. However, there are exceptions. One example is P.O.V., a female patient operated on by Dr. Mark Rayport of the Medical College of Ohio. The patient reported frequent dramatic signs of interhemispheric competition for at least three years after surgery. "I open the closet door. I know what I want to wear. As I reach for something with my right hand, my left comes up and takes something different. I can't put it down if it's in my left hand. I have to call my daughter."[8]

Another case is a young man in Georgia who continued to show some profound problems two years after his operation.[9] In working at his father's grocery store he had tremendous difficulty performing stocking and shelving tasks. For example, in stocking canned goods, one hand would place a can in its proper spot on a shelf and the other hand would remove it. These conflicting hand movements persisted even when he thought he was "really" concentrating on the task. His physical and occupational therapists tried many times to practice similar tasks with him, but were unable to stop the problem in real life contexts.

Cases such as these support the concept that the cerebral commissures transmit a good deal of information that is inhibitory in nature—that is, activity in one hemisphere leads to callosal transmissions that serve to moderate, decrease, or stop certain activity in the other. Creating efficient new function through the balance of competitive or "opponent" processes is very common in biological systems. All locomotion, for instance, is based on the action of opposing muscle groups, and all postures depend on a careful balance of such muscle groups. In the central nervous system, opponent processes seem to underlie, for example, geometric illusions where the same drawing can be viewed in two different ways and appears to alternate dramatically between them.

With respect to hemispheric interaction, research with animals has indicated that the cerebral commissures pass information that can either excite or inhibit activity.[10] Colwin Trevarthen reported that split-brain baboons at times reached for an object with both forelimbs at the same time, presumably because no inhibitory processes were available to establish unilateral control over the action.[11] Other work demonstrated that monkeys whose corpus callosum was cut reached to grasp presumably hallucinated objects when the occipital region of one hemisphere was electrically stimulated.[12] This did not occur in animals with the commissures intact, suggesting that in normal animals the unstimulated hemisphere would "disconfirm" the hallucination through inhibitory information passed via the callosum.

It seems likely, thus, that inhibition mediated by the corpus callosum is an important process in maximizing efficiency in behavioral performance and perhaps even in producing new kinds of functions. It is very apparent, however, that these functions are quickly masked by some compensatory mechanisms in most split-brain patients. In fact, in a large majority of cases the two sides of the body appear to work in a coordinated fashion. Perhaps the rarity of patients with persistent disconnection effects indicates that more than callosal damage is necessary in order for the patient to be unable to adjust to the commissurotomy.

For the most part, a battery of sophisticated tests specifically designed to identify a commissurotomy patient would be needed for anyone to know the operation had occurred. Much more common, however, are reports of subtle changes in behavior or ability after surgery. Although some of the reported changes have not held up when carefully studied, others do appear to be verifiable consequences of the operation.

## Subtle Deficits Following Surgery

Several patients have reported great difficulty learning to associate names with faces after surgery. Verification of this came from a study in which subjects had to learn first names for each of three pictures of young men.[13] This procedure was only incidental to the main purpose of the study, but it proved to be a major stumbling block for the subjects. The investigators reported that subjects eventually learned the name–face associations by isolating some unique feature in each picture (for example, "Dick has glasses") rather than by associating the name with the face as a whole. This suggests that the deficit in the ability to associate names and faces may be due to the disconnection of the verbal naming functions of the left side of the brain from the facial-recognition abilities of the right side.

Deficits in the ability to solve geometrical problems have been anecdotally linked to the absence of the corpus callosum. Patient L.B., a high school student with an IQ considerably above average, was transferred out of geometry into a class in general math after he experienced inordinate difficulty with the course. Another report told of a college student who had exceptional difficulty with geometry despite average grades in other courses. Research with split-brain patients studying the ability of each hemisphere to match two- and three-dimensional forms on the basis of common geometrical features showed the right hemisphere to be markedly superior, especially on the most difficult matches.[14] Thus, as in the preceding example, the patient's deficits may be the result of the disconnection of the speaking left hemisphere from the right-hemisphere regions specialized for such tasks.

Another complaint of some split-brain patients is that they no longer dream. Because dreaming is primarily a visual-imaging process, investigators have speculated that it might be the responsibility of the right half of the brain. The operation would serve to disconnect this aspect of the patient's mental life from the speaking left hemisphere and would result in verbal reports that the patient does not dream.

This idea, however, has not been confirmed by further research. Split-brain patients were monitored for brain-wave activity while sleeping and were awakened whenever the recordings indicated they were dreaming. They were then asked to describe the dreams they had just been having. In contrast to the prediction that they would be unable to do so, the patients provided the experimenters with descriptions of their dreams.[15]

Other anecdotal evidence has pointed to poorer memory after surgery. These reports were apparently supported by a study of memory abilities in which several split-brain patients were compared with other epilepsy patients and were found to have poorer scores on a variety of memory tests.[16] A major problem with this type of study, though, is that we really do not know much about split-brain patients' preoperative memory abilities. We can compare their performance after surgery with that of epileptic control subjects who have not had surgery, but we have no way of knowing if the memory skills of the split-brain patients before their surgery were really comparable to the memory skills of the control group. Perhaps they had poorer memories to begin with!

The best approach is to compare memory abilities before and after surgery in the same patient. This was done informally in five patients in the Rayport series. When tested for attention, memory, and sequencing abilities, four showed noticeably impaired performance when tested five to 38 months after surgery. A male patient, J.A.C., reportedly prepared for a shower by removing his clothes, only to put them on again without getting wet. P.O.V., the female patient mentioned earlier, became forgetful to the point of being unable to keep track of her own medication or remember simple directions and arrangements even for a few hours.[17]

This pattern apparently is not found in all or even most patients, however. In the case of patient D.H. operated on by Dr. Donald Wilson of the Dartmouth Medical School, memory performance improved considerably after surgery.[18]

The most likely explanation for this finding is that D.H.'s true abilities were suppressed by drugs and his general condition before surgery. The operation did not miraculously improve his memory; instead, it allowed his true abilities to emerge. In any case, this single-subject study shows that memory deficits do not *necessarily* follow split-brain surgery, and it indicates that further work will be needed to answer the question of whether the operation affects memory and, if so, in which way. It also points to the importance of appropriate controls in studies looking for changes in split-brain patients.

Overall, it is not clear why a few patients seem to show persistent patterns of deficit after commissurotomy, whereas the majority of patients do not. Important differences among patients in their preoperative condition and surgical treatment probably exist, although we do not yet know what they are. There are some consequences of commissurotomy, however, that are dramatic and quite consistent across patients but are short lived.

### Acute Disconnection Syndrome

The *acute disconnection syndrome* is probably due to the surgical division of the commissures as well as to the general trauma resulting from the surgeon's having to squeeze or compress the right hemisphere to gain access to the nerve tracts between the hemispheres.

Patients are often mute for a time after surgery and sometimes they have difficulty controlling the left side of the body, which may at first seem almost paralyzed and then work very awkwardly. As the patient recovers use of the left hand, competitive movements between the left and right hands sometimes occur. This problem usually passes quickly.

After recovering from the initial shock of major brain surgery, most patients report an improved feeling of well-being. Less than two days after surgery, one young patient was well enough to quip that he had a "splitting headache." Within a few weeks, the symptoms of the acute disconnection syndrome subside, making it necessary to use carefully contrived laboratory tests to reveal what had taken place earlier in the operation.

## CROSS CUING

As the study of split-brain patients continued, certain inconsistencies in the findings began to occur with greater frequency. Patients previously unable to identify verbally objects held out of sight in the left hand began to name some items. Some pictures flashed in the left visual field (to the right hemisphere) were also correctly identified verbally. One interpretation of these results is that over time, the right hemispheres of the patients acquired the ability to talk. Another is that information was being transmitted between the hemispheres by way of pathways other than those that were cut.

Although these were interesting and exciting possibilities, Michael Gazzaniga and Steven Hillyard were able to pinpoint a much simpler explanation for their findings.[19] They coined the term *cross cuing* to refer to patients' attempts to use whatever cues are available to make information accessible to both hemispheres. Cross cuing is most obvious in the case where a patient is given an object to hold and identify with his or her left hand, which is out of the line of vision and thus disconnected from the verbal left hemisphere. If, for example, the left hand is given a comb or a toothbrush to feel, the patient will often stroke the brush or the surface of the comb. The patient will then immediately identify the object because the left hemisphere hears the tell-tale sounds.

Cross cuing provides a way for one hemisphere to provide the other with information about what it is experiencing. The direct channels of information transfer are eliminated by the surgery in most instances leaving the patient with indirect cues as the only means of interhemispheric communication. Cross cuing can often be quite subtle, testing the ingenuity of investigators seeking to eliminate it from the experimental situation.

A good example of this is the patient who was able to indicate verbally whether a 0 or a 1 had been flashed to either hemisphere. The same patient was unable to identify verbally pictures of objects flashed to the right hemisphere, nor was he able to identify most objects held in his left hand. This suggested that he lacked the ability to speak from the right hemisphere. Instead, the investigators proposed that cross cuing was involved when the patient reported the numbers flashed to the right hemisphere. They hypothesized that the left hemisphere would begin counting "subvocally" after a presentation to the left visual field and that these signals were picked up by the right hemisphere. When the correct number was reached, the right hemisphere would signal the left to stop and report that digit out loud.

To test this idea, the patient was presented with an expanded version of the task: the digits 2, 3, 5, and 8 were added without his knowledge. At first the subject was very surprised when a new number was presented. His response to the first unexpected number presented to the right hemisphere was, "I beg your pardon." With a little practice, however, he was able to give the correct answer for all the numbers presented to the right hemisphere, but with hesitation when the number was high. In contrast, responses to the same digits presented in the right visual field (to the left hemisphere) were quite prompt.

These findings fit well with the idea that the left hemisphere began counting subvocally after a digit was presented to the right hemisphere. The larger the number of potential digits, the longer the list of numbers the left hemisphere had to go through before reaching the correct one.

Cross cuing generally is not a conscious attempt by the patient to trick the investigator. Instead, it is a natural tendency by an organism to use whatever information it has to make sense of what is going on. This tendency, in fact, contributes further insight into why the common, everyday behavior of split-brain patients seems so unaffected by the surgery.

Careful testing procedures that prevent cross cuing, however, can lead to striking "disconnection" effects, such as those described in the case of patient N.G. In these situations, the patient is unable to tell what picture was flashed to the right hemisphere, although the left hand can point to the correct object. If blindfolded, the patient cannot verbally identify an object held in the left hand but can select with that hand other objects related to it (for example, selecting a book of matches after having held a cigarette).

To an observer unfamiliar with the patient's surgical history, these findings give the impression that the left arm has a mind of its own. They are less mysterious when we realize that the split-brain operation has disconnected the patient's right hemisphere from the centers in the left hemisphere that control speech. The left hand, thus, is the primary means through which the right hemisphere can communicate with the outside world.

## LANGUAGE AND THE HEMISPHERES

Split-brain research has dramatically confirmed that, in most persons, control of speech is localized to the left hemisphere. We have seen that the typical split-brain patient is unable to identify verbally pictures of common objects flashed in the left visual field (to the right hemisphere), although the patient has no difficulty identifying the same pictures presented in the right visual field (to the left hemisphere). The right hemisphere *knows* what the picture represents, however, for it can guide the left hand to select a similar item from among several objects placed behind a screen out of the subject's sight.

The ability to talk, then, is strongly localized in one hemisphere in the split-brain subject as well as in clinical patients. But what about other language abilities? How well can the right hemisphere understand language, either written or spoken? The earliest split-brain studies to consider these questions flashed printed words to the left or the right hemisphere. However, the brief presentation time necessary to ensure that the stimuli reached only one hemisphere placed severe limitations on the kinds of words that could be used.

This problem was eliminated with the development of a new method of restricting visual stimuli to one hemisphere. Developed by Eran Zaidel, who worked extensively with two of the patients in the original California series, it utilizes a device known as the Z *lens*, which is illustrated in Figure 2.5.[20] The Z lens is a contact lens that permits the patient to move his or her eyes freely when examining something, but at the same time ensures that only one hemisphere of the patient's brain receives the visual information. The Z lens makes it possible for the subject to view a stimulus for as long as he or she wants, yet it allows the investigator to present the stimulus to one hemisphere alone.

Zaidel's strategy was to test the comprehension abilities of each hemisphere by using a variety of stimuli that had been used previously both with children and with aphasic patients. The goal was to obtain data that would allow him to compare the abilities of the right hemispheres of split-brain patients with the right-hemisphere abilities of the two groups for which norms were already available.

In tests of auditory vocabulary, two split-brain patients heard a single word spoken by the experimenter and then viewed a display of three pictures through the Z lens. Each patient's task was to select the picture that corresponded with the word. Because the pathways of the auditory system are arranged so that each ear sends information to both hemispheres, under ordinary conditions it is not possible to tell whether one or both hemispheres have understood a spoken message. The Z lens, however, allowed Zaidel to lateralize the response alternatives to one hemisphere so that he could determine how well each half of the brain matched a spoken word to its written counterpart.

The same procedure was also used with the Token Test, in which the subject was asked to arrange plastic shapes of different colors and sizes according to verbal instructions, such as, "Put the yellow square under the green circle." Again, instructions were delivered orally while the objects to be arranged were viewed through the Z lens. The Token Test is commonly used as a test of damage to left-hemisphere language zones, as it is sensitive to impairments not picked up by other aphasia tests.

Zaidel's work revealed a surprising degree and array of comprehension abilities in the right hemisphere.[21] The pattern of results was complex, though, and it was not possible for Zaidel to make a simple

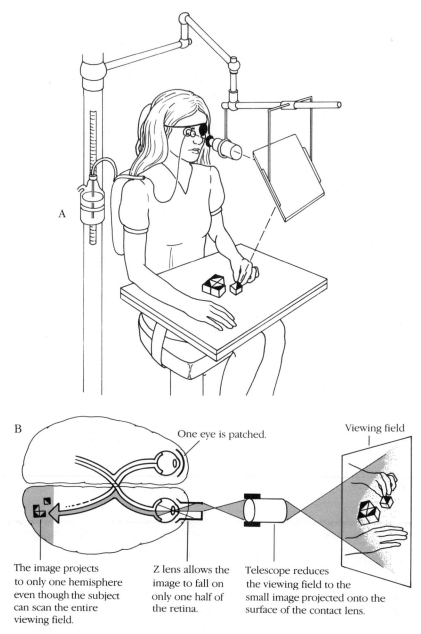

The image projects to only one hemisphere even though the subject can scan the entire viewing field.

Z lens allows the image to fall on only one half of the retina.

Telescope reduces the viewing field to the small image projected onto the surface of the contact lens.

One eye is patched.

Viewing field

**Figure 2.5** The Z lens. A. The Z lens setup keeps the patient's field of view lateralized to one hemisphere. B. One eye is patched, and the image is projected to only one half of the retina of the other eye. [Part A. adapted from Zaidel, "Language Comprehension in the Right Hemisphere Following Cerebral Commissurotomy," in *Language Acquisition and Language Breakdown: Parallels and Divergencies*, ed., A Caramazza and E. Zurif, Fig. 12.2, p. 233, (Baltimore, Md.: The Johns Hopkins University Press, 1978)]

summary statement about the right hemisphere's linguistic "age" or "health." On the vocabulary tests, the right hemisphere generally performed at least as well as a normal 10-year-old, although with the Token Test items it experienced difficulty characteristic of aphasic impairments.

The language asymmetries we have reviewed so far are those found in typical split-brain patients, if it is appropriate to talk of "typical" patients in view of their varied neurological history. The question of how findings from these patients bear on the division of functions between hemispheres in the normal brain is highlighted when we consider how neurological histories can produce dramatic departures from this picture.

## Conversing with the Right Hemisphere

P.S., a right-handed male 16 years of age at the time of surgery, has a preoperative history suggesting considerable damage to the left hemisphere early in life. Studied extensively by Michael Gazzaniga and Joseph LeDoux, P.S. began to use spoken language to identify words and objects flashed to the right hemisphere about three years after surgery.[22] After ruling out cross cuing and inadequate lateralization of stimuli to one hemisphere as possible explanations, Gazzaniga and LeDoux then considered regeneration of the fibers that normally transfer visual information as a basis for P.S.'s newly found ability. Other tests eliminated this explanation as well, providing stronger support that P.S. was indeed "talking" from his right hemisphere.

For example, P.S. was able to compare two stimuli only if they both appeared in the same visual half-field. If half of the information was presented to the right hemisphere and half to the left, his performance dropped to chance level. In other tests, complex scenes were briefly presented in the left visual field. A picture of a man holding a gun, for example, produced the response "Holdup." When questioned about details, however, the patient provided an inaccurate description of the picture. The investigators concluded that the simple response was correctly generated by the right hemisphere, while the more talkative (and ignorant of the picture) left hemisphere provided the erroneous elaboration.[23] Figure 2.6 illustrates these tests.

Although P.S. represents the first split-brain patient to acquire the ability to speak from the right hemisphere, we should perhaps not be

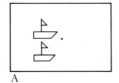 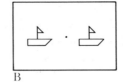 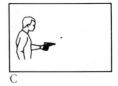

A                                    B                                    C

**Figure 2.6** A. The stimuli to be compared are presented within the same visual field. B. The stimuli require comparison across visual fields. C. An example of a complex scene flashed in either the left or right visual field.

too surprised at this occurrence in light of his history of left-hemisphere damage. For many years, some neurologists have argued that the recovery of language function following severe damage to the language hemisphere in some cases is a result of a process by which the intact hemisphere assumes many of the functions of the damaged one. The intriguing questions are why some people can do this while others cannot, and whether language is learned by the intact hemisphere after the injury or has been present, but lying dormant, for much of the patient's life.

## The Right-Hemisphere Language Controversy

On the basis of his review of research dealing with the role of the right hemisphere in language, Gazzaniga argues that the normal right hemisphere is nonlinguistic.[24] Signs of linguistic ability in the right hemisphere of split-brain patients are attributable, he claims, to early left-hemisphere damage resulting in reorganization of language functions to the right hemisphere. Patient P.S. is a good example. Gazzaniga notes that only three of the 28 patients tested in the Wilson patient series, including P.S., showed evidence of right-hemisphere language to some degree and that in each of these cases signs of early left-hemisphere injury were present. He further notes that only two patients from the California series, L.B. and N.G., showed evidence of right-hemisphere language, that these were the same patients extensively studied by Zaidel using the Z lens, and that both are suspected of having left-hemisphere injury. Citing these factors, Gazzaniga argues that evidence for the role of the right hemisphere in language in split-brain patients cannot be extended to the normal brain.

Zaidel disagrees with Gazzaniga's conclusions.[25] He claims that six, not two, California split-brain patients have shown evidence of right-hemisphere language and that there is little reason to believe that L.B. and N.G. have the kind of left-hemisphere lesion that would result in right-hemisphere takeover of language function. He further points to clinical data suggesting a role for the right hemisphere in language, citing right-hemisphere recovery of some language functions in aphasia and the fact that selective language deficits do occur following right-hemisphere lesions in right-handers. He suggests that differences among aphasic patients in the degree to which the right hemisphere takes over language functions result from variability in the amount of interference to the right hemisphere caused by different kinds of left-hemisphere lesions. He also notes that there may be inherent variability among right-handers in the language functions of the right hemisphere.*

It is clear that existing data are not sufficient to clarify the very important question of the nature and extent of right-hemisphere involvement in language in the normal brain. The issue is one of considerable theoretical as well as practical significance, however, and is currently the focus of a great deal of research.

## Some Cautions About Interpreting Data

The preceding controversy points to the need for caution in extending any research finding with split-brain subjects to normal subjects. Both the factors that produced the epilepsy in the first place and the epilepsy itself may have produced changes in the brains of split-brain patients, making their brains fundamentally different from those of normal subjects. Neurologist Norman Geschwind noted that some commissurotomy patients probably suffered epilepsy as a result of brain lesions occurring in utero. Such prenatal lesions have been shown to result in significant reorganizations of the brain that differ from those occuring after birth during childhood. Geschwind also pointed out that long-standing epilepsy may itself produce major changes in brain organization. Perhaps the epilepsy has modified the use of brain pathways making the patients different from the unaffected adult population.

Summarizing his views on this issue, Geschwind observed that "many of the arguments in the literature between different investigators as to the effects of callosal section probably do not reflect a real difference in the adequacy of the data, but simply arise because the investigators have been studying patients in whom the patterns of

*See Chapter 6 for a more extensive discussion of the role of the right hemisphere in language and in recovery from aphasia.

brain development and connections are simply not equivalent."[26] Some researchers would dismiss split-brain research because of the problems in interpreting results. A better approach, we think, is to continue to learn what we can about the brain from the study of split-brain patients, remembering that such research will be but one of several tools needed to complete the picture.

## VISUO-SPATIAL FUNCTIONS IN THE HEMISPHERES

The older literature on damage to the human brain provided split-brain investigators with good clues about the kinds of tasks likely to be performed better by the right hemisphere. On the basis of split-brain studies, the most general statement that can be made about right-hemisphere specializations is that they are nonlinguistic functions that seem to involve complex visual and spatial processes.

The perception of part–whole relations, for example, seems to be superior in the right hemisphere. In one task, patients viewed line drawings of geometric shapes that had been cut up and the pieces slightly separated. Their task was to decide which of three solid alternatives felt with one hand out of view was represented by the fragmented figure. The left hand was far superior on this task; the right hand showed chance performance in six of seven patients. In another study, commissurotomy patients were shown arcs (sections of circles) presented to either the left or the right visual field. After each presentation, they were asked to choose which circle from a set of different-sized circles would be formed by the arcs they saw. The patients performed much better when their judgments were based on arcs presented to the left visual field (right hemisphere).[27]

One of the most dramatic demonstrations of right-hemisphere superiority in visuo-spatial tasks was recorded on film by Gazzaniga and Sperry while they were testing W.J., the first patient of the California series. W.J. was presented with several cubes, each containing two red sides, two white sides, and two half-red and half-white sides divided along the diagonal. His task was to arrange these blocks to form squares with patterns identical to those shown on a series of cards. Figure 2.7 illustrates the task.

The beginning of the film shows W.J. readily assembling the blocks with his left hand to form a particular pattern. When he tries to form a pattern with his right hand, however, he experiences great difficulty. Slowly and with considerable indecision, the right hand arranges the blocks. At one point, the left hand moves into the picture and begins to assemble the blocks in the correct pattern. It is gently but firmly removed from the table by the investigator, while the right hand continues to fumble, unaided by the more skillful left.

Other evidence pointing to right-hemisphere superiority in visuo-spatial ability comes from differences in the abilities of the two hands of the split-brain patient to draw a figure of a cube. Invariably, the left hand produces a better drawing. Examples are shown in Figure 2.8.

What is the basis for the right hemisphere's superior abilities in these visuo-spatial tasks? Two possibilities suggested themselves to investigators. First, the right hemisphere could be dominant for the expression of visual understanding, just as the left hemisphere is dominant for the expression of language understanding, although both halves of the brain might be equally skilled in *perceiving* spatial relationships. This view emphasizes an asymmetry in the ability to perform the complex motor acts required by the tasks. An alternative interpretation holds that there are true differences in perceptual abilities between hemispheres.

LeDoux and Gazzaniga conducted several experiments that they claim demonstrate a manipulative basis for right-hemisphere superiorities. They argue that the right-hemisphere advantage in tasks like block design depends on the involvement of manual activities. In one series of experiments, they presented split-brain patients with draw-

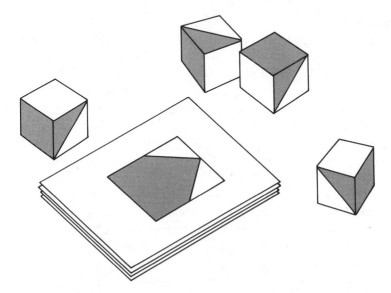

**Figure 2.7** A block-design task. The subject is asked to arrange the colored blocks to match the sample pattern.

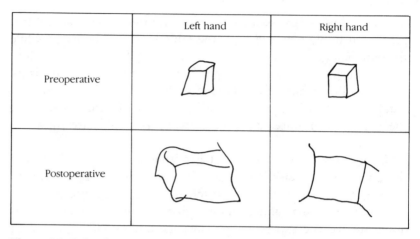

|  | Left hand | Right hand |
|---|---|---|
| Preoperative |  |  |
| Postoperative |  |  |

**Figure 2.8** Cube drawings before and after commissurotomy. Preoperatively, the patient could draw a cube with either hand. Postoperatively, the right hand performed poorly. The patient was right-handed. [From Gazzaniga and LeDoux, *The Integrated Mind*, Fig. 18, p. 52 (New York: Plenum Press, 1978)]

ings of various block-design patterns. These drawings were flashed to the left hemisphere via the right visual field. After each presentation, the patients were asked to choose a similar pattern from among several patterns displayed on a table. The patients' left hemispheres were able to do this quite well, despite not being able to form similar patterns with blocks when the patients were asked to do so using the right hand.

LeDoux and Gazzaniga argue that once the manipulative aspect of solving a visual pattern was removed, the left and right hemispheres performed equally well; thus, the right-hemisphere advantage is due, not to a general visuo-spatial superiority, but to a superiority in being able to manipulate spatial relationships in the environment. They further suggest that this manipulative skill is indicative of a developed awareness on the part of the right hemisphere of the relationships among the body, body movements, and the spatial environment.[28]

Although there may be considerable validity to the concept that right-hemisphere superiority is a *manipulo-spatial* superiority, another interpretation of these experiments is possible. The format in which the left hemisphere did well on the problem was in a simple match-to-sample test—the left hemisphere saw a pattern and then had to choose one like it. Hand manipulation of blocks was not involved, but neither was any *mental* manipulation of the patterns. If the left hemisphere had to choose its answers from pictures of block patterns presented in some spatially altered form (for example, tilted, turned upside down, or slightly separated) it might fail again, relative to the right hemisphere, despite not having to manipulate any blocks. Some evidence for this comes from another experiment by Laura Franco and Roger Sperry.

Franco and Sperry tested each hand of right-handed commissurotomy patients and normal control subjects on matching unseen objects by touch with geometric shapes presented in free vision. They found that the left hands of the split-brain subjects performed consistently better than the right hands. Furthermore, this left-hand (right-hemisphere) superiority increased as the shapes became less geometric and more free-form. When the sets of objects to be matched consisted only of free-form contours, the right hand (left hemisphere) performed barely above choice level. Normal subjects did equally well with each hand on these tasks.[29]

One can argue that left-hemisphere difficulty increased as the objects became less describable verbally or, perhaps, less structurally constrained. In either case, the results show that matching such objects by touch and visual perception requires the involvement of the right hemisphere, for it seems that simply disconnecting the two half-brains results in a severe breakdown in the performance of the preferred right hand. What seems most important in solving the matching tasks is not the tactile manipulation and sensations from the fingers of the hand but "knowing what kind of shaped object to feel for . . . this in turn requires being able to subjectively visualize what the seen figure would look like if folded up."[30] Thus, the right-hemisphere superiority is not just in spatially related hand activities but also in visual–mental manipulations. We shall discuss some further implications of this issue in Chapter 12.

## IMAGERY

The subject of visual–mental imagery has enjoyed a recent increase in interest as investigators have sought to understand how it is generated and what parts of the brain are involved in it. Although the visual, nonverbal nature of imagery initially suggests greater involvement of the right hemisphere, a recent review of the neuropsychological evidence found little support for this idea.[31] Reports of deficits in imagery, for example, were just as likely to follow left-sided brain damage as right-sided damage. One possible explanation of this is that imagery depends on a number of components, each of which may or may not be lateralized. If this view is correct, a particular imagery task may show more left- or more right-hemisphere specialization depending on the precise component processes involved in it.

Split-brain patients appear to be close to ideal subjects in which to study some of these ideas. With this in mind, Martha Farah and her colleagues presented J.W., a male patient who is part of the Wilson series, with upper case letters in the left or right visual field and asked him to indicate whether their lower case counterparts were tall or short by pushing one of two buttons. For example, lower case versions of B, D, and F are tall, whereas lower case versions of A, C, and E are short. J.W.'s task was to image the lower case form of the letters as each was presented and to respond appropriately. J.W. did well when the stimuli were presented in the right visual field (left hemisphere), but he could not make these judgments above chance level when the stimuli were presented in the left visual field (right hemisphere).[32]

Psychologist Michael Corballis, working with patient L.B., one of the early California series of patients, also obtained a right visual field (left hemisphere) advantage in a similar test with letters, although L.B.'s right hemisphere performed somewhat above chance level.[33] When L.B. was tested in a task requiring mental rotation, however, the results were strikingly different. His task was to decide if a letter was in its normal form or backward, i.e., mirror imaged. The letters, flashed individually to the left or right visual field, were presented at different orientations.

Previous research has shown that neurologically normal subjects performed this task by mentally rotating a letter to its upright position and then making the judgment of normal or backward. The evidence for this is elegantly simple. The speed with which a subject responds to a given letter turns out to be a function of the letter's orientation. The farther it is from upright, the longer it takes the subject to decide if it is normal or backward.

When L.B. was tested in this task, both hemispheres showed a pattern of response times consistent with mental rotation. However, the right hemisphere was dramatically more accurate and faster in making the judgments.

The results of these studies are consistent with the idea that mental imagery is not a single, unitary process, and that the two hemispheres may contribute differently to the subprocesses involved in different tasks. Tasks involving simply visualizing may be handled differently than those involving manipulation of the images. The studies reinforce the importance of looking at the components of tasks, and of not making simple, a priori assumptions about hemispheric involvement in complex activity.

## PARTIAL COMMISSUROTOMY

Since the split-brain operations of the early 1960s, several neurosurgeons have attempted to control intractable epilepsy with a procedure less radical than the severing of all the forebrain commissures. The idea was to limit the surgery to the areas of the corpus callosum and anterior commissure most likely to transmit epileptic discharges in any particular patient. If the source of the epileptic discharges could be localized to some specific region of the brain, they reasoned, then cutting only those fibers connecting that area with the opposite hemisphere should help control the epilepsy.

This was what Van Wagenen had attempted in the first human split-brain operations of the 1940s. His results, however, did not consistently bring relief from the spread of seizures. The success of complete commissurotomy two decades later encouraged neurosurgeons to attempt partial surgical procedures once again. The results have been quite good, from both a medical and a scientific viewpoint. The growing number of subjects with only specific parts of the interhemispheric commissures cut has allowed investigators to study the function of specific regions of the commissures.

One question asked is what kinds of information are transferred across particular regions of the commissures. Gazzaniga and his associates have studied a group of partial-commissurotomy patients operated on by Dr. Donald Wilson to answer this question. Work with these patients has suggested that there is a high degree of specificity of function within the cerebral commissures of humans.

Parts of the front region of the corpus callosum are responsible for *somatosensory*, or touch, transfer. The rear third of the corpus callosum, the *splenium*, transfers visual information. Recent data suggest that the anterior commissure also transfers visual information in some, but not all, patients.[34]

A patient with the front half of the callosum cut will not be able to tell what he or she has in the left hand but will be able to tell what was flashed in the left visual field. The tactile information is not accessible to the verbal left hemisphere, whereas the visual information gets across. A patient with only the splenium cut may or may not show any sensory disconnection, depending on whether the anterior commissure is capable of transferring visual information in that patient. Tactual identification, in any case, would be normal.

Patients who have undergone partial commissurotomy show interesting capabilities for visual and tactile matching even though the transfer of one or the other modality is disconnected by the operation. A patient is asked, for example, to hold an object out of sight with the right hand. He or she then views an object flashed in his or her left visual field and decides whether they are the same. A patient split either tactually or visually can do this task well. In the first case, the left hemisphere apparently bases the decision on a match of tactual information with the visual information transferred from the right hemisphere. In the second case, the right hemisphere makes the match by comparing visual information with tactile information transferred across the callosum from the left.

Partial commissurotomy has proved itself to be quite effective in alleviating epilepsy in some patients. In addition, the procedure is of considerable interest from a research standpoint. It has helped, and will continue to help, refine our knowledge about the role of different parts of the interhemispheric fibers and the brain regions they connect. Because the anatomical projections of the fibers are known, one can estimate what regions are connected by the fibers that remain after partial commissurotomy. Patients' abilities and inabilities to perform and transfer lateralized tasks can then give an indication of which parts of the brain are involved in a particular task.

## INFORMATION PROCESSING
## IN THE TWO HEMISPHERES

As research into the specialized functions of the two hemispheres continued, the pattern of results suggested a new way to conceptualize hemispheric differences. Instead of a breakdown based on the type of tasks (for example, verbal or spatial) best performed by each hemisphere, a dichotomy based on different ways of dealing with information in general seemed to emerge.

According to this analysis, the left hemisphere is specialized for language functions, but these specializations are a consequence of the left hemisphere's superior analytic skills, of which language is one manifestation. Similarly, the right hemisphere's superior visuo-spatial performance is derived from its synthetic, holistic manner of dealing with information. Much of the work that led to this reanalysis of hemispheric differences was conducted by Jerre Levy and her colleagues working with the California series of patients.

One of the first suggestions that the two hemispheres have different information-processing styles came from a study in which split-brain patients were asked to match small wooden blocks held in the left or the right hand with the appropriate two-dimensional representation selected from drawings of blocks shown in "opened-up" form. Overall, the left hand was considerably better than the right at this task, but the most interesting finding was that the two hemispheres appeared to use different strategies in approaching the problem.

An analysis of errors showed that the patterns the right hand (left hemisphere) found relatively easier to deal with were the patterns that were easy to describe in words but difficult to discriminate visually. For the left hand (right hemisphere), the reverse was true. Thus, the left hemisphere appeared to make its matches on the basis of verbal descriptions of the properties of the blocks and the two-dimensional patterns. It seemed unable to fold up the two-dimensional representation mentally so that a match could be made on the basis of overall appearance.[35]

Other work has shown that the two hemispheres differ in the kinds of information they pick up from visual stimuli. We will discuss these studies at greater length in a later section of this chapter. For now, we need only point out that pictures that can be matched either by their functions (such as a cake on a plate matched with a spoon and a fork) or, by their appearances (such as a cake on a plate matched with a hat with brim) are handled differently by the two hemispheres. See Figure 2.9 for examples of the stimuli. With ambiguous instructions simply to match similar stimuli, the left hemisphere of the split-brain patient matches by function, and the right hemisphere matches by appearance.

Levy concluded that the left hemisphere's strategy in dealing with incoming information is best characterized as analytic, while the right hemisphere appears to process information in a holistic manner.[36] There are other ways to interpret the differences we have just considered, but the analytic–holistic distinction has been the most influential in moving thinking about hemispheric differences away from the verbal–nonverbal dichotomy. The latter is clearly too simplistic to explain all the results found with brain-damaged, split-brain, and (as we shall see in the next chapter) normal subjects.

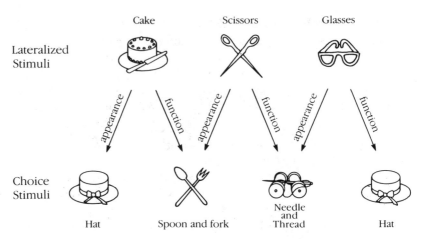

**Figure 2.9** Function and appearance matches by split-brain patients. The stimuli in the top row are visually presented to one hemisphere at a time. The patient is instructed to pick the best "match" from the choice stimuli. When the left hemisphere sees the stimuli it tends to match by function. When the right hemisphere sees the stimuli it tends to match by appearance. [Adapted from Levy and Trevarthen, "Metacontrol of Hemispheric Function in Human Split Brain Patients," Fig. 1, p. 302. *Journal of Experimental Psychology*, 1976, (American Psychological Association), Reprinted by permission.]

## VISUAL COMPLETION

Patient N.G. sits in front of a screen. Once again, she is asked to gaze at a spot marked in the middle. A strange picture appears briefly on the screen. It is a split face made up of the left half of one face and the right half of another, joined down the middle. On the right is half of the face she has been taught to identify as "Dick"; on the left, the face belonging to "Tom." A split stimulus such as this is known as a *chimeric figure*. It is named after Chimera, a mythical monster made up of parts of different animals.

N.G. is asked to report what she saw. She says she saw "Dick." When questioned further, she denies that there was anything odd about the picture. Later, the same composite picture is flashed on the screen. This time she is asked not to say anything. Instead, she is shown several faces in full view and is asked to point with either hand to the one she saw. This time she points to the picture of "Tom."

This experiment, shown in Figure 2.10, again shows that each half of the brain is blind to what the other side is seeing. What is particularly striking is that in this split-face study, each half of the

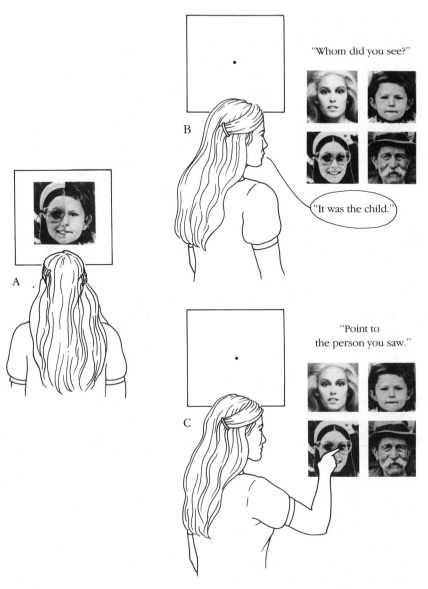

**Figure 2.10** Chimeric-stimuli tests with split-brain patients. A. The subject is told she will see a picture. She is asked to fixate on the center of the screen; a composite picture is flashed. The subject is asked to identify the picture, either B verbally or C by pointing with one hand or the other. Split-brain patients seem unaware that the chimeric stimuli are incomplete or conflicting. When asked to vocalize the answer, they choose the picture from which the right-field half of the composite was made. When asked to point, they choose the picture from which the left-field half was made. [Adapted from Levy, Trevarthen, and Sperry, "Perception of Bilateral Chimeric Figures Following Hemispheric Disconnection," Fig. 4, p. 68. *Brain* 95 (1972).]

brain seemed to see a normal, symmetrical face, despite the unusual composition of the stimuli. In addition, the patient's report of what she sees changes with the nature of the response she is asked to make. The patient shows no sign of conflict when this occurs.

*Completion*, the tendency for split-brain patients to see as whole what are really partial figures falling at the visual midline, was first noted when patients showed the ability to identify accurately a square flashed briefly in the center of the visual field. Because the left half of the square is projected to the right hemisphere and the right half to the left hemisphere, the fact that the patients reported seeing a normal square meant that the left hemisphere had "completed" the partial figure presented to it. The right hemisphere also perceived a normal square, for the left hand would draw a complete figure when a patient was asked to sketch what he or she saw with that hand.[37] Later studies have shown that chimeric figures such as the composite pictures presented to patient N.G. also give rise to visual completion.

The completion phenomenon is seen in some patients who have unilateral damage to the visual regions of the brain, as well as in split-brain patients. It is not well understood in either case, but it is clearly one of the reasons split-brain patients report that the world appears normal. In conjunction with eye movements that bring information to both hemispheres, completion helps bring to visual experience a unity that extends across the visual field.

## The Evidence from Chimeric-Figures Studies

The use of chimeric figures with split-brain patients has advanced the study of how the two hemispheres accomplish their division of labor when the subject is presented with a task. Although we cannot be sure that the intact brain works in the same way, it is well worth our time to review what has been learned about the dynamics of hemispheric interaction from split-brain patients.

Jerre Levy and her colleagues have extensively studied chimeric stimuli with the split-brain patients in California. In the first study, they used chimeric faces formed from pictures of three young men.[38] Subjects were told that they would see a picture flashed briefly on a screen and then would be asked to point to the picture seen from among several presented in a display viewed in free vision. Subjects fixated on a dot in the center of their visual field, and the chimeric face was flashed for 150 milliseconds to ensure that each half of the face would reach only one hemisphere. Regardless of the hand they used to point with, the patients overwhelmingly selected the face going to the right hemisphere. Double responses, as well as left-hemisphere-only responses, were rare.

This is evidence that the right hemisphere can control the right hand as well as the left hand in a simple pointing task. Up to now, we considered only the crossed, or *contralateral*, nerve fibers that allow each hemisphere to control the hand opposite to it. However, a much smaller number of same-side, or *ipsilateral*, fibers allow each hemisphere to exert some control over the hand on the same side of the body. Ipsilateral motor control, though, is generally quite coarse and limited to movements of the whole arm or hand. Fine finger movements require the use of the contralateral hemisphere and generally cannot be controlled by the ipsilateral hemisphere.

In the present task, the right hemisphere, better at recognizing faces than the left, exercises its limited ability to control the right hand via the ipsilateral fibers. When subjects are asked to identify verbally what they saw, however, the error rate goes up, and the majority of the responses are to the face that went to the left hemisphere.* When the facial recognition task is set up so that the left hemisphere is forced to play a role (for example, by requiring a verbal response), we get evidence that it can do the task, but it does not do as well as the right hemisphere.

Another study using pictures of common objects (a rose, an eye, and a bee) divided in half to form chimeric stimuli produced almost identical results. When pointing, patients matched the object seen by the right hemisphere. When asked to report verbally what they saw, they gave more left-hemisphere responses but made more errors. These results extend the generality of the right hemisphere's superior skills in dealing with nonverbal visual stimuli.

## Dominance and Capacity

Levy concluded that two factors are at work in determining the outcome of these tasks.[39] The first is *dominance*, the tendency for one hemisphere to process information and control responding. The

---

*Most, but not all, verbal responses were to the faces presented to the left hemisphere. A greater-than-chance number of right-hemisphere faces were also reported. The investigators suggest that the right hemisphere may be controlling speech in these instances. A more likely explanation, however, is that lateralization of the inputs was not perfect and that stimuli to the left visual field occasionally reached the left hemisphere.

other is *capacity*, the ability of a hemisphere to perform a task when the experiment requires it to do so. In the two chimeric-figures studies just considered, the left hemisphere showed the capacity to recognize faces and objects when the subject was required to respond verbally. However, it was not dominant in the task; the overwhelming majority of responses came from the right hemisphere in the manual, free-response situation.

The concepts of dominance and capacity are further illustrated in another chimeric-figures study.[40] This experiment used the rose, eye, and bee stimuli in a task where subjects were instructed to respond on the basis of phonetic (sound) similarity between the stimulus and choice items. After seeing a chimeric object, they were told to point to the picture that rhymed with what they saw. Toes, a pie, and a key were the choices. In this situation, over 82 percent of the matches were to the item presented to the left hemisphere, regardless of the hand used. In contrast, when subjects were asked to do direct visual matching with the same stimuli, they pointed to the object seen by the right hemisphere.

To see whether the right hemisphere had any capacity at all in this task, the investigators flashed a single complete picture of the rose, the bee, or the eye in the left visual field and asked the patients to select the figure that rhymed. Performance was at a chance level.

These results are interesting for two reasons. First, they suggest that the right hemisphere lacks the ability to deal with speech at a phonetic, or sound, level. This finding contrasts with results obtained by Zaidel and the Z lens. Zaidel's work pointed to the apparent ability of the right hemisphere to understand connected speech. Second, Levy's results provide an example in which the left hemisphere is dominant for a task that the right hemisphere appears totally incapable of performing.

## HEMISPHERIC "DISPOSITION": WHO IS IN CHARGE HERE, ANYWAY?

In the studies we have considered up to now, the hemisphere controlling the response in a free-response situation was always the one with the greater capacity for that particular task. This makes good intuitive sense. If the two hemispheres have unequal abilities in a given situation, the superior hemisphere should assume responsibility for responding. More recent work, however, has suggested that this is not always the case and that the hemispheres can differ in their disposition to respond at particular times.

Jerre Levy and Colwyn Trevarthen constructed chimeric figures from drawings of common objects and asked subjects to point to a similar picture from an array viewed in free vision.[41] Objects could match on the basis of their function or on the basis of their appearance. Functional and appearance matches for stimuli to both the left and right hemispheres were included among the choices on each trial. This allowed the investigators to see whether each hemisphere had a preferred "mode" for making matches. The investigators hypothesized that functional matches would be best performed by the left hemisphere and appearance matches would be the specialty of the right.

This prediction was supported by the data from one patient who was given ambiguous instructions to match "similar" objects. Responses to left-hemisphere stimuli were overwhelmingly functional, while responses to right-hemisphere stimuli were on the basis of appearance. The investigators then specifically instructed the same subject and other patients to perform matches on the basis of function or appearance. In general, function instructions elicited function matches to left-hemisphere stimuli, and appearance instructions elicited appearance matches to right-hemisphere items.

A large number of responses, however, deviated from the expected pattern. In some cases, appearance instruction resulted in a response to the right-hemisphere stimulus, but the subject made a function match. Similarly, function instructions sometimes resulted in a response to the left-hemisphere stimulus that was based on appearance. In these cases, the hemisphere appropriate to the instructions responded, but in an "inappropriate" way. The reverse also occurred: the hemisphere inappropriate in terms of the instructions sometimes controlled the response, using the "appropriate" processing strategy. For example, the right hemisphere might respond under "function" instructions, making its decision on the basis of function, or the left hemisphere might respond under "appearance" instructions, with the response based on appearance.

These results show that a given hemisphere does not always do the tasks for which it is thought superior, nor in performing a task does it always process information in the manner expected of it. This surprising result led Levy to speculate that "hemispheric activation does not depend on a hemisphere's real aptitude or even on its actual processing strategy on a given occasion, but rather on what it *thinks* it can do."[42]

## SEPARATED AWARENESS AND
## UNIFYING MECHANISMS

Under certain conditions, each hemisphere of a split-brain patient appears to function as an independent processor, producing results reminiscent of the behavior of two separate individuals. As Sperry has observed:

> Each hemisphere . . . has its own . . . private sensations, percep-
> tions, thought, and ideas all of which are cut off from the corre-
> sponding experiences in the opposite hemisphere. Each left and right
> hemisphere has its own private chain of memories and learning expe-
> riences that are inaccessible to recall by the other hemisphere. In
> many respects each disconnected hemisphere appears to have a sepa-
> rate "mind of its own."[43]

Yet, most casual observers would not notice anything unusual about most split-brain patients shortly after commissurotomy. In fact, a patient who recovered from the operation without complications could probably go through a routine medical checkup a year or two later without giving away his or her surgical history to anyone not already acquainted with it. Speech, language comprehension, person-ality, and motor coordination are remarkably preserved in patients without a corpus callosum and other commissures.

What keeps the two separate hemispheres acting as a unit during the everyday activities of these patients? A variety of unifying mecha-nisms, some of which we have already considered, seem to compen-sate for the absence of the cerebral commissures. Conjugate eye movements, as well as each eye's projecting to both hemispheres, play an important role in establishing unity of the visual world. The eye movements initiated by one hemisphere to bring an object into direct view serve to make that information available to the other hemisphere as well. Much of the conflict that would result from having the two hemispheres view different halves of the visual field is thus avoided.

The operation of ipsilateral as well as contralateral fibers in the touch modality was mentioned in the context of the chimeric-figures studies. It provides another means by which each hemisphere is made aware of stimulation from both sides of space. The ipsilateral infor-mation is generally incomplete and inadequate to enable a patient to identify verbally an object held in the left hand. However, the ipsilateral pathways do provide partial information.

Still another way information is made available to both hemispheres is by commissures located in the lower regions of the brain. A great deal of the brain below the cortex is not split by the commissurotomy procedure. The human split-brain operation severs the nerve bundles connecting the cortical levels of the brain. These are the major fibers connecting the hemispheres, but other, smaller commissures remain intact. These other commissures connect paired structures that are part of the brain stem. They are shown in Figure 2.11.

One such structure, the *superior colliculus*, is involved in the location of objects and the tracking of their movement. The colliculus is believed to process the "where" aspects of the visual world, as opposed to the "what," or finely detailed, aspects of vision. The left and right superior colliculi communicate through the commis-

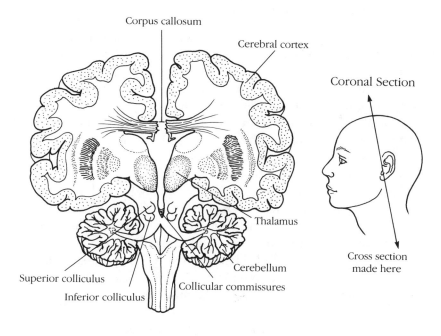

**Figure 2.11** Extent of separation of the brain after forebrain commissurotomy. The structures of the midbrain remain connected by the collicular commissures. [From Sperry, "The Great Cerebral Commissure," Scientific American, Inc., 1964. All rights reserved.]

sures connecting them, so each hemisphere is provided with information about the location of objects regardless of where the objects fall in the visual field. Such crude location information could explain the phenomenon of visual completion mentioned earlier.

The brain stem is also believed to play a role in the process whereby the two hemispheres share emotional reactions. Emotional changes induced by presenting something to only one hemisphere are thought to spread partly into the other hemisphere through brain-stem routes. The flow of emotional change is difficult to isolate, however, because emotion involves so many external changes controlled by and accessible to both hemispheres. The overt bodily changes produced by one hemisphere may be read as cues by the other (cross cuing); in addition, it is possible that there is more direct transfer of emotional "tone" between the two cerebral hemispheres through brain-stem commissures.

## Evidence for Information Shared by the Disconnected Hemispheres

Most recently, a series of studies with split-brain patients has suggested that both hemispheres may have access to selected aspects of a stimulus presented to one hemisphere alone. The stimulus used in one study looking at visual attention consisted of a three-by-three-cell grid located to the left or the right of the subject's point of fixation.[44] On each trial, one of the target digits was presented for 150 milliseconds in one of the nine cells; the subject's task was to indicate whether the target was odd or even by depressing one of two response keys. On within-field trials, before the onset of the target an X (spatial cue) appeared either briefly in one of the nine cells in the grid or was superimposed on the central fixation point. When it appeared in one of the nine cells, it occurred either in the cell corresponding to the position of the target digit to follow or in a different cell. On between-fields trials, two grids appeared, one in each field, with the X appearing in a cell in one field and the target presented subsequently in a cell in the other field. Figure 2.12 illustrates this.

Earlier work with this procedure had shown that reaction time is faster when the spatial cue indicates the target's subsequent location, allowing the subject to direct his or her attention to the appropriate location prior to the onset of the target. Correspondingly, reaction time is longer when the spatial cue directs the subject's attention to an incorrect location. The question explored in this study was

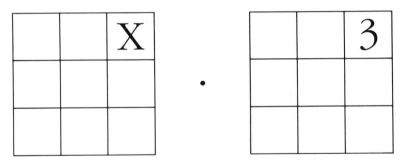

**Figure 2.12** Example of stimuli for a trial in the between-fields condition. For the first part of each trial, two empty grids were presented on either side of a fixation dot. Next, the spatial cue (X) appeared for 150 milliseconds in one of the grid cells. After a 1.5-second interval in which only the empty grids were shown, the target digit was presented in the opposite grid in either the same relative position as the cue or in a different position. This figure illustrates a valid cue (same position) trial.

whether this effect would be found in split-brain patients when the task required access to information from both hemispheres (between fields). Results were quite clear: for each of the two split-brain subjects tested, reaction time decreased when the subject had prior information about the target's spatial location in both the between-fields and within-field conditions and increased when an invalid cue was presented.

A second experiment using the same approach showed that ex-plicit information about the location of a stimulus presented in one visual field is not available to the other hemisphere. In the within-field condition, an X appeared briefly in one of the grid cells, followed later by an X in the same cell or in a different cell. In the between-field condition, the two Xs appeared in the same or differ-ent cells on different grids. The subject's task was to indicate by a key press whether the Xs appeared in the same positions or in different positions.

One of the two patients tested did not perform better than at a chance level in the between-fields task, while the second patient's responses were at a level somewhat better than chance. Recall, however, that both patients benefited from the spatial cue in the first experiment. The investigators suggest that these data provide evi-dence for distinguishing between stimulus information needed for explicit identification of spatial location and stimulus information needed to direct visual attention. They argue that different neural pathways may be involved in these two functions and that commissurotomy does not disrupt the access of either hemisphere to information needed to direct visual attention.

Another study suggesting that both hemispheres may have access to selected aspects of a stimulus presented to one hemisphere alone focused on semantic processing, or extraction of meaning. In normal subjects, processing the meaning of a word can have a significant effect on judgments about subsequent words. This effect is called *semantic priming.* In a task in which a subject is required to determine whether a letter string is a real word or a nonword, presentation of a semantically related word beforehand results in shorter reaction time than does presentation of a semantically unrelated word.

Adapting this procedure for use with split-brain patients, John Sidtis and his colleagues presented one patient with a series of common nouns flashed to the left or to the right of a central fixation point.[45] The subject's task was to indicate whether each target word referred to something natural or to something manufactured. Each target word was preceded by either an unrelated word in the same category (for example, ship–gate) or a related word in the same category (ship–boat). The preceding word appeared in either the same visual field as the target (within field) or in the visual field opposite the one in which the target was presented (between fields.)

Although left-hemisphere performance was more accurate overall than right-hemisphere performance, the effects of semantic relatedness were found in both the within-field and between-fields conditions. The investigators concluded that the right and left hemispheres maintain access to a functionally common semantic system, although neither hemisphere can verbally name words presented to the right hemisphere. Thus, we have a situation where semantic priming of one hemisphere facilitates a subsequent judgment by the other hemisphere, although the activation does not provide sufficient information for explicit naming.

These two sets of findings suggest additional ways in which the two disconnected hemispheres share information. The mechanisms underlying this shared access are not clear, however, and additional work needs to be done to extend these findings to larger samples of patients. These studies are good examples of the importance of isolating individual components or stages in the processing of a stimulus for study: different results are found depending on which stage or component is looked at.

## WHAT DO THE CEREBRAL COMMISSURES REALLY DO?

We started this chapter with an account of the mystery surrounding the function of the corpus callosum. Are we now any nearer to understanding it? A simple answer would be to say, yes, we know that the cerebral commissures transfer information obtained by one hemisphere over to the other hemisphere. Although this is true, it is not a particularly revealing or complete answer. At the very least, we want to know the nature of the information that is transferred and how it is used by the hemispheres.

Some investigators have suggested that it is primarily sensory information that transfers across the callosum, providing a complete representation of all sensory input in each hemisphere. We do not know, however, that a separate representation of the world in each hemisphere is really necessary. After all, a split-brain animal or human patient does very well in a normal perceptual environment outside of contrived laboratory tests.

Perhaps, then, the corpus callosum transfers more complex, processed information and performs a function other than simply providing a duplicate representation of sensory input. Before we deal further with these issues, however, let's briefly consider the possible basis for asymmetries in human brain function and their consequences. It is likely that an understanding of the role of the cerebral commissures will require an understanding of the nature of hemispheric asymmetry.

### A Model of Brain Asymmetry

It has been postulated that in the course of evolution the functions of the left and right hemispheres began to diverge. Areas in the left hemisphere became more adept at generating rapidly changing motor patterns, such as those involved in fine control of the hands and the vocal tract. They also became more skilled at processing the rapidly changing auditory patterns produced by the vocal tract during speech.

Further speculation has led to the idea that the left hemisphere is skilled at sequential processing in general and, therefore, is the more analytic of the two hemispheres. This analytic mode of information processing is thought to apply to all incoming information, not just to speech. Visual information, for example, would be treated in an analytic manner by being broken up and reorganized in terms of features.

Areas of the right hemisphere, by contrast, became more adept at simultaneously processing the type of information required to perceive spatial patterns and relationships. Some investigators have claimed that the right hemisphere's specialties are an outgrowth and elaboration of the processes considered basic to vision and visual memory. Further speculation has led to the idea that the right hemisphere is the more holistic and synthetic of the two in handling all kinds of information.

Although some of these labels describing the functions of the left and right hemispheres are vague and await further work to clarify them, it is clear that differences along these lines do exist. Some investigators have argued that a basic incompatibility between the mechanisms generating these processing styles accounts for their evolutionary development in different hemispheres.

A question that immediately comes to mind is how the two hemispheres share control of behavior in everyday situations. The first possibility investigators have considered is that one hemisphere, usually the left, dominates the control of behavior. The original concept of cerebral dominance was based on this idea. It gained support from early findings with split-brain patients showing that the left hemisphere assumed control of responding in situations where there were simultaneous and different inputs to the two hemispheres. What was overlooked was the fact that these tests generally involved linguistic stimuli (words, for example) and often required a verbal response. Given these conditions, it is not at all surprising to find the language-rich hemisphere "dominating."

An alternative idea, that there is a constant vying for control between the hemispheres, is an outgrowth of subsequent work with split-brain patients. As a wider variety of tasks was employed, including some that could be performed better by the right hemisphere, some interesting results emerged. In the chimeric-figures studies, for example, we have seen that it is not always possible to predict which hemisphere will control a response, despite instructions specifically designed to "engage" one hemisphere. Observations of this sort have led to speculation that there is a delicate balance between the hemispheres, with one or the other taking over depending on the task and other as yet unspecified factors.

Some investigators have suggested that the corpus callosum and other commissures play an important role in achieving interhemispheric harmony in the normal brain, serving to integrate the verbal and spatial modes of thinking into unified behavior. How is this harmony achieved? Is it simply a matter of ensuring that the two hemispheres have the same information available to them, or does it also involve a more complex system of inhibition or suppression of activity in the hemispheres?

## The Commissures as Interhemispheric Integrators

This brings us back to the question of the role of the cerebral commissures. There are no definitive answers yet. At this point, the role of the callosum and other commissures can perhaps best be seen as that of a conduit through which the hemispheres exchange information and perhaps handle the problems associated with conflicts among independent processing units. Because the commissures are simply bundles of nerve fibers, they cannot in and of themselves *control* anything. But they can serve as channels through which synchronization of hemispheric function occurs and duplication or competition of effort is prevented.

Perhaps this integration is accomplished by the callosum's simply serving as a sensory "window," providing a separate and complete representation of all sensory input in each hemisphere. More likely though, is the possibility that more complex, processed signals normally traverse the commissures, informing each hemisphere about events in the other and, to an extent, controlling their respective operations. This would allow the whole brain to supersede individual hemispheric competencies.

Early in the course of evolution and in the development of bisymmetric bodily organization, the continuous transmission of sensory information from one side to the other may have been the one essential function of interhemispheric pathways. It seems likely, however, that with the development of asymmetries in brain function, the role of these pathways became more profound.

If this is the case, why do we not see evidence of serious problems in split-brain patients? We have previously discussed at least part of the answer, including the fact that the hemispheric disconnection in these patients is never really complete. Another possibility is that the role of the commissures is most important in the early developmental period following birth. Severing them later in life may not be overly critical because hemispheric differences and interhemispheric relationships have already been established. We will delve further into models of callosal function in Chapter 12.

## Agenesis of the Corpus Callosum

What would happen if the cerebral commissures were severed at birth? Although there are no cases of split-brain surgery performed in infants, reports of several cases of a congenital absence, or *agenesis*, of the callosum might provide insight into its role in development.

George Ettlinger and his colleagues compared the performance of a small number of patients having partial or total developmental absence of the corpus callosum with that of control subjects on a variety of tasks sensitive to hemispheric disconnection.[46] Their results revealed a surprising absence of impairments, even in patients with total agenesis, although the total-agenesis group was deficient in matching arrays of dots of different densities presented in the left and right half-fields of vision. They concluded that callosal agenesis patients utilize noncallosal commissural pathways that compensate for the absence of the corpus callosum but that these extracallosal pathways have some limitations in their ability to transmit information from one side to the other.

Similar results were obtained in a study testing one patient with complete absence of the corpus callosum on tasks developed for use with split-brain subjects.[47] No evidence of hemispheric disconnection was found. In contrast, some earlier work with a small number of cases of agenesis showed impairment compared, with normal subjects, on tasks requiring two-handed manipulation and coordination.[48]

It is difficult to interpret the findings with callosal agenesis patients because the patients vary so widely. In addition, the majority of agenesis cases are below average in intelligence, and it is not clear how this may contribute to particular patterns of performance. Although it is tempting to see a causal link between depression of intelligence and the failure of the corpus callosum to develop, it is possible that lowered intelligence may be due to a more widespread pathology created by the same unidentified factors that lead to callosal agenesis.

## IN SUMMARY

Our review of data from split-brain subjects has led us to the conclusion that hemispheric specialization is not an all-or-none phenomenon but, rather, falls on a continuum. Recent work with split-brain patients has revealed that each hemisphere is capable of handling many kinds of tasks but often differs from the other hemisphere in both approach and efficiency. Almost any human behavior or higher mental function, however, clearly involves more than the actual specialties of either hemisphere and utilizes what is common to both hemispheres.

In research with split-brain subjects, language continues to stand out as the most salient and profound difference between the left brain and the right brain. Some investigators have claimed that all other hemispheric differences are manifestations of the verbal asymmetry.[49] They argue that the region of the left hemisphere that developed specialization for language would no longer be available to handle the processing of spatial information formerly controlled by either half of the brain. The right hemisphere, then, would appear specialized for spatial skills, although its specialization was really a result of the left hemisphere's deficit rather than the right hemisphere's superiority. This argument provides an interesting perspective on the problem of how lateralization developed, although it would be exceedingly difficult to "prove" in the usual sense.

CHAPTER 3

# Studying Asymmetries in the Normal Brain

Fortunately, most people are neurologically normal, having two undamaged hemispheres connected by intact commissures. What does evidence about the left brain and right brain from studies of brain-damaged and split-brain patients tell us about the role of the two hemispheres in the rest of humanity?

We have already considered some of the problems involved in trying to draw conclusions about the normal brain from clinical studies. We have seen how a specific deficit resulting from damage to a particular region of the brain does not necessarily mean that the damaged area once controlled the disrupted function. We noted as well the striking adaptability of the brain, which complicates the interpretation of studies with brain-damaged and split-brain subjects.

Because of these problems, it is not possible to draw firm conclusions about the workings of the normal brain from what we have learned in the brain-damage clinic alone. The clinical work can suggest what to look for, but rigorous conclusions about normal functioning require the confirmation of research with normal brains. The problem is to devise ways of studying the contribution made by each half of the brain to behavior in an intact system.

The investigation of asymmetries in normal subjects has been carried out in several ways. One of the oldest and most extensively used techniques takes advantage of the natural split in human visual pathways. This split neatly divides our visual world into two fields, each of which projects to one hemisphere. By flashing material very briefly to the left or the right of the point on which a subject is fixating, investigators are able to lateralize inputs—that is, to present them to one hemisphere only. Because of the connections between the hemispheres, this one-sided presentation lasts only a fraction of a second, but it appears to be sufficient to allow investigators to compare the abilities of one hemisphere with those of the other.

Similarly, it has been discovered that simultaneously presenting different auditory information to each ear leads to the initial lateralization of auditory stimuli. Information presented to the left ear appears to project first to the right hemisphere, and information presented to the right ear is lateralized to the left hemisphere. This procedure, known as _dichotic listening_, has allowed investigators to study differences and similarities in the way the two hemispheres handle speech as well as other types of auditory information.

More speculative but nevertheless intriguing approaches to the study of asymmetry in normal subjects have involved the careful observation of overt behavior while subjects engage in different tasks. For instance, a person's eye movements to one side or the other have been used to show which hemisphere is more active when the subject is solving a problem or playing a mental game. In another technique, investigators observe the consequences of performing several tasks at the same time. The idea is that tasks interfering with each other the least are likely to be controlled by different parts of the brain—in some cases, perhaps by different hemispheres.

In this chapter we review data collected from normal subjects with whom such techniques have been used.

## VISUAL FIELD ASYMMETRIES

The investigation of visual asymmetries in normal subjects often resembles the testing situations used with split-brain patients. Visual stimuli flashed briefly in the left visual field project first to the right hemisphere; stimuli flashed in the right visual field project initially to the left hemisphere. In split-brain patients, this initial lateralization to one hemisphere or the other is maintained because the connections between the hemispheres have been cut. In a normal subject, however, the connections are intact and can transfer information presented to either hemisphere. Nevertheless, it was found that differences could be detected in a person's performance on certain tasks, depending on whether the task was presented to the right or the left visual field.

### Visual-Field Differences: The Result of Reading Habits or a Sign of Hemispheric Asymmetry?

In the early 1950s, Mortimer Mishkin and Donald Forgays demonstrated that normal right-handed subjects were better at identifying English words briefly presented to the right of fixation than they were at identifying words flashed in the left visual field. However, when Yiddish words were presented in the same way to subjects who could read Yiddish, a slight advantage in favor of the left visual field was found. The authors concluded that experience with reading produces a "more effective neural organization [which] is developed in the corresponding cerebral hemispheres (left for English, right for Yiddish)." In other words, acquired directional reading habits result in better processing of written English in the right visual field, while Yiddish, a language that uses the Hebrew alphabet and reads from right to left, is processed more accurately in the left visual field.[1]

This explanation enjoyed widespread acceptance for several years, although it did not address the question of why the advantage for the right visual field with English words was considerably greater than that for the left visual field with Yiddish words. A decade later, however, the publication of work with the California split-brain subjects suggested a reason for the lack of parallelism in the size of the visual-field differences.

Split-brain subjects, as we have seen, showed dramatic differences in their ability to report printed English words in the left and the right visual fields. Those differences were interpreted as a reflection of the functional differences between the hemispheres for language. Perhaps, investigators began to think, the asymmetries found in the split-brain patients contribute to the visual-field differences found in normal subjects as well. Mishkin and Forgays' findings, then, may have been due to two factors operating simultaneously: (1) the biases in favor of one visual field due to acquired reading habits in a particular language *super-imposed* on (2) an advantage for the right visual field resulting from differences between the left brain and the right brain.

An important test of this two-factor interpretation came from later studies investigating visual-field asymmetries with English or Yiddish words presented vertically to minimize the possible role of directional scanning. With the effects of directional scanning reduced, the two-factor interpretation predicts that the functional differences between the hemispheres should produce a right-visual-field advantage for both Yiddish and English words. Precisely this result was found.[2]

These findings, as well as a variety of other data that we will consider, lend support to the idea that visual-field differences in normal subjects reflect brain asymmetries in those subjects. This conclusion is an exciting one, for it suggests that differences between the left brain and the right brain found in clinical and split-brain subjects apply to the normal brain as well and that these differences can actually be studied in normal subjects.

### Why Does Lateralized Presentation Result in Asymmetric Performance?

Before we turn to other evidence supporting the conclusion that visual-field differences reflect brain asymmetries in normal subjects, we should first address a fundamental issue. Even if there are functional differences between the hemispheres in normal subjects, why are they reflected in differences in performance for the two visual fields? Despite the initial lateralization or one-sided presentation, both hemispheres have access to all incoming information. Very brief presentations to one side of fixation ensure that a stimulus initially is projected directly to only one half of the brain, but the connections between the hemispheres can transmit information about the stimulus to the other side almost instantaneously. Why, then, do we find differences in performance between the visual fields?

There are two models of hemispheric asymmetry that are widely considered. The first, known as the direct access model, assumes that information will be processed by the hemisphere that first receives it, regardless of the differences in ability that may exist between the hemispheres. This is illustrated in Figure 3.1a. In other words, the first hemisphere to receive a task will be the one to handle it, although it may not be the one best equipped to do the job. The direct access model, thus, predicts an advantage in performance for information that reaches the appropriately specialized hemisphere first, since processing by that hemisphere presumably would be better than processing by the other hemisphere.

The relay model, on the other hand, assumes that information is always processed by the hemisphere best equipped to deal with it. Material presented initially to the nonspecialized hemisphere, in this model, would have to reach the specialized hemisphere via the commissural fibers before processing could take place. If this transfer results in some loss of clarity of information, as illustrated in Figure 3.1b, an advantage would be found for stimuli reaching the specialized hemisphere directly.

In both models, asymmetries in performance between the visual fields emerge in tasks where the hemispheres do not have equal capacities to begin with. And in both, information presented directly to the hemisphere specialized for a specific function would be expected to produce better performance—that is, more accurate or faster responding—than one in which information goes first to the other half. They differ, however, in their view of the participation of the nonspecialized hemisphere, and in the role played by the cerebral commissures.

Perhaps the strongest evidence that visual-field asymmetries in normal subjects reflect underlying hemispheric differences is the similarity between these findings and what has been found in research with brain-damaged and split-brain patients. Although a right-visual-field advantage is found with normal subjects in a variety of tasks using words and letters, subjects show a left-visual-field advantage for stimuli that are thought to be handled by the right hemisphere.

For example, several studies have demonstrated that subjects recognize faces presented in the left visual field more quickly than those presented in the right visual field.[3] Other work has shown that subjects more accurately remember the locations of dots presented on a card when the material is presented initially to the right hemisphere.[4] These findings provide strong support for the idea that

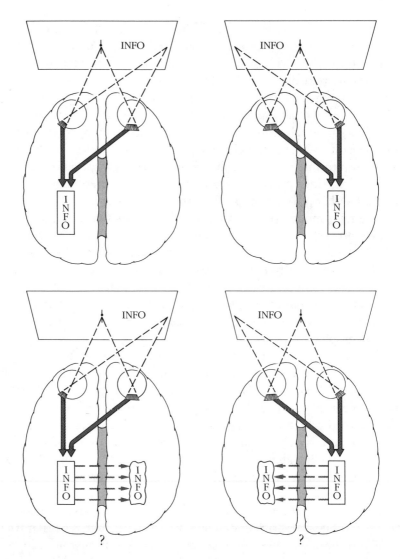

**Figure 3.1** A. In the direct access model, the hemisphere to receive information first is the one that will process that information, regardless of its ability to do so. B. In the relay model, information is processed by the hemisphere specialized to deal with it, regardless of the hemisphere to which it is initially presented. A hemisphere receiving information indirectly via callosal transfer may be at a disadvantage because of time loss, limitation on what aspects of the information are transferred, and inhibitory processes between the hemispheres.

visual-field differences reflect hemispheric differences: the right-visual-field advantage reflects left-hemisphere specialization for language functions, and the left-visual-field superiority results from right-hemisphere specialization for the processing of visuo-spatial stimuli.

We should point out, though, that studies using nonverbal stimuli have not produced results as consistent as those found with words or letters. Some studies using nonsense forms and geometric shapes have shown no differences for the two visual fields; other studies have reported differences in performance.[5] For the most part, however, the studies that do obtain differences between fields show the left visual field to be superior. The problem is that many studies that use stimuli believed by investigators to be processed by the right hemisphere do not find any differences between visual fields. This is reminiscent of the problems encountered when investigators started to look for evidence of special right-hemisphere functions in studies with brain-damaged patients. The functions of the right hemisphere proved to be much more elusive than those of the left. A similar picture has emerged in studies with neurologically normal subjects.

We discuss these and other findings later in this chapter when we consider what has been learned about the nature of hemispheric asymmetries from visual-field and dichotic-listening studies.

## USING AUDITORY STIMULI TO STUDY ASYMMETRIES

Techniques to lateralize auditory information have also been used to study hemispheric differences. Doreen Kimura, working at the Montreal Neurological Institute, noticed that under certain conditions, subjects were more accurate at identifying words presented to the right ear than they were at identifying words delivered to the left ear. Kimura was using the dichotic listening procedure, in which subjects listen to two different spoken messages simultaneously, one message to each ear. She wanted to compare the performances of brain-damaged subjects and normal subjects in a task involving an overload of information.

### Dichotic Listening

The stimuli used by Kimura consisted of pairs of spoken digits, for example, "one" and "nine." The members of each pair were aligned for simultaneity of onset and were recorded on separate channels of audio tape. Subjects listened through headphones to trials consisting of three pairs of digits presented in rapid succession. After each trial, the subject was asked to recall as many of the six previously presented digits as possible, in any order.

Kimura found that patients with damage to the left temporal lobe did more poorly than patients with damage to the right temporal lobe, but regardless of where the damage was located, subjects typically reported the digits presented to the right ear more accurately. This right-ear advantage was also found in normal control subjects.[6]

The finding that patients with damage to the left hemisphere performed more poorly overall than did patients with damage to the right hemisphere was predictable. The dichotic listening task involves the abilities to understand and to produce speech, both of which are primarily left-hemisphere functions that might be disrupted to some extent in patients with damage on the left side. The observation that the ears performed asymmetrically, however, was surprising.

A little anatomy reveals why the asymmetry was unexpected. Unlike the retina, which sends projections contralaterally to the brain from one half of its surface and ipsilaterally from the other half, each ear sends information from all its receptors to both hemispheres. Thus, complete information about a stimulus presented to the right ear is represented initially in both hemispheres, and vice versa. Even if speech stimuli could be processed in only one hemisphere, we would not expect to see any evidence of the asymmetry, because each ear has direct access to both hemispheres.

### Kimura's Model of Ear Asymmetry

To explain her findings, Kimura noted evidence from animal studies suggesting that the contralateral projections from ear to brain are stronger than the ipsilateral pathways.[7] She also proposed that when two different stimuli are presented simultaneously to each ear, the difference in the strengths of the pathways is exaggerated so that information sent along the ipsilateral route is suppressed. Given these assumptions, it was then possible to explain the right-ear advantage.

Under dichotic presentation conditions, the stimulus to the left ear may reach the left hemisphere in one of two ways: over the suppressed ipsilateral route or over the contralateral pathways to the right hemisphere and then across the cerebral commissures. The stimulus to the right ear, however, has a simpler task. It gains access to the left hemisphere along the contralateral route. Because it is likely to arrive at the left hemisphere for processing in better form than its left-ear counterpart, a small right-ear advantage emerges. Kimura's model is depicted in Figure 3.2.

Some support for Kimura's ideas has come from studies showing that there is basically no difference between the two ears in a subject's ability to detect or identify stimuli presented one at a time. Individual subjects may have hearing loss in one or both ears, but overall, when data are collected from large numbers of subjects, the two ears perform similarly.[8] This suggests that ordinarily, without any competition from the contralateral pathways, the ipsilateral fibers are sufficient to produce good performance. This point has been confirmed in work with split-brain subjects.

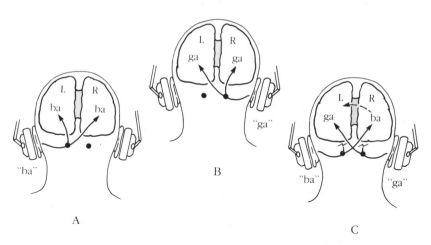

**Figure 3.2** Kimura's model of dichotic listening in normal subjects. A. Monaural presentation to the left ear is sent to the right hemisphere by way of contralateral pathways and to the left hemisphere by way of ipsilateral pathways. The subject reports the syllable ("ba") accurately. B. Monaural presentation to the right ear is transmitted to the left hemisphere by way of contralateral pathways and to the right hemisphere by way of ipsilateral pathways. The subject reports the syllable ("ga") accurately. C. In dichotic presentation, ipsilateral pathways are suppressed, so "ga" goes only to the left (speech) hemisphere and "ba" to the right hemisphere. The syllable "ba" is accessible to the left (speech) hemisphere only through the commissures. As a consequence, "ga" is usually reported more accurately than "ba" (a right-ear advantage).

### Dichotic Listening in Split-Brain Subjects: Testing Some Assumptions

Split-brain patients show a normal pattern of response when speech stimuli are presented to one ear at a time. They can identify words equally well in either ear, just as neurologically intact subjects do. This shows that the ipsilateral path from the left ear to the left hemisphere is functional under conditions of monaural presentation. If, however, speech stimuli are presented dichotically to split-brain subjects, a dramatic, highly exaggerated version of the ear asymmetry found in normal subjects occurs. The typical split-brain patient reports the right-ear items accurately, but the left-ear report is at a chance level. In fact, the patients frequently have to be coaxed into guessing about the identity of left-ear items because they report that they hear only one stimulus.[9]

This situation with split-brain patients is consistent with Kimura's model and helps confirm it. With the corpus callosum cut, communication between the hemispheres is disrupted, but both the ipsilateral and the contralateral projections of each ear are left intact. (These pathways are subcortical and are not cut during surgery.) If, as Kimura suggested, the ipsilateral pathways are suppressed under dichotic stimulation, each ear would send its half of the information to the opposite hemisphere only over the contralateral pathway. The right hemisphere would receive input from the left ear, and the stimulus to the right ear would reach the left hemisphere. Because the right hemisphere is very limited verbally, it would not be able to talk about the word it received from the left ear. At the same time, information about the left-ear word could not transfer into the left hemisphere because the corpus callosum was cut. As a result, the left-ear items would not be identified. Figure 3.3 shows how Kimura's model of ear asymmetry would operate in split-brain patients.

The split-brain patient is able to report only the right-ear words in a dichotic presentation. If the presentation is not dichotic (that is, if the words go to one ear at a time), both ipsilateral and contralateral pathways do function so that left- as well as right-ear words reach the left hemisphere. The patient can then report words presented to either ear, and the dramatic ear asymmetry disappears.

In summary, simultaneous presentation of different words to both ears of the split-brain subject results in the patient's reporting only the right-ear words. Neither the contralateral nor the ipsilateral

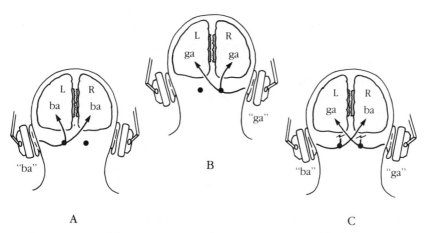

**Figure 3.3** Dichotic listening in split-brain subjects. A and B. Monaural presentations operate as they do with normal subjects. Because both ipsilateral and contralateral pathways are unaffected by commissurotomy, the patient can accurately report a signal to either ear. C. In dichotic presentation, the ipsilateral pathways are suppressed (as in normal subjects), but "ba" is not accessible to the left (speech) hemisphere because the commisures are cut. Only "ga" is reported (a complete right-ear advantage).

auditory pathways are affected by the split-brain operation, lending support to the idea that ipsilateral pathways are suppressed by such dichotic presentation. In normal subjects, the ear asymmetry with dichotic presentation is not so dramatic, because information can transfer across the callosum. Nevertheless, there is an advantage for incoming information that does not have to transfer across interhemispheric commissures for processing. This is reflected in a small advantage for right-ear words, because they project most directly to the verbal left hemisphere.

## Does Ear Asymmetry Really Reflect Hemispheric Asymmetry?

Other support for Kimura's model comes from the finding that the ear advantage reverses in subjects who have been shown to have speech controlled by the right hemisphere instead of by the left. Patients tested with sodium amobarbital to determine the hemisphere controlling speech have been given the dichotic listening task to see whether the ear asymmetry is related to hemispheric asymmetry. Those with left-hemisphere speech centers typically show a right-ear advantage; those with right-hemisphere speech show a left-ear advantage.[10] The sodium amobarbital test allows a direct assessment of speech lateralization without having to infer it from the patient's handedness. Thus, in the rare cases of right-handers with right-hemisphere speech, a left-ear advantage would generally be found. These data are very important in establishing the validity of the dichotic listening test as a measure of brain asymmetry.

A more recent study using a similar approach has shown results that are even more encouraging.[11] Patients whose speech centers were previously determined by the amobarbitol test were asked to monitor a sequence of dichotically presented word pairs for the occurrence of a specific target word appearing randomly in the series. Each time the patients heard the target word they were to press a button. The results were scored in terms of the number of target words correctly detected in each ear, as well as the speed with which they were detected. By incorporating both percentage correct identification and reaction time scores in the data analysis, the researchers were able to correctly classify 95 percent of the patients in terms of the hemisphere controlling their speech.

More data are needed, but these results suggest that dichotic monitoring performance is a better predictor of hemispheric speech representation than the standard task where subjects are asked to report all they hear. Why this might be the case is not clear; however, the findings provide additional evidence that ear asymmetries, indeed, are reflective of hemispheric asymmetry for speech.

Finally, research has demonstrated that the ear asymmetry found in a given subject differs as a function of the nature of the stimuli that are presented. A left-ear advantage has been found with stimuli believed to be processed by the right hemisphere—stimuli such as musical chords and melodies. The dichotic listening procedure serves to lateralize auditory inputs in the normal brain in the same way that tachistoscopic presentation lateralizes visual inputs. If an input goes first to the hemisphere specialized for processing it, responses are more accurate than if the stimulus must be transferred to the other hemisphere. Because two stimuli must be presented at once to produce this lateralization, the dichotic procedure differs from the visual case. This difference, though, appears to be a consequence of anatomical differences between the auditory and visual systems and does not represent any fundamental difference in the nature of the asymmetries, themselves.

## Is It Necessary to Present Stimuli Dichotically?

An assumption critical to Kimura's model of the ear-asymmetry effect is that ipsilateral transmission of information is suppressed when stimuli are delivered dichotically. Kimura's own efforts to demonstrate an ear asymmetry when material was delivered to only one ear at a time were unsuccessful, suggesting to her that the ipsilateral left ear/left hemisphere route is comparable with the contralateral right ear/left hemisphere route under monaural presentation.

Although the importance of dichotic presentation in obtaining asymmetries has been supported in a number of studies,[12] other investigators have reported success obtaining ear asymmetries with monaural stimulation, particularly in tasks using reaction time as a measure.[13] In these tasks, the experimenter measures how quickly the subject is able to make a decision about a stimulus. The reasons for the differences among studies are not clear. Should monaural ear asymmetries prove to be reliable phenomena, however, Kimura's model would need only a minor adjustment to account for them.

# WHAT HAS BEEN LEARNED FROM VISUAL AND AUDITORY ASYMMETRIES?

During the last decade, a great many studies have been conducted using the techniques of dichotic listening and lateralized tachisto-scopic presentation with normal subjects. As in the research with split-brain patients, there has been a gradual evolution of ideas about the nature of hemispheric asymmetries as new data suggest different interpretations of earlier work.

## The Verbal–Nonverbal Distinction

Much of the early work on the left brain and right brain in normal subjects led investigators to believe that the two hemispheres differ basically in terms of the types of stimuli they are best prepared to deal with. A typical visual task involved the lateralized presentation of stimuli that the subject was asked to identify. A similar procedure was employed with dichotic stimuli as well: two items were presented simultaneously, and the subject was asked to report what was heard. Sometimes the basic task was modified so that the subject was required to recognize a specific stimulus, rather than identify each item, and sometimes the experimenter was interested primarily in how quickly a subject could respond to a stimulus instead of how accurate the response was. Often, both speed and accuracy were measured in the same study.

Stimuli were said to show a left-hemisphere advantage if performance was superior when items were presented to the right ear or in the right visual field. A right-hemisphere advantage was assumed if performance was superior when items were presented to the left ear or in the left visual field. Differences in performance between sides were quite small—frequently, just a few percentage points better in identification or a few milliseconds faster in response—but anywhere from 70 to 90 percent of the right-handed subjects tested in a typical study would show the asymmetry.

Most of the early studies showing a right-side advantage used stimuli that were language-related in a very obvious way. Tachistoscopically presented words and even single letters produced a right-visual-field advantage.[14] Dichotically presented spoken digits and words also resulted in an advantage to the left hemisphere.[15] The advantage, though, was not limited to meaningful spoken utterances.

Studies have shown that nonsense syllables such as "pa" and "ka" also produce a right-ear advantage and that speech played backward produces a right-ear superiority in recognition as well.[16] Backward speech can be produced by reversing the position of the playback and take-up reels on a tape recorder and then rewinding and playing the tape. The result sounds like an exotic Scandinavian language. Taken together, the results of these studies suggest that stimuli do not have to be meaningful to produce a left-hemisphere advantage but should be language-related or verbal in some way.

The picture for the right hemisphere is more difficult to summarize. A wide variety of visual stimuli have produced left-visual-field or right-hemisphere superiorities. We have mentioned studies that used faces and dot displays as stimuli and obtained a left-visual-field advantage. The dichotic listening studies that result in a right-hemisphere advantage are also diverse. One of the earliest demonstrated a left-ear superiority in the recognition of melodic excerpts.[17] Two different four-second piano melodies were presented simultaneously on each trial. The subject was asked to indicate which of the four sequentially presented excerpts played immediately thereafter had been members of the pair delivered dichotically. Other studies revealed a left-ear advantage when familiar environmental noises were presented dichotically.[18] In a typical trial, the subject would be asked to identify a pair of sounds, such as a dog barking and a train whistling.

All these "right-hemisphere" stimuli share the attribute of being nonverbal, and many investigators have argued that the distinction between the functions of the two hemispheres lies along this verbal–nonverbal dimension. In this view, all language-related stimuli are dealt with primarily in the left hemisphere, and the right hemisphere is specialized for handling certain types of nonverbal stimuli. This appears to be a neat, reasonably satisfying summary of the data we have reviewed so far. However, problems that have emerged in more recent work have led researchers to seek another explanation of the fundamental differences between the left brain and the right brain.

## The Information-Processing Approach

Consider the following experiment. The subject is given a short list of letters to memorize and then briefly views a familiar object in the left or the right visual field. The subject's task is to decide whether the first letter of the name of the object is among the letters in the memorized list. Which visual field would lead to a faster response?

Suppose that the subject viewed single letters instead of pictures and had to decide whether the letter was among those that had been memorized. What could be predicted about the speed of response in this case?

It would be reasonable to expect a left-visual-field superiority in the first case and a right-visual-field superiority in the second. Pictures, after all, are nonverbal stimuli, and letters clearly fall in the verbal domain. In fact, the results obtained were the complete reverse. Picture stimuli resulted in faster performance when they were presented to the left hemisphere, and the letters were responded to more quickly when they were projected initially to the right hemisphere.[19] Why?

Studies such as this provide fairly compelling evidence that an analysis of hemispheric differences simply in terms of verbal and nonverbal stimuli is inadequate. What seems to be more important than the nature of the stimulus is what the subject does with the stimulus. In the case of the supposedly nonverbal pictures, the subject was asked to identify each picture and recover the initial letter of its name, a clear-cut language function. The single-letter stimuli, on the other hand, were verbal in nature but in this task did not have to be approached as verbal stimuli. The subject could readily perform the task by matching the mental image of the letter against the images of the set of memorized letters. Theoretically, the subject could do this without ever knowing the name of the letter presented.

This kind of explanation emphasizes the task to be performed by the subject rather than the nature of the stimulus per se. It reflects a shift away from left- and right-hemisphere stimuli to left- and right-hemisphere modes of processing information.

Another study that highlights this information-processing approach to brain asymmetry was one that took advantage of the fact that there are alternate ways for subjects to remember pairs of words. One is to rehearse the words by repeating them out loud or subvocally; a second is to form an image of the two items interacting in some way. For example, faced with the task of remembering "flag" and "chicken," subjects can repeat the words over and over again, or they can form an image of the two words, such as a chicken carrying a flag. (The use of images of this type has been shown to be a very effective memory aid.)

The researchers hypothesized that verbal and imagery strategies would involve different cerebral hemispheres. They proposed that this difference would be tapped by having subjects indicate whether a picture flashed to the left or the right visual field corresponded to one of the words previously presented. Results showed that when subjects were told to remember the word pairs by subvocal rehearsal, response time was faster for probes to the right visual field. When subjects were asked to form images of the pairs to be remembered, response time was faster for the left visual field.[20] These findings were in keeping with the predictions.*

The way a subject approaches a particular task, then, has important consequences for the outcome of studies investigating differential hemispheric involvement. The two studies we have just reviewed directly manipulated the subject's strategy with specific instructions to deal with the stimuli in a certain way. Perhaps the strategies different subjects naturally bring to bear on a particular task can affect the outcome as well.

---

*In Chapter 2 we discussed the problems associated with thinking of imagery as a left-hemisphere only or right-hemisphere only task. The data reviewed there suggested that the precise nature of the task was critical in determining the outcome. Given the results obtained in the study under present discussion, it appears that the authors were fortunate in selecting an imagery task that showed right-hemisphere specialization.

Still further evidence for information-processing differences between the hemispheres comes from studies using languages other than English. In Japanese, there are two writing systems, *Kana* and *Kanji*. The Kana system is sound-based: a symbol represents the sound of a syllable without any meaning. The Kanji system is meaning-based. Kana and Kanji also differ in terms of their graphic complexity, Kanji characters generally being more complex. Examples are given in Figure 3.4.

There are two versions of Kana, with 69 symbols each; these are usually mastered by the end of the first grade. The number of Kanji characters is much greater. A minimal set of 1,850 Kanji has been adopted by the Ministry of Education in Japan, although knowledge of 3,000 Kanji is needed to read such material as newspapers. Kana and Kanji also differ in that Kana characters have a one-to-one correspondence with a syllable, while each Kanji character has several alternative meanings, with the number of syllables ranging from one to four or more depending on the meaning.[21]

Studies of Japanese aphasic patients have suggested some interesting differences in the way these two types of linguistic symbols are processed in the brain. Sumiko Sasanuma has shown that a sizable number of patients exhibit selective impairment of Kana processing whereas the ability to process Kanji remains relatively well preserved or almost intact. A much smaller number of patients show selective impairment of Kanji with Kana processing relatively unaffected.[22]

| MEANING | KANA | KANJI |
|---------|------|-------|
| INK | インキ<br>(INKI) | 墨 |
| UNIVERSITY | ダイガク<br>(DAIGAKU) | 大學<br>(GREAT LEARNING) |
| TOKYO | トウキョウ<br>(TOKYO) | 東京<br>(EAST CAPITAL) |

**Figure 3.4** The two separate forms of writing in Japan. Kana is syllabic, with words articulated syllable-by-syllable. Kanji is ideographic, with each character simultaneously representing a sound and a meaning.

Analysis of the errors made by aphasic patients suggests that different strategies are used for the two types of symbols: visual processing for Kanji, as opposed to phonologic, or sound-based, processing for Kana.[23]

These observations have led Sasanuma and colleagues to tests of the hypothesis that Kana and Kanji represent different modes of linguistic processing differentially involving the two hemispheres.[24] To test this hypothesis with neurologically normal Japanese subjects, sets of Kana and Kanji nonsense words were prepared and presented briefly one at a time in the left or the right visual field. Results showed that subjects showed a significant right-field superiority for identification in the Kana task and a left-field, but no significant, superiority for the Kanji task. The investigators concluded that Kana and Kanji characters are processed differently in the two hemispheres; further, Kanji processing is particularly complex because both visual and verbal functions likely play a role, depending on the specific task. Whether Kanji would show a left- or a right-visual-field superiority might depend on, among other things, the strategy used by the subject and the mode of response (verbal or nonverbal).

Taken together, the findings on Kana and Kanji point to the importance of the kind of processing a subject must perform in determining hemispheric asymmetries. Additional discussions of how differences among languages may be related to cerebral asymmetry are found in Chapter 8, where bilingualism is considered from the perspective of the development of asymmetry, and in Chapter 11, where language is viewed from the perspective of possible cultural differences in hemispheric utilization.

## THEORETICAL ISSUES IN INTERPRETING BEHAVIORAL STUDIES

Tachistoscopic presentation and dichotic listening studies have served as the basis for much of our current theorizing about the nature of the left brain and right brain in normal subjects. Several important issues about these techniques remain unresolved, however.

### What Are the Tests Measuring?

One concern is that these behavioral tests typically underestimate the incidence of left-hemisphere speech in right-handers found with sodium amobarbital (Wada) testing. Studies generally find that approximately 80 percent of right-handed subjects show a right-ear or right-visual-field advantage for language stimuli; sodium amobarbital testing, in contrast, indicates that more than 95 percent of right-handed individuals have left-hemisphere language. What causes this discrepancy?

One possibility is that the tests are not a pure measure of brain asymmetry and that other factors are involved. Perhaps individual differences in the neural pathways connecting the eyes and ears to the brain play a role in the outcome of the studies.

The strategies that subjects adopt in these tasks may also contribute in a major way to performance.[25] In dichotic listening, for example, subjects can actively shift their attention to the left-ear or the right-ear stimulus. If the left-ear items are at a disadvantage because of hemispheric asymmetry, some subjects may choose to direct their attention to the weaker ear, thereby producing a smaller right-ear superiority than might be found otherwise. Other subjects, in contrast, may focus their attention on the clearer of the two stimuli on any trial, without trying to identify both of them. These subjects would show a larger right-ear advantage than one would expect. At the present time, we do not have really good way to deal with this potential problem.

We should also note that the discrepancy between the results of Wada testing and behavioral measures of asymmetry may be due to the possibility that each is tapping a different aspect of functional asymmetry. The Wada test is used to determine the hemisphere that controls speech output. Perhaps tachistoscopic and dichotic listening tasks, which are basically tests of perception and not production, reflect functions that are less lateralized.*

Another problem is that visual and dichotic measures of lateralization are not highly correlated with each other. If these tests are measuring the same lateralized functions, it would be reasonable to expect them to produce results that are highly related to each other. Studies that have compared asymmetries in dichotic listening and tachistoscopic tasks in the same subjects have found some degree of relationship, but not a high one.[26] Why? Perhaps these tests are not measuring the same thing after all.

---

*The terms *lateralized* and *lateralization* are frequently used to refer to the division of functions between the hemispheres, as well as to the restriction of information to one hemisphere.

Another concern, one that has implications for the preceding two as well, is that repeated testing of the same subjects does not always produce the same results. A test is reliable to the extent that repeated administrations yield similar results. Some studies have found the reliability of the dichotic listening and tachistoscopic tests to be lower than one might expect.[27] For example, some subjects who, when first tested, showed a right-ear advantage for dichotically presented speech shifted to a left-ear advantage when tested a week later. Presumably, the organization of an individual's brain is a stable characteristic and does not change over short periods of time. Signs of variability within an individual may mean that the laterality tests are tapping functions, such as the formation of strategies to be used in performing the tasks, which can shift over brief intervals of time.

### What Do the Tests Tell Us About the Nature of Asymmetries?

Yet another issue raised by dichotic and tachistoscopic studies is whether hemispheric differences are absolute or relative. Does a difference in performance between visual fields mean that only one hemisphere is capable of performing the task? Or does it simply reflect the fact that one hemisphere is better at the task than the other? The typical study with normal subjects does not allow us to tease apart these alternatives because performance in the "inferior" visual field may be the result of either less efficient processing by the nonspecialized hemisphere or processing by the specialized hemisphere after transfer of information across the commissures. In either case, we would expect the same results: a difference in performance between the two sides.

A related issue is whether the size of the asymmetry found in different subjects can tell us anything about the degree of lateralization for certain functions in particular subjects. We mentioned earlier that a subject's strategies may play a role in determining the size of the asymmetry effects, independent of lateralization per se. Is it also possible that differences in the size of the asymmetry can tell us something about the extent of lateralization? Is a subject with a large right-ear advantage more lateralized than a subject with a smaller right-ear advantage? This intriguing problem has many investigators

looking for ways to transform scores reflecting a subject's performance into a meaningful index of lateralization.*

## CAN ATTENTIONAL BIAS ACCOUNT
## FOR ASYMMETRIES?

The last issue we consider here is the absence of general agreement
about the basis of the lateral asymmetries found in normal subjects.
When we introduced tachistoscopic and dichotic listening work, we
argued that asymmetries reflected the initial lateralization of stimulus
input to the hemisphere best able to deal with the material. This type
of explanation has been characterized as a "wiring" account of the
difference because the asymmetries result from the wiring of the
nervous system and processing differences between the hemispheres.
Information lateralized to the hemisphere *not* specialized for it was
at a disadvantage because it had to traverse callosal pathways in
order to get to the more appropriate hemisphere. Another quite
different explanation has also been offered for these results.

Marcel Kinsbourne has proposed that asymmetries observed in
dichotic listening and tachistoscopic studies reflect covert shifts in
attention to one side of space following the activation of one hemisphere.[28] He argues that the hemisphere specialized for a particular
task becomes differentially active, or "primed," when appropriate
material is presented to a subject, and that this activation, or priming, "spills over" to the centers controlling attention to the opposite
side of space.

For example, in Kinsbourne's view, the right-ear advantage in
tasks with dichotically presented speech is a consequence of the
activation of the left hemisphere, followed by greater attention to
the contralateral, or right ear. A left-ear advantage in a dichotic
music task would reflect differential right-hemisphere involvement
and a concomitant shift of attention to the left side of space.

---

*The issue of how to compute measures of lateralization from scores on behavioral tests is
important and complex. In tests where percent correct is the dependent variable, it is
possible to use difference scores (left minus right, or variations thereof) as the index of
lateralization. Such scores are not independent of overall performance, however. Some
investigators have claimed that a laterality measure should be independent of how well
someone does; others have argued that information on overall performance may itself be
related to lateralization.

Kinsbourne's model of asymmetries is similar to the wiring account in that it begins with the assumption that there are basic functional differences between the hemispheres. It differs from the wiring model in its explanation of how hemispheric differences give rise to the performance differences that are studied in behavioral tests.

Kinsbourne's attentional model of asymmetries has received some support from a variety of different studies. In a series of interesting experiments, Kinsbourne and his colleagues showed that tasks not normally showing a visual-field asymmetry could be made to show a right-side advantage if subjects were asked to rehearse subvocally a short list of words while they viewed the laterally presented stimuli.[29] The rehearsal is presumed to activate the left hemisphere and produce a shift in attention to the right side, resulting in more accurate performance in that visual field.

Other evidence consistent with the attentional model comes from studies showing that the context in which stimuli are presented affects the type of asymmetry that is observed. For example, the right-ear advantage in speed of responding to certain dichotically presented syllables becomes a slight left-ear advantage when the subject is required to compare a brief melody presented immediately before each syllable pair with a melody presented immediately after.[30] An attentional view would claim that the musical stimuli "primed" the right hemisphere so that the shift in attention to the left ear would cancel out the shift to the right ear that ordinarily occurs when speech is presented.

We should note, though, that some attempts to replicate and extend work based on the attentional model have not been successful, and few investigators believe it is a complete explanation for asymmetries observed in lateralized testing. At the same time, some researchers question the adequacy of the wiring account of these asymmetries and are inclined to think that both views may play some role in the phenomena we have been considering. Both models can be combined, for example, if we assume that priming one hemisphere serves to facilitate the processing of stimuli that are presented directly to it.[31]

Although there are still questions to be resolved about inconsistencies, dichotic and tachistoscopic techniques have confirmed that much of the split-brain and clinical data do reflect processes in the normal brain. There is a striking correspondence between many of the hemispheric differences shown in normal subjects through these indirect techniques and the ideas gleaned from the brain-damage clinic by several generations of neurologists and neuropsychologists.

Although the development of thought about the implications of the split-brain data has been similar to the development of ideas about the implications of the normal data, research with normal subjects using dichotic listening and tachistoscopic techniques has made contributions that go beyond the verification of clinical evidence. Many of the contributions are theoretical and help to sharpen the focus of research into laterality by pinpointing important issues.

We turn now to discussions of two other behavioral techniques that have become popular in research with normal subjects.

## LEFT-LOOKERS AND RIGHT-LOOKERS

According to poets, the eyes are windows to the soul. To some neuropsychologists, they are windows to the left brain and right brain as well. We are all familiar with the patterns of looking at and away from others that characterize social interaction. A listener generally will look directly at a speaker when asked a question but will look away while answering.

In the course of his practice, clinical psychologist M. E. Day noticed that patients tended consistently to look to the left or to the right when answering questions. On the basis of further work, Day suggested that the direction of these *lateral eye movements* (*LEMs*) might be associated with certain personality characteristics.[32] Five years later, psychologist Paul Bakan of Simon Fraser University, in Canada, published data supporting Day's ideas and went on to propose that the eye movements are related to hemispheric asymmetry as well.[33]

### The Direction of Lateral Eye Movements The Result of Individual Differences or Question Types?

Bakan's hypothesis was based on the well-established fact that eye movements to one side are controlled by centers in the frontal lobe of the contralateral hemisphere. He suggested that cognitive activity occurring primarily in one hemisphere would trigger eye movements to the opposite side and, therefore, eye movements could be viewed as an index of the relative activity of the two hemispheres in an individual. Accordingly, left-lookers, or persons who typically make eye movements to the left, are those for whom the right hemisphere predominates; right-lookers are persons who have greater left-hemisphere involvement in overall functioning.

Bakan viewed the direction of lateral eye movements as a stable characteristic of each individual. Later investigations exploring LEMs as an index of hemispheric activity began to consider the role played by the type of question used to elicit eye movements.[34] Questions requiring verbal analysis, it was reasoned, will tend to activate the left hemisphere in most right-handers; questions involving an analysis of spatial relationships will activate the right hemisphere. The differential activation of the halves of the brain would then be reflected in right LEMs and left LEMs, respectively.

The predicted association between the nature of the question and the direction of eye movement has been reported in many studies. To engage the left hemisphere, subjects have been asked to interpret proverbs, spell words, provide definitions, do simple arithmetic (solve 144/6 times 4), and solve logical problems (Al is smarter than Sam, and Al is duller than Rick. Who is smarter?). Questions involving visualization (How many edges are there on a cube?), spatial relations (If a person is facing the rising sun, where is south with respect to him or her?), and musical skills (identifying piano melodies) have been used to activate the right hemisphere. When differences in direction are found, right LEMs predominate in response to questions in the first group, and left LEMs follow questions of the second type.[35]

Gary Schwartz and his colleagues at Yale have also looked at lateral eye movements in response to emotional questions. In addition to verbal and spatial questions of the sort just described, verbal emotional questions (For you, is anger or hate the stronger emotion?) and spatial emotion questions (When you visualize your father's face, what emotion first strikes you?) were studied. Results showed that verbal questions produced more right LEMs overall than did spatial questions, in keeping with earlier findings; emotional questions produced more left LEMs overall. These findings have been taken as support for greater right-hemisphere involvement in the processing of emotional information.[36]

The first studies relating the direction of lateral eye movement to hemispheric asymmetry generated a great deal of excitement. The notion that there were individual differences in *hemisphericity*, the tendency to rely on the processes of one half of the brain, was appealing to many investigators. Lateral eye movements seemed to be a very straightforward, quick, and harmless measure of these differences in normal people.

Later studies indicating that the direction of eye movements is related to the nature of the question posed to the subject had great appeal to those who were interested in studying functional differences between the hemispheres. The work suggested that it is possible to explore the abilities of the left brain and the right brain in normal subjects quite directly, without using dichotic listening or tachistoscopic procedures.

For these reasons. LEM research has been very attractive and has generated considerable interest. Important issues that have serious implications for the interpretation of these studies remain unresolved, however. Why have some studies indicated that the tendency to be a left-looker or a right-looker is a stable characteristic of each person, whereas other studies show that the direction of eye gaze is a function of the type of question posed to the subject? One possible explanation is suggested by the work of Ruben and Raquel Gur, who proposed that factors in the experimental situation may account for these results.[37]

## Eye Movements and the Location of the Experimenter

In the earlier work suggesting stable differences in lateral eye movements among subjects, the experimenter typically faced the subject when asking a question and then manually recorded the direction of the eye movements that followed. Later studies frequently employed a camera to videotape all eye movements, and in these cases the experimenter sat out of view behind the subject or in another room.

Perhaps, the Gurs reasoned, the presence or absence of another person in full view of the subject affects the pattern of eye movements. They postulated that the experimenter-present situation may be more threatening and anxiety-provoking and that under these conditions the anxious subject will reveal certain characteristic modes of response: the subject may show greater activation of the hemisphere most compatible with his or her cognitive style, although that hemisphere might not be appropriate for a particular type of question. In the experimenter-absent condition, the level of anxiety would be lower, permitting the differential hemispheric activation to reflect the nature of the question posed to the subject.

A study by Gur and Gur used the same set of questions to compare directly the eye movements that occurred when an experimenter sat in front of the subject with the subject's LEMs when the experimenter was out of sight. The results confirmed their prediction. When the experimenter was facing them, the subjects typically looked to the left or to the right regardless of the nature of the question. When the experimenter was positioned behind the same subjects, their eye movements were linked to the type of question posed.

### Do LEMs Really Measure Brain Activation?

The Gurs' findings point to an important procedural factor that may account for some of the conflicts between studies, but they leave unresolved a major problem: do lateral eye movements really reflect differential hemispheric activity, or can they be explained in other ways? What exactly is the evidence linking LEMs to hemispheric asymmetry? A recent review of work in this area has noted that the link is an indirect and weak one, based primarily on investigators' conceptions of what constitutes a left-hemisphere or a right-hemisphere question.[38]

Questions requiring an analysis of words or meanings are believed to engage the left hemisphere; questions involving spatial relations or musical skills are considered right-hemisphere tasks. When eye movements in the predicted direction follow these questions, the results are generally seen as supporting the link between eye movements and differential hemispheric activity. The problem, however, is that there is little in the way of direct evidence outside of the eye-movement research to support this association.

Especially troublesome is the fact that approximately half of the studies in this area have failed to find the predicted differences. A priori, the questions used in these studies seem just as "left hemisphere" or just as "right hemisphere" as those employed in the studies reporting success. The logical problem of establishing a relationship between eye movements and brain asymmetry becomes somewhat circular if one must define left- or right-hemisphere activity in terms of the questions that produce the expected results.

Unfortunately, we have no eye-movement data on split-brain patients engaged in various tasks, nor do we have any information about eye movements in the presence of direct electrical stimulation. In the absence of independent verification that eye movements are related to differential hemispheric activity, it would be wise to interpret results of LEM studies cautiously. In particular, it may be premature to postulate conclusions about brain asymmetries and the processing of different kinds of questions on the basis of the direction of eye movements.

Despite these cautions, the LEM work is interesting and definitely worthy of further study. In certain situations, people do differ in the way they characteristically shift their gazes, and in other situations the pattern of shifts is related to the nature of the questions posed to the subjects. The link between eye movements and brain asymmetry may eventually prove to be a firm one. At the present time, however, it is important to keep its fragility in mind.

## DOING TWO THINGS AT ONE: MAPPING FUNCTIONAL CEREBRAL SPACE

We all know that certain combinations of tasks are relatively easy to do together, while other tasks seem to interfere with each other. For example, many people can listen to music and read simultaneously, although the same people are unable to follow a conversation as they read. Intuitively, it seems as if tasks that call on different areas of the brain show less interference when performed together than tasks that rely on the same general areas. Perhaps, then, it would be possible to study patterns of brain organization in normal subjects by seeing how tasks interfere with each other.

Marcel Kinsbourne has taken precisely this approach in a number of interesting studies investigating what he refers to as "functional cerebral space."[39] He proposes, first, that the distance between brain areas controlling different movements is reflected in the extent to which there is competition or cooperation when several movements are attempted simultaneously. He notes that the two arms are better at performing cooperative movements than is an arm–leg combination, but they are worse at performing competitive tasks. It then follows, according to Kinsbourne's model, that the brain area controlling an arm is closer to the brain area controlling the other arm than it is to the brain area controlling the leg.

Kinsbourne's studies to map functional cerebral space have concentrated on observing subjects vocalizing and doing something with one of their limbs at the same time. In one of the first studies utilizing this approach, right-handed subjects were asked to balance a dowel rod on their index fingers under two conditions: in silence and while repeating short sentences. Results indicated that when the subject was speaking, the right hand could not maintain balance as well or for as long as it could when the subject was silent. This was not the case with the left hand, however, which performed equally well in both conditions.[40]

Although there are no direct connections between the speech-control center and any limb-control center, Kinsbourne assumed that the control region for speech is closer to the control center for the right arm than to the left-arm control center. This idea is reasonable enough anatomically in view of the contralateral rule (the right hand is controlled by the left brain) and the fact that the speech area is in the left hemisphere. What is unique about Kinsbourne's work is that his model of functional cerebral space led him to make predictions about interference of speech and dowel balancing that were borne out by the data.

A later study showed that the difficulty of the spoken material affected the degree of disruption in the right hand's performance. More difficult material produced shorter right-hand balancing times than easier material. Left-hand balancing times were unaffected by the difficulty of the verbalization. Interestingly, left-handers showed disruption in the balancing times of both hands under the verbalization condition, in keeping with evidence suggesting that left-handers as a group have less clearly lateralized verbal functions.[41]

Work using this approach has also been extended to split-brain subjects and children. These studies employed a task in which subjects were required to tap at a fixed rate with the index finger of one hand. In one condition, subjects performed verbal tasks while they tapped; in the control condition, the subjects tapped in silence. For both groups, disruption of tapping was greater for the right hand.[42]

The experiments investigating so-called functional cerebral space are clever and quite interesting, although some important reservations remain about this approach. First, there is no validation of functional space that is independent of the study used to demonstrate it. If two tasks interfere with each other, they are assumed to be closer in functional space than two tasks that interfere less or not at all. Standing by itself, this type of reasoning is too circular for comfort.

Second, phenomena of this type have not proved to be as robust as one might wish: there have been numerous reports of failures to replicate basic findings. The reasons some investigators have been unsuccessful are not clear, but it is obvious that the outcome of these studies is influenced by many factors.

A third problem is that certain reasonable predictions about functional cerebral space have not been confirmed by experimentation.

For example, many sources of evidence indicate that the right hemisphere plays a crucial role in singing. However, singing does not differentially disrupt left-hand performance. Why not? We need answers to this as well as to the other questions raised here before we can evaluate the functional cerebral space approach to the study of asymmetry.

## IN SUMMARY

In this chapter we reviewed researchers' efforts to explore hemispheric differences by studying the behavior of normal subjects in special testing situations. This general approach is commonly termed *behavioral* because directly observable behavior is what is being measured. Overall, the data fit well with the picture of hemispheric differences that emerged from studies of brain-damaged and split-brain patients.

In tracing the history of behavioral investigations of laterality in normal subjects, we have seen an increasingly complex picture unfold. We have seen that attentional factors may play a role in producing asymmetry in behavior. It is also clear that differences between the hemispheres go beyond the kinds of stimuli they are best equipped to deal with. As in the research with split-brain patients, we see that basic differences lie in the processing strategies of each hemisphere.

The appeal of work with normal subjects is unmistakable. First, the limitations placed on clinical and split-brain research by the scarcity of subjects are avoided. Second, work with neurologically normal subjects offers the investigators more freedom in the kinds of experiments that can be devised. Third, and perhaps most important, work with normal subjects permits the study of asymmetries in the same system one is ultimately trying to understand: the normal human brain.

# Measuring the Brain and Its Activity: Some Physiological Correlates of Asymmetry

Perhaps the most direct way to investigate differences between the hemispheres is to measure the activity of the brain itself. This strategy contrasts with the approaches considered in Chapter 3, where inferences about the brain were drawn from behavior in special testing situations. More direct measurements of brain activity bypass the need for many of the assumptions that are made in behavioral studies. They also make it possible to study special groups of subjects, such as infants or animals, who might not be able to respond in the manner required by behavioral tests.

There are many different ways to measure brain anatomy and to monitor brain activity. With respect to anatomy, perhaps the most obvious is to measure the size and shape of the hemispheres or compare areas within each hemisphere. Anatomy can also be examined at a more microscopic level to determine whether differences exist in the nature of cells or cell density in equivalent ("homologous") regions of the two hemispheres.

Cerebral activity is very complex, encompassing various chemical and electrical processes along a continuum from microscopic to macroscopic function. The metabolic processes of neurons require that blood bring oxygen and glucose to brain tissue and remove waste products. Thus, the flow of blood to the two sides of the brain is a useful measure of brain activity. Differences in the metabolism of specific nutrients such as glucose can be monitored as well, permitting an even finer analysis of relative activity on each side as well as within small regions of the brain. Neurometabolic processes also result in electrical activity that can be recorded from electrodes placed on the scalp. The "brain waves" recorded at various sites on the head and even weak magnetic fields produced by neural activity can be studied for differences within and between hemispheres.

In this chapter, we review evidence using these different measures to study more directly the activity of the left brain and the right brain.

## ELECTRICAL ACTIVITY IN THE LEFT BRAIN AND THE RIGHT BRAIN

In 1929, an Austrian psychiatrist named Hans Burger discovered that patterns of electrical activity could be recorded from electrodes placed at various points on the scalps of human beings. These patterns were called the *electroencephalogram* (*EEG*), literally meaning "electrical brain writing." Although the EEG is monitored from the scalp, Burger was able to demonstrate that some of the activity it records originates in the brain itself and is not simply due to scalp musculature.

Devices to record the EEG soon became commonplace in clinical settings as investigators demonstrated that brain abnormalities such as epilepsy and tumors are accompanied by distinctive patterns of electrical activity. Its potential as a research tool was also quickly recognized, and innumerable studies looking for EEG correlates of personality, intelligence, and behavior were undertaken.

## Using the EEG to Study Asymmetry

Until the late 1960s, EEG recordings were typically made from electrodes placed at different points along the top of the head or on one side of the head only. It was assumed that activity would be identical on the two sides. A few studies did report EEG asymmetries, however, when electrodes were placed on each side. The asymmetries seemed to be related to hand preference, but not in any simple way. David Galin and Robert Ornstein, of the Langley Porter Neuropsychiatric Institute in San Francisco, were two of the first investigators to study these asymmetries in detail and to relate them to the nature of the task performed by the subject while the EEG was being recorded.

The rationale for their approach is nicely stated in this excerpt from one of their papers:

> Although the split brain work has shown that the verbal and spatial cognitive systems can function independently, there are few studies which attempt to evaluate their interaction in normal people. Our opinion is that in most ordinary activities we simply alternate between cognitive modes rather than integrating them. . . . Therefore, in a subject performing a verbal or a spatial task, we expected to find electrophysiological signs of differences in activity between the appropriate and inappropriate hemispheres.[1]

They recorded EEG activity from symmetrical positions on either side of the head while subjects performed verbal tasks, such as writing a letter, and spatial tasks, such as constructing a memorized geometric pattern with multicolored blocks. Results were analyzed in terms of the ratio of right-hemisphere EEG power (R) to left-hemisphere EEG power (L). Electroencephalogram power is simply the amount of electrical energy being produced per unit of time. Galin and Ornstein found that the R/L power ratio was significantly greater in the verbal than in the spatial tasks.

They were thus successful in showing a link between the amount of EEG activity in the hemispheres and the type of task performed by a subject. At first glance, though, these results seem to be the precise opposite of what one would predict on the basis of what is known about the relationship between tasks and hemispheres. Letter writing is a left-hemisphere task and should produce relatively more left-hemisphere activity than a task involving blocks. This "problem" is readily resolved by considering the composition of the EEG activity.

Several different rhythms of activity have been identified as constituents of the EEG record. The first one discovered is also the most famous: the alpha rhythm. Alpha activity is a rhythmic cycling of electrical activity occurring from 8 to 12 times per second. It is the predominant activity present in the EEG when the subject is resting quietly with closed eyes. Other rhythms that are part of the EEG are also identified by Greek letters. Figure 4.1 shows EEG waveforms for five different brain states.

An analysis of Galin and Ornstein's results showed that the predominant rhythm in the EEG records was alpha. Because alpha reflects a resting brain state, *less* alpha activity would be expected to follow *greater* involvement in a particular task. It then follows that the left hemisphere should show relatively less alpha when a subject is performing a language task in contrast with the amount of alpha activity present when the subject is doing a spatial task like the block-design problem. This is precisely what was found.

## Advantages and Disadvantages of the EEG

Electroencephalographic measures of asymmetry have been popular with many investigators. Because they do not rely on an overt response from the subject, they can be used to study brain asymmetries in infants, aphasic patients, and other subjects from whom it might be difficult to obtain such responses. In addition, EEG is a

---

Figure 4.1 Typical electroencephalograms. The "head" to the left of each record shows the approximate placement of the electrodes. A. At rest with eyes open. B. At rest with eyes shut. The large-magnitude waves occurring at a frequency of eight to 12 per second are the alpha waves. C. The dramatic spiking associated with an epileptic seizure. D. "Brain death" or "cerebral death." Even though the heart may be beating, the electrically quiet record shows the patient is clinically dead. E. Simultaneous recording of left- and right-temporal EEG activity while the subject performs a block-design task. The graph to the right of each hemisphere's record is an analysis of the relative "power" of various frequencies in the EEG waveform. Notice that the left recording contains a greater amount of alpha, evident from the 8- to 12-cycle peak in the frequency graph. During speaking and writing, more alpha is recorded on the right. The degree and direction of asymmetry varies with the task. [Part E adapted from Galin and Ornstein, "Lateral Specialization of Cognitive

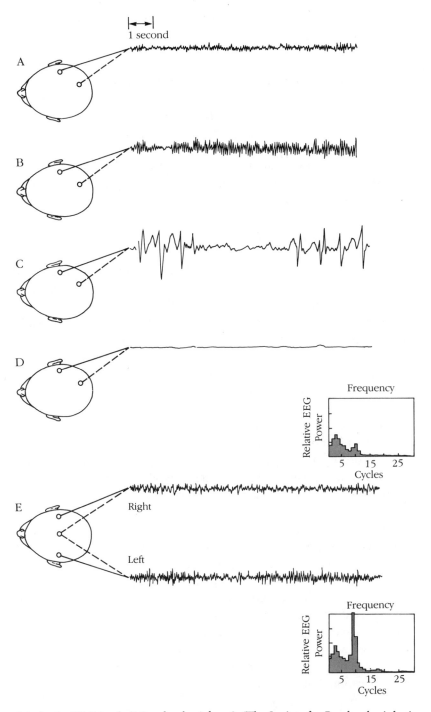

Mode: An EEG Study," *Psychophysiology* 9, (The Society for Psychophysiological Research), 1972, Fig. 1, p. 417, and from Doyle, Ornstein, and Galin, "Lateral Specialization of Cognitive Mode: II. EEG Frequency Analysis," Fig. 1, p. 571. *Psychophysiology* (1974) 11 (The Society for Psychophysical Research). Reprinted with permission from the publisher.]

continuous measure over time and can be used to study ongoing activity in the brain while the subject performs long, complex tasks.

Although the latter feature of the EEG measure is quite useful in some studies, it poses a problem for others. The EEG is an overall, continuous measure of brain activity. Thus, it is difficult to see changes in the EEG that relate to the occurrence of specific stimulus events. In fact, the complex EEG waveforms do not appear to change very much during different kinds of sensory input but, rather, seem to reflect the general arousal level of the brain.

## The Evoked Potential

A searching analysis of the EEG, however, reveals that specific changes do occur in response to the presentation of a stimulus such as a flash of light. The problem is that these changes are hidden by the overall background activity of the brain. In order to make visible the change in response to a specific stimulus, a computer is used to average the waveform records following repeated presentations of the same stimulus. Electrical activity that is random with respect to the stimulus presentation will tend to be canceled out by this process, whereas electrical activity occurring in a fixed time relation to the stimulus will emerge as the potential evoked by the stimulus.

Figure 4.2 shows how an *evoked potential* (EP) emerges from an EEG record by averaging the waveforms that follow successive presentations of the same stimulus. The evoked potential consists of a sequence of positive and negative changes from a baseline and typically lasts about 500 milliseconds after the stimulus ends. Each potential can be analyzed in terms of certain components or parameters, such as *amplitude* or *latency* (the amount of time from the onset of the stimulus to the onset of the activity).

The nature of the stimulus is one of the factors that affects the precise form of the evoked potential. As a whole, auditory evoked potentials differ from visual evoked potentials, which differ from evoked potentials produced by touch stimulation. In addition, the region of each hemisphere generating maximum activity differs for each type of stimulus. Figure 4.3 shows some representative EPs to stimuli in different modalities.

Of primary concern is whether the EP generated by a stimulus is the same when recordings are made from equivalent locations on the two sides of the head. Are there differences between the hemispheres in the electrical activity evoked by various stimuli and, if so,

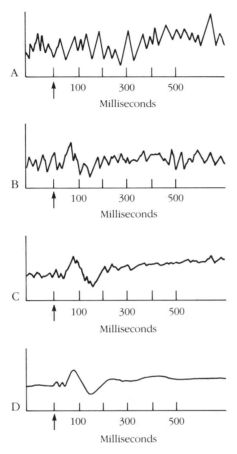

**Figure 4.2** A single evoked response is seen emerging from the background noise of an EEG after averaging the EEG patterns obtained from successive stimulations. The stimulus, an auditory click, occurs at the time indicated by arrow. A. EEG response of a single stimulus. B. Average of two responses. C. Average of 16 responses. D. Average of 64 responses.

what can such differences tell us about the roles of the left brain and the right brain in normal subjects?

A number of studies have recorded EPs from each hemisphere while subjects were presented with simple stimuli, such as clicks or blank flashes of light.[2] Some of these studies have reported asymmetries in the amplitude or latency of the EP. Of greater interest, however, are the studies in which subjects were presented with more complex stimuli or tasks that presumably engaged the specialized functions of the hemispheres.

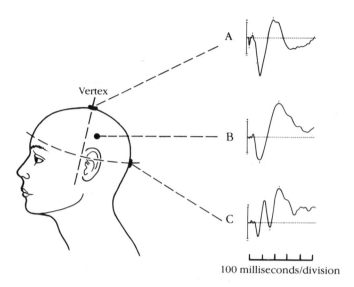

Vertex

A

B

C

100 milliseconds/division

**Figure 4.3** Typical evoked potentials for A. auditory, B. somatosensory, and C. visual stimulation. The dotted lines indicate the approximate location on the scalp from which the most pronounced peaks are recorded. [Adapted from Thompson and Patterson, eds., *Bioelectric Recording Techniques*, (New York: Academic Press, Inc.)].

In a study by Monte Buschbaum and Paul Fedio of the National Institutes of Health, for example, differences were observed in EPs while subjects viewed verbal and nonverbal stimuli flashed in the left or the right visual field.[3] The verbal stimuli were three-letter words; the nonverbal items were nonsense stimuli composed of an artificial alphabet of letters. When recordings were made from the occipital lobes, results showed greater differences between the EPs to the two types of stimuli in the left hemisphere than in the right.

Asymmetries using auditory stimuli have been reported as well. Psychologist Dennis Molfese and colleagues have collected extensive data on evoked potentials to speech and nonspeech stimuli.[4] In one study, they found that the amplitude of part of the EP to speech stimuli was greater in the left hemisphere than in the right hemisphere. This difference was seen even when the subject merely listened to the stimuli and did not try to identify them. Nonspeech stimuli, however, produced larger amplitude activity in the right hemisphere.

Several studies have looked at how asymmetries are affected by the task the subject is performing while the EP is recorded. In one such study, subjects were presented with a sequence of synthetically produced spoken syllables that could differ in initial syllable ("ba" versus "da") or in pitch (high or low).[5] In one half of the trials, subjects were instructed to listen for each occurrence of "ba," regardless of its pitch. In the other half, the subjects were instructed to listen for high-pitched syllables, independent of their names.

Evoked potentials to the high-pitched "ba" were recorded from the left and right hemispheres in each case. This procedure enabled the investigators to study the effect of the task performed on EP asymmetry using exactly the same stimuli in the two conditions. The only difference between conditions was the kind of mental activity the subjects had to perform when the stimuli were presented.

Results showed a difference in the EPs produced during the naming and pitch tasks, but only in the left hemisphere. The evoked potentials recorded from the right hemisphere were not different for the two conditions. These findings led the researchers to suggest that there are hemispheric differences in the ability to identify a syllable but no differences in the ability to determine the pitch of the syllable.

## Probe Evoked Potentials During Mental Activity

Standard EP experiments were limited to recording responses to short, usually simple stimuli. The *probe evoked potential* is a more recent development that greatly expanded the applications of EP methods to studying brain–behavior relationships involving more complex mental activity. Instead of examining the response to repeated stimulation against a resting-state background, the experimenter asks the subject to perform a task, of any complexity, during which some irrelevant "probe" stimulus (for example, a click or a light flash) is repeatedly introduced. What is of interest is to what extent is the EP, which is normally excited by the probe stimulus, suppressed by activity or task the subject is performing. It is presumed that the brain can do well only so many things at one time. Thus, the more complex the background task, the greater the reduction of the brain's normal response to some intermittent probe stimulus. The change in the probe EP amplitude is thought to be determined by how demanding the task is. Probe EPs can be recorded from different regions of the brain simultaneously during the performance of any task. By analyzing which region or regions affect the probe response, inferences can be made about what areas are involved in the task performance.

In the first study using this method to demonstrate hemispheric specialization, EPs to flashes of light were recorded while subjects were engaged in spatial or linguistic tasks like those used by Galin and Ornstein in their EEG work (for instance, writing and block design). Electroencephalogram power was also analyzed in this experiment, allowing the investigators to compare EP and EEG as indicators of lateralized mental functions. Results showed that the probe EP reflected asymmetrical brain activity during verbal-versus-spatial tasks similar to the asymmetries in activity found using EEG recordings.[6] Some inconsistencies were observed, however, probably owing to probe EP sensitivity to nonlateralized aspects of the tasks used, such as differences in motoric output involved (for example, the hand movement).

More recent studies have applied probe EP methods to study hemispheric contribution to specific tasks while attempting to limit artifactual problems by keeping stimulation and response requirements consistent. In one study, the relative engagement of temporal and parietal regions of the left and right hemispheres was monitored during an arithmetic task and a visuo-spatial task by recording EPs to a probe tone presented through earphones.[7] In all conditions, the subjects viewed the same series of stimuli, consisting of fragmented segments next to a whole geometric shape, with numbers printed inside each fragment as well as inside the complete shape. In the visuo-spatial run, the subjects signaled with a finger movement if the fragments would create the intact geometric shape presented next to them. In the arithmetic trials, the subjects signaled if the numbers inside the fragments added up to the number inside the completed shape.

The amplitude of the EPs to the tone probes varied according to which task the subjects were performing. Probe EPs were significantly reduced, compared with controls, in the left temporal area during arithmetic calculations. The visuo-spatial task resulted in greater probe reduction in the right parietal region. These results confirm, of course, left-hemisphere involvement in "serial-analytic" operations, such as those involved in speech and calculation, and right-hemisphere involvement in certain visuo-spatial processes. In addition, this study is a good example of newer experimental design strategies in brain–behavior research, in which instructions to the subject are varied in tasks involving identical stimuli and identical responses. This allows investigators to better isolate the changes in brain function that result purely from differences in psychological or mental function.

Similar experiments using probe EPs have been used to carefully investigate hemispheric involvement in recognizing emotional tone in speech.[8] Subjects listened to the same conversations under two task conditions, one in which they had to report, at the end of the presentation, how many times the syllable "na" occurred. In the other condition, the subjects had to report the emotions communicated by each speaker during the conversation. Evoked potentials were recorded to a click sound repeated throughout the two trials. Probe EP reduction was greater in the left hemisphere during the syllable-detection condition and greater in the right during the emotional-tone judgments. Thus, the same conversation was shown to be processed to a greater extent by the left hemisphere when attention to speech sounds was required and by the right hemisphere when emotional-tone judgments were necessary. (Further discussion of the role of the right hemisphere in emotion is found in Chapters 6 and 10.)

## NEUROMAGNETOMETRY

Neural activity generates not only electrical fields but produces magnetic fields as well. Both electrical and magnetic phenomena are consequences of the movement of charge. In biological systems, the charge consists of ions that move across cellular membranes, generating the neural impulses that are transmitted from neuron to neuron. The electrical fields produced by the ion movement have been extensively studied and form the basis for the research reviewed in the previous section. In recent years it has become technologically possible to record and isolate the magnetic fields that accompany the electrical fields generated by neuronal activity within specific regions of the brain. Magnetic fields created by the activity of single neurons are extremely small but under certain conditions the magnetic fields of a number of simultaneously active neurons combine to produce fields that are sufficiently strong to be measured at the surface of the head. Such a recording is called a *magnetoencephalogram* (MEG), the magnetic counterpart of the EEG.

Calculations based on MEG measurements permit three-dimensional localization of the cell groups generating the measured field. Thus, a major advantage of this technique over the EEG is its ability to better localize within the brain the source of the activity being recorded. Figure 4.4 illustrates the equipment.

Special superconducting coils are needed to pick up the very weak brain magnetic fields and measurements routinely are done within elaborate magnetically shielded rooms. The heart of a MEG probe is a sensing instrument called the *superconducting quantum interference device (SQUID)*, which is kept immersed in liquid helium. By either moving a probe about the head or using multiple probes placed in different positions about the head, the MEG procedure creates "isocontour maps," concentric circles representing different intensities of the magnetic field (see Figure 4.5). Based on such maps, a three-dimensional location of the neurons generating the field can be calculated.

Researchers initially attempted to use MEG to establish the location and depth of the electrical currents underlying discharges in epileptic tissue with greater accuracy than possible with EEG alone. They were very successful; for example, in one patient epileptic activity was localized to an exact region 10 to 11 millimeters beneath the subject's scalp.[9]

### Evoked Fields

Response to external stimulation can be measured with MEG using an analog of the EP. We have seen how a repeated auditory, somatosensory, or visual stimulus will generate a measurable response or change in averaged EEG waveforms. The same stimulus results in a characteristic waveshape in the magnetic field recorded over specific cerebral regions, the source of which is much more localizable than the source of an EP. For example, the source of magnetic field patterns evoked by repeated clicks (*evoked fields* or *EFs*) has been clearly localized to the auditory temporal cortex of each hemisphere.[10]

Investigators are just starting to measure localized magnetic phenomena reflecting more complex psychological or cognitive processes. In one study a procedure analogous to the probe EP technique was used.[11] In a control condition, auditory EFs over both hemispheres were recorded in subjects listening to repeated click stimulation. In the other condition, the click stimulation was maintained but the subjects also listened to a tape-recorded series of foreign language words and were asked to respond only when they heard a specific syllable within a word, the sound "na." The amplitude of the EF waveform recorded to the repeated click stimulation and originating in the left temporal cortex was greatly reduced by the linguistic target task, indicating interference, or masking, due to the

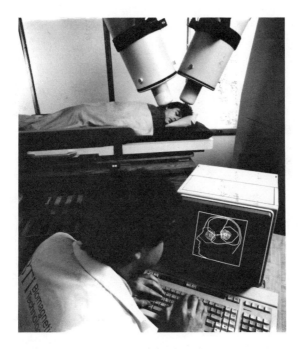

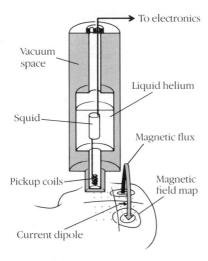

Figure 4.4 A. A patient undergoing a brain scan using a 14-channel neuromagnetometer. The process tracks the electrical function of the brain by detecting magnetic fields generated by the electrical current within the brain. [Courtesy of Biomagnetic Technologies, Inc., San Diego, CA.] B. Brain magnetic fields are measured using a superconducting amplifier (SQUID; see text) coupled to special coils. The liquid helium keeps the system at a low temperature, necessary for superconductivity. [Courtesy, Dr. Jackson Beatty, University of California, Los Angeles, CA.]

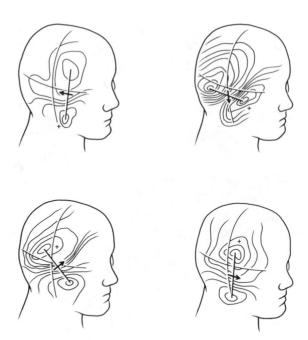

**Figure 4.5** Examples of isocontour maps displaying the magnetic fields gener-ated by epileptic activity in a patient's right hemisphere. Such MEG recordings allow precise localization of the sources of the seizure activity. This patient's recordings indicated multiple sources within the right temporal lobe. [From Beatty, Barth, Richer and Johnson, "Neuromagnetometry," Figs. 2–10, p. 38. in Psychophysiology; ed., Coles, Donchin, and Porges, Guilford Press, 1986]

concurrent verbal processing. The EF waveform originating in the right temporal cortex was not affected. Thus, it was mostly left-hemisphere resources that were being utilized by the task.

## BLOOD FLOW IN THE HEMISPHERES

The flow of blood through the tissues of the body varies with the metabolism and activity in those tissues. The blood flow, which provides necessary nutrients and removes waste products, turns out to be very sensitive and responsive to minute changes in cellular activity. In fact, changes in the activity in various regions of the brain appear to be reflected in the relative amount of blood flowing

through those regions. This discovery has made it possible to identify and study the interaction of various areas of the brain during
ongoing human behavior by measuring regional changes in blood
flow.

A modern technique of measuring blood flow in an awake and
functioning human was developed by Niels Lassen and David Ingvar [12] and others. They injected a special radioactive isotope
(Xenon-133) into an artery leading to the brain and monitored the
flow with a battery of detectors arranged near the surface of the
head. (The low level of gamma radiation emitted by the isotope is
not considered harmful and washes out of the bloodstream within
15 minutes.) The technique, originally used with patients requiring
the test for medical reasons, has since been refined to the point
where subjects can breathe a special air–xenon mixture and have
their blood flow monitored by placing their heads next to a machine
housing the special detectors.

The results of a host of studies measuring cerebral blood flow
during different kinds of physical and mental activity have been quite
impressive. Classic predictions about brain areas involved in psychological functions have been brought to life. The regions of each
hemisphere involved in vision, for example, show increased blood
flow if the subject is looking at a moving pattern. Speech stimuli
increase blood flow in the auditory areas of each side.

Although the most striking patterns of blood flow show differences from front to back across the whole brain, differences between the hemispheres have also been found using techniques that
permit the study of regional blood flow in the two hemispheres
simultaneously. Jarl Risberg compared the blood-flow pattern of
right-handed male volunteers during two tasks, one a verbal analogies test and the other a test of perceptual "closure." In the closure
task, the subjects had to view very sparsely drawn pictures and figure
out what they were.[13]

Small but highly significant hemispheric differences in blood flow
of about 3 percent were found in the two conditions. As expected,
the mean left-hemisphere flow was greater during the verbal analogies task, and the mean right-hemisphere flow was greater during the
picture-completion task. Risberg was able to measure which regions
within each hemisphere contributed the most to interhemispheric
blood-flow differences. The largest differences were found in the
frontal, fronto-temporal, and parietal regions for the verbal tests. In
the resting state, differences between corresponding regions of the
hemispheres were very small.

A more recent series of experiments was conducted to compare several tasks thought to involve primarily right-hemisphere processing.[14] Nineteen right-handed subjects performed three tasks: judgment of line orientation, mental rotation of three-dimensional cube arrays, and a fragment puzzle task. Examples of the visually presented stimulus material are shown in Figure 4.6.

In the *rotation* condition subjects judged whether projected drawings of two three-dimensional arrays of cubes were identical but only rotated in space. In the *puzzles* task, subjects judged whether fragmented figures could form a simultaneously presented whole figure. In *line orientation* a slide showing a line pair was presented for four seconds, followed by presentation of a fan array of lines with arrows pointing at two. The subject had to decide whether the angle

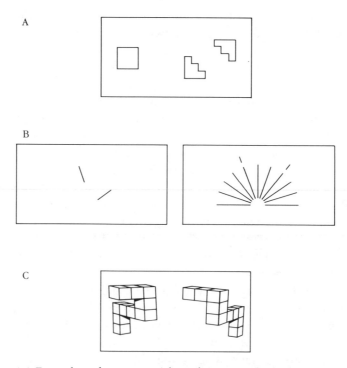

**Figure 4.6** Examples of test material used in a cerebral blood flow study comparing three visuo-spatial tasks. A. Fragment-puzzle task (Will the fragments on the left form the figure on the right?). B. Line-orientation task (Is the angle formed by the two lines the same as the angle formed by the lines at which the arrows point?). C. Mental-rotation task (Mentally rotate either of the two figures to see if they are identical.). [From Deutsch, et al., 1988]

formed by the lines at which the arrows pointed was the same as in the previously presented pair. Response to these tasks was a right index finger movement for "yes" and a left index finger movement for "no." All tasks began before the blood flow scan and continued throughout the 11-minute scan duration.

Asymmetries in hemispheric flow (right side greater) were observed only in the line orientation and rotation conditions. The magnitude of the asymmetry was greater in the rotation task in which blood-flow increases were especially prominent in parietal areas. Based on these results the authors suggest that mental rotation uses more exclusively right-hemisphere "skills" than the other tasks surveyed. Whether the nature of these skills is revealed more by the rotation task than the line orientation task, of course, is another issue. Mental rotation does involve "mental manipulation" in space, a concept mentioned previously in the context of right-hemisphere superiority for certain tasks attempted with split-brain patients (see Chapter 2).

It is of interest that a recent review of research concerning sex differences in spatial ability concluded that large differences are found consistently only on measures of mental rotation with males performing considerably better than females as a whole.[15] In the cerebral blood flow study just described, the investigators did report a sex difference in performance consistent with these general findings, but they reported that both men and women nevertheless showed the right asymmetry in activation. If anything, the extent of right-hemisphere activation seemed greater in women. The authors suggested that this may reflect the necessity of a "greater effort" on the part of the women in performing the mental rotations required. If this is true, it could also explain why another study using line orientation judgments found significant blood-flow asymmetries only in women.[16] In any event, the cerebral blood flow data, though very supportive of a strong role of the right hemisphere in certain visuo-spatial tasks, is not as supportive of sex differences in hemispheric asymmetry in function. It leaves open the possibility that any sex differences in performance are not due so much to how "lateralized" but rather to how efficient (within a hemisphere) talents can be.

Blood-flow investigators Lassen, Ingvar, and Skinhoj report that they have been most impressed by the striking similarity in the blood-flow patterns in the two sides, even during such highly lateralized activities as speech.[17] Hemispheric differences in activity seem to be much more subtle than the changes that occur in both hemispheres. This suggests that hemispheric differences are but one of several different organizational schemes in the brain. The work on cerebral blood flow shows that complex tasks typically involve increased patterns of activation in many areas of each hemisphere.

Notable left–right asymmetries in blood flow continue to be reported, however, with interesting theoretical implications. One study has provided some evidence that there is a greater amount of gray matter in the left hemisphere than in the right.[18] The term *gray matter* refers to areas of the brain where neuronal cell bodies are located—brain tissue that normally has a grayish tint to it. The cerebral cortex is mostly gray matter, consisting of billions of tightly packed neurons with relatively short interconnections (cell processes, or "nerve endings"). *White matter* refers to regions of the brain consisting mainly of neural tracts, that is, the long, fat, coated "nerve" fibers that interconnect gray matter areas and form the "wiring" extending out from the brain. Because the blood flow in gray matter is almost four times that in white matter, it is possible to separate these two in cerebral blood-flow measurements and calculate the relative proportion of each.

Thirty-six right-handed males, ages 18 to 22, underwent cerebral blood-flow scans while in a resting state. Analysis of the results revealed that there was more gray matter relative to white matter in the left hemisphere than in the right, particularly in the frontal and precentral regions. The investigators suggest that the existence of more tissue containing dense interconnected neurons in the left hemisphere may subserve a left-hemisphere organization that emphasizes processing or transfer *within* regions, whereas right-hemisphere organization depends on information transfer *across* regions and utilizes more white matter.

Regional blood-flow measurements have also shown that the extent of hand-movement-induced change in blood flow in the hemispheres depends on which hand is tested. Blood-flow measurements were made using normal right-handed volunteers at rest and during movement of either hand. Left-hand movement resulted in a prominent focal flow increase in the motor region of the right hemisphere. Right-hand movement, however, resulted in a much smaller increase in the left-hemisphere motor area. The investigators speculate that motor organization differs for preferred and nonpreferred hand movements. It is also possible that the larger blood-flow increase in the right hemisphere is due to a greater effort required for right-handers to move their left hands.[19]

Isak Prohovnik and associates have looked at the extent of coupling between blood flow in equivalent (homologous) regions of the two hemispheres during different stimulation conditions.[20] They found that anatomically equivalent regions of the two hemispheres tend to change flow rates simultaneously during variations in the subject's rest state and during simple sensory and motor activities. When tasks become more complex, involving higher-level mental activity, flow rates increase less symmetrically, with different regions of each hemisphere showing the greatest change. The investigators feel that these data show that metabolic activity is more closely coupled between regions of the two hemispheres supporting simple sensory—motor activities, whereas regions involved in higher-level processing are free to function more independently. (See the Appendix for a review of basic concepts of functional neuroanatomy.)

Another study examined data from 121 regional cerebral blood-flow studies conducted under a variety of conditions involving different stimuli, response modes, and task requirements.[21] These were compared to scans conducted while subjects were at rest. Figure 4.7 illustrates how closely coupled blood flow is in equivalent regions of the two hemispheres at rest. Significant hemispheric differences were found in the frontal regions when all tasks were combined. Right flow was greater than left, especially in the more demanding tasks. The study concluded that the right frontal activation observed may be due to general attentional demands and not limited to tasks usually thought to involve the right hemisphere. This finding suggests a very general role for the right hemisphere in attention or vigilance and is especially interesting in light of the clinical data on the neglect syndrome and other disorders associated with right-hemisphere lesions (see Chapter 6).

## METABOLIC SCANNING

Cerebral blood-flow techniques do have some limitations as measures of brain activity. The studies described above do not provide accurate information about the deepest regions of the brain. Most of the observed patterns are at the cortical levels. In addition, measuring blood flow is an indirect way of measuring cerebral metabolism. Although the relationship between blood flow and metabolism is well established, blood flow may not always be responsive enough to rapid variations in brain activity. There are also occasions when

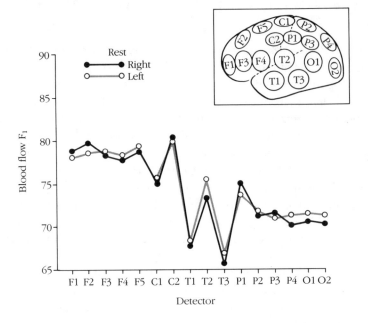

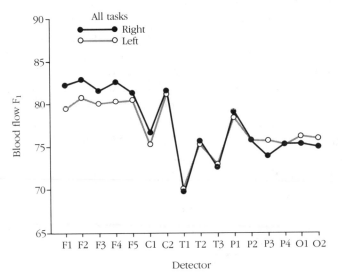

**Figure 4.7** Graphs show mean cerebral blood flow for 16 detector positions in each hemisphere for subjects at rest (upper graph) and while performing various demanding tasks (lower graph). The inset shows approximate detector positions. F, frontal; C, central; T, temporal; P. parietal; O, occipital. Note how coupled left and right flow is across equivalent regions of the two hemipsheres at rest. The greater flow in frontal and lower in posterior regions is a typical finding in scans of normal subjects. The posterior flow increases due to sensory stimulation during most tasks. There appears to be a greater right frontal increase during most attention-demanding tasks. The right–left asymmetry is significant for detectors $F_1$, $F_2$, and $F_4$ in the lower graph. [From Deutsch, et al., 1987.]

blood flow and metabolism are not well correlated, as in patients who have sustained severe head injury.

Cerebral metabolism on a microscopic scale can be monitored by measuring the rate at which radioactively labeled glucose or other nutrients are taken up by different regions of the brain. It has been shown that the metabolic rate within small regions of the brain changes in a consistent pattern during specific behavioral activity.[22] Originally, such measurements required sacrificing the animals involved in the experiment and slicing brain tissue. New techniques have been developed that allow measuring the distribution of special metabolic tracers in an alive and functioning brain.

### Emission Tomography

Emission tomography is a visualization technique that yields an image of the distribution of a radioactively labeled substance in any desired cross section of the body or head. In *single photon emission tomography (SPECT)* biochemicals of interest are labeled with radioactive compounds that emit gamma rays in all directions. These substances, called *radiopharmaceuticals*, are injected into the bloodstream of subjects. As the radiopharmaceuticals reach the brain, detectors surrounding or rotated about the head pick up these emissions and computer programs are used to "reconstruct" what the distribution of the labeled substance must have been to generate the pattern of emissions sensed by the detectors. So far, SPECT procedures have been used to measure cerebral blood flow and blood volume in three-dimensional cross sections of the brain.

*Positron emission tomography (PET)* utilizes the properties of the special radiation generated by positron emitting substances, which generate pairs of photon traveling in exactly opposite direction, thus aiding in the exact localization of the distribution of any specially labeled substance.

Positron emission tomography is the only technique developed so far that can produce regional three-dimensional quantification of glucose or oxygen metabolism in the living human brain. Glucose metabolism is a more direct measure of the function of neural tissue than cerebral blood flow, especially in patients with cerebral injury or disease that may affect normal vascular regulatory mechanisms. Most of the work with PET pertaining to normal brain function up to now has been in scanning metabolism during simple sensory stimulation. Figures 4.8 and 4.9 illustrate how PET images have

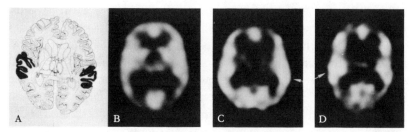

**Figure 4.8** Positron emission tomographs of the brains of subjects listening to a factual story with only one ear. Bright areas correspond to regions with higher cerebral metabolic rate for glucose; darker areas represent lower metabolic rates. A. The primary auditory cortex is schematically indicated in black on the brain outline. B. Unstimulated control subject with symmetrical temporal metabolism. Monaural auditory stimulation resulted in metabolic rate increases in the temporal cortex contralateral to the stimulated ear, as in C. Left ear stimulated. D. Right ear stimulated. The region of activation also seemed more extensive than merely the primary auditory cortex (arrows in C and D). [From Reivich and Gur, "Cerebral Metabolic Effects of Sensory Stimuli," Fig. 1, p. 332, in *Positron Emission Tomography* ed., Reivich and Alavi, Alan R. Liss, Inc., 1985]

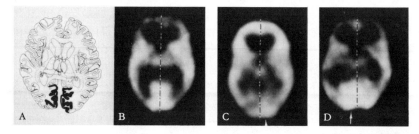

**Figure 4.9** Positron emission tomographic images of the brains of subjects stimulated visually. A dotted line defines the midline of each image. A. Schematic representation of a horizontal section through the brain with the striate (primary visual) cortex indicated in black. B. In a blindfolded, visually unstimulated subject, glucose metabolism in the visual cortex of the occipital pole is symmetrical. C. Left-visual hemifield stimulation causes asymmetrical glucose metabolism, with the right striate cortex 25 to 30 percent more active than the left. D. Stimulation of the right-visual hemifield causes this pattern to reverse, with the left striate cortex having a metabolic rate 18 percent greater than a homologous area in the right hemisphere. [From Reivich and Gur, "Cerebral Metabolic Effects of Sensory Stimuli," Fig. 2, p. 332, in *Positron Emission Tomography* ed. Reivich and Alavi, Alan R. Liss, Inc., 1985]

clearly delineated areas in the temporal cortex associated with auditory stimulation and areas in the occipital lobe that are active during visual stimulation.

Investigators only recently are attempting to use PET to study higher mental function, including hemispheric asymmetries during different cognitive tasks. One reason for this delay has been the problem that scanning of positron emitter labeled glucose compounds takes about 45 minutes, too long a period during which to maintain a reliable mental state or most task conditions. Newer radiopharmaceuticals allow the measurement of regional cerebral oxygen consumption and blood flow with PET in a matter of several minutes.

A recent study attempted to distinguish brain areas activated by specific language functions by repeated PET scans during a four-level progression of tasks in 7 normal subjects.[23] The base state was visual fixation on a symbol (+) presented on a video monitor. Observation of single nouns was the second level. Vocal repetition of cue words added motor output. In the final condition the subject had to respond to a presented object noun with a verb describing some use of the object, thus adding a semantic processing demand to the condition.

By subtracting the blood-flow pattern measured during one level of task from another task level, the investigators tried to isolate some of the changes induced by relatively specific mental activity. The investigators found that vocalization showed *bilateral* flow increases in the sensory-motor strip and several frontal-lobe regions. The semantic task did show an asymmetrical activation of the lower left frontal lobe compared with the control condition (vocal repetition alone). Perhaps most interesting was the fact that despite the attempt to isolate the activity due to stimulation from that of cognitive processes, the investigators still found some lateralized activity in association areas of the left hemisphere associated with "just looking" at words. The researchers suggested that the subjects were reflexively performing some linguistic analysis of the stimulus cue words even though there was no language task demand per se. The level of activity did not change in these areas of the left hemisphere during active reading/vocalization or the semantic task, supporting the idea that the subjects had already automatically done some form of linguistic analysis during passive presentation of the cue words.

This study is just a preliminary example of the kinds of experiments that will have to be conducted with techniques such as PET in order to tease apart the many stages and confounding variables

involved in studying even basic brain activity–behavior relationships. Studies with PET are only starting to explore their potential in
mapping brain activity during different behavioral states.[24] It is
hoped that these techniques will provide a great deal of new insight
into the functions of the hemispheres in the near future.

## ISSUES RAISED BY TECHNIQUES MEASURING
## BRAIN ACTIVITY

Electrophysiological measures, studies of regional blood flow, and
other measures of metabolic processes all offer investigators the
opportunity to study relationships between brain activity and behavior. They have been of great value in validating physiologically some
of the insights about brain function gleaned from psychological
research with brain-injured as well as normal subjects.

At the same time, measures of brain activity during task performance have raised some questions about the most exaggerated claims
for hemispheric asymmetry. There is little to support the notion that
either one or the other hemisphere turns on to perform a specific
task all by itself. Each of the measures we have discussed points to
the involvement of many areas of the brain in even the simplest task.
There are asymmetries in activity between the hemispheres, to be
sure, but they can be very subtle, a fact that should lead us away
from thinking about hemispheric specialization in overly simple
terms.

## ANATOMICAL ASYMMETRIES IN THE
## TWO HEMISPHERES

A 1968 report by Norman Geschwind and Walter Levitsky demonstrated unequivocal anatomical asymmetries in the two hemispheres
of the human brain in the regions important for speech and language.[25] Published in a journal widely read by scientists in a number
of different disciplines, their paper generated a great deal of excitement among those interested in hemispheric asymmetry of function.

Geschwind and Levitsky were not the first investigators to notice
such asymmetries in the brain, however. Asymmetries had been
reported sporadically as far back as the second half of the nineteenth
century. In general, at that time the differences were considered

trivial and insufficient in size to account for functional differences between the left brain and the right brain.

By the late 1960s, however, the time was ripe to reconsider the possibility that functional asymmetries between hemispheres might have a physical basis on a nonmicroscopic, anatomical level. Since the publication of Geschwind and Levitsky's paper, several other investigators have studied the problem and extended the search for asymmetries to neonates and non-human primates as well.

Here we review the evidence pointing to asymmetries in the adult human brain. We reserve discussion of work with neonates and non-human primates for Chapters 8 and 9, respectively.

## Measuring the Hemispheres

The asymmetries found by Geschwind and Levitsky were in the length of the temporal plane, the upper surface of the region of the temporal lobe behind the auditory cortex. Of the 100 brains measured at postmortem, 65 were found to have a longer temporal plane in the left hemisphere than in the right, 11 had a longer temporal plane in the right hemisphere, and the remaining 24 showed no difference. On the average, the temporal plane was one-third longer on the left than on the right. Figure 4.10 shows the location of these asymmetries.

Although the size of these asymmetries is impressive, their location is more significant. The temporal plane is part of Wernicke's area, a region named after Karl Wernicke, who first noted that damage to this area frequently results in a variety of aphasic symptoms. Geschwind and Levitsky suggested that the asymmetries they observed were compatible with the functional asymmetries believed to be controlled by this region.

Several studies using various procedures to measure the temporal plane have confirmed Geschwind and Levitsky's observations.[26] Direct measurements on a total of 337 brain specimens (including the 100 brains studied by Geschwind and Levitsky) have been reported. Seventy percent showed asymmetry favoring the left hemisphere in length or area of the temporal plane.

*Does the left get bigger or the right get smaller?* In a recent re-evaluation of the anatomical data used by Geschwind, neurologist Albert Galaburda and associates found an interesting relationship between the degree of asymmetry and the size of each temporal plane. Geschwind previously had assumed that the asymmetry he observed was a

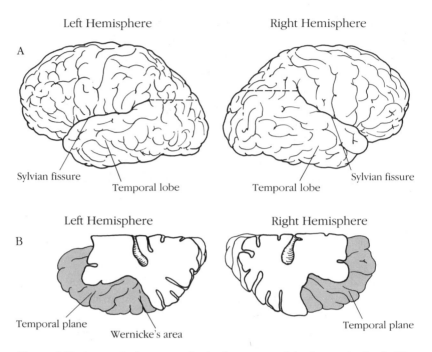

**Figure 4.10** Anatomical asymmetries in the cortex of the human brain. A. The sylvian fissure, which defines the upper margin of the temporal lobe, rises more steeply on the right side of the brain. B. The temporal plane, which forms the upper surface of the temporal lobe, is usually much larger on the left side. This region in the left hemisphere is considered part of Wernicke's area, a region involved in language. [From Geschuind, "Specializations of the Human Brain," Scientific American, Inc., 1979. All rights reserved.]

result of greater or more rapid development of the left side. He predicted that symmetrical brains resulted from a less developed left side.

Galaburda found that the left planum remains roughly constant in size (corrected for variability in total brain size) but that the right planum is larger in symmetrical and smaller in asymmetrical brains.[27] Thus, symmetrical brains tend to have two large plana, whereas most asymmetrical brains have a large left and a small right planum. Galaburda speculated that whatever factors play a role in the development of these asymmetries act by controlling the extent of development of the right side in most individuals.

*Callosal size and functional asymmetry* Canadian biopsychologist Sandra Witelson conducted postmortem examinations of the brains of 42 terminally ill subjects whose hand preference was accurately tested on a number of tasks while alive. The corpus callosum was larger by about 75 square millimeters, or 11 percent, in left-handed and ambidextrous people than in those with consistent right-hand preference ("extreme right handers"). Witelson suggested that because left and mixed handers tend to show greater bihemispheric representation of cognitive functions, this may be associated with greater anatomical connection between the hemispheres. It is unlikely that this greater connectivity is a result of the growth of more axons during development because of greater bimanual experience, because all evidence indicates that the number of axons are maximal at birth. A more plausible hypothesis concerns the rate of naturally occurring neuronal/axonal death. Developmental neurobiology indicates that naturally occurring "regressive" events, such as the death of neurons and the elimination of certain axonal connections, play a major role in late stages of fetal development (neurogenesis), reducing what amounts to an earlier overproduction of neurons and fibers. The corpus callosum has markedly fewer fibers at maturity than in fetal and newborn stages. Very right-handed people may lose considerably more interhemispheric connections through neural elimination than those who become more functionally bilateral.[28]

The mechanisms governing this neuronal loss are unknown and the reasons that have been proposed are completely speculative. It is possible that very lateralized brains do not need as many interhemispheric fibers as those that have a more bilateral distribution of most functions. It is a fairly new idea in neurobiology that the actual degeneration of certain neurons and their connections is part of the organizing mechanisms of the brain. In a later section we discuss a technique that can be used to measure the size of neural fiber bundles, such as the corpus callosum, in live subjects.

*Which hemisphere develops faster?* It is possible to notice the presence of anatomical asymmetry in the middle of gestation in the human fetus.[29] Although controversial, there is some evidence that the right hemisphere develops earlier and faster than the left. A number of anatomists have noted that "folding" of the cortex into the familiar sulci takes place earlier on the right side. The assumption is that folding occurs as the brain grows, and growth takes place earlier on the right in several regions including the vicinity of the sylvian fissure. It is believed that part of the folding/growth involves the *loss* of neurons and axons; therefore, it is possible that the earlier appearance of cortical markings on the right (perisylvian area) reflects the earlier or more marked loss of neural elements. As we noted above, because the right temporal plane is smaller than expected in asymmetrical brains (rather than the left being larger), it is conceivable that a right temporal plane undergoing excessive or accelerated cell loss during development folds earlier and achieves a smaller final size.

Some recent microanatomical work, indeed, suggests that the relatively larger right planum in symmetrical brains is a result of the preservation of neurons, which normally would be lost during development, and that the standard asymmetrical pattern is a result of neuronal and axonal loss by the right planum during fetal development and the first few years after birth.[30] Microscopic examination of areas around the temporal lobe defined by specific cell types (architectonic areas) shows a reduced number of neurons on the nondominant side. In symmetrical cases, the two sides are both large with comparable numbers of neurons. Thus, it appears that unilateral neuronal loss leads to asymmetry.

## Measurements in the Living Brain

The anatomical studies considered up to this point have involved measurements taken from brains examined at postmortem. Other evidence suggests that it is also possible to find asymmetries in the living brain.

One technique takes advantage of the fact that the paths of the large blood vessels in the brain reflect the anatomy of the surrounding brain tissue. In particular, the middle cerebral artery courses through the language-critical region of the temporal lobe. For many years, neurologists have used a procedure known as cerebral angiography to visualize this major blood vessel to determine whether the brain regions surrounding it have been damaged. A dye injected into the internal carotid artery in the neck (the same artery used in the Wada procedure) flows into the middle cerebral artery, making the artery visible when a skull x-ray is taken. Majorie LeMay and her colleagues have evidence suggesting that left–right asymmetries consistent with those found in postmortem brain measurements may be observed with the angiographic procedure.[31]

Another technique used to measure asymmetry in the living brain is *computerized tomography*, or *CT*, scan. In a CT scan, an x-ray source is revolved in a plane around the head as detectors continuously monitor the intensity of the x-ray beam passed through to the other side. A computer stores this information and then uses it to reconstruct an image of a slice of brain. By adjusting the angles

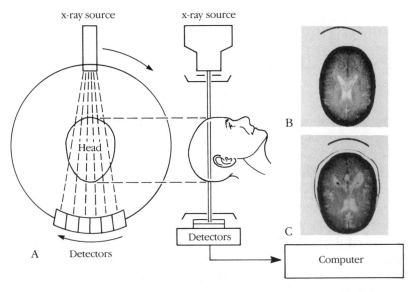

**Figure 4.11** A. Computerized tomography (CT) scan uses an x-ray beam and an array of detectors revolving around the subject's head to calculate the density of tissues in a particular slice of the brain. A computer reconstructs a two-dimensional picture of what the brain looks like in the plane swept by the x-rays. The CT pictures shown here are B. normal, with no evidence of pathology, and C. abnormal, with enlargement of the ventricles (fluid-filled spaces—the light central areas), especially on the right, moderate atrophy, and right fronto-temporal infarct (stroke).

through which the x-rays pass, the appearance of any slice of the brain is made available. Figure 4.11 shows a representative CT scan. This technique has been used extensively to pinpoint the locations of lesions in cases of brain damage. LeMay and her colleagues have also been active in using CT scan data to study asymmetries, with some success.[32]

## Nuclear Magnetic Resonance

All of the scanning techniques used to measure either the function or the structure of the brain depend on radiation, generated either by an x-ray machine on the outside of the head or by chemical tracers distributed inside the head. A new brain-imaging technique using *nuclear magnetic resonance (NMR)* is now capable of generating fine cross-sectional images of brain structure without using penetrating radiation. The technique uses a combination of radio waves and a strong magnetic field (generated by a large electromagnet) to detect the distribution of water molecules in living tissue (the hydrogen atoms in the water "resonate" due to the combined effect of the radio waves and magnetic field). In this way, brain tissue densities can be very accurately calculated, and a fine pictorial image can be generated by computer.[33] Figure 4.12 shows an example of the resolution achieved by NMR imaging.

In a preceding section we discussed how anatomical measurements were used to compare the size of the corpus callosum in postmortem examination of patients with well-documented hand preference. Because of its sensitivity to the fatty myelin sheaths of nerve bundles, NMR is an excellent technique for precisely imaging the corpus callosum in living subjects. One recent study reported no differences in callosal size between right-handers and left-handers as measured by NMR.[34] It should be noted, however, that this study did not use the same rigorous criteria for handedness used in the Witelson study, where the significant effect (smaller callosal size) was noted only in "consistent" or extreme right-handers. Witelson, as it turns out, has also reported NMR findings on two living subjects documented to be consistent left-handers.[35] These individuals,

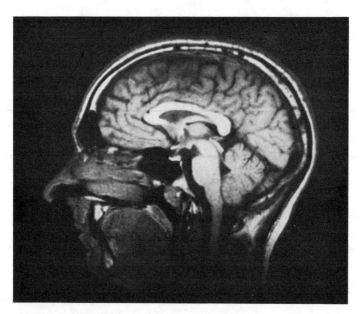

**Figure 4.12** Nuclear magnetic resonance (NMR) scan. A computer-reconstructed image of a cross section of a normal brain, using data derived from the NMR of hydrogen in the water molecules of a subject's head. [Reproduced with permission from General Electric Co.]

Witelson reports, also have larger callosums than consistent right-handers, supporting a model of handedness in which even extremely left-handed individuals are not simply mirror image versions of right-handers in terms of hemispheric organization.

NMR remains a very convenient tool for the study of such issues. We are sure to see many more anatomical studies using this technique in the near future. Research is underway to allow the NMR technique to also image metabolism in the human brain. When this becomes possible, it will open up a whole new approach to studying hemispheric asymmetry of function — one that will provide not only three-dimensional information about this function but will be safe enough to allow studies on many more subjects than is currently possible.

## Microscopic Asymmetries

We have dealt up to now with evidence for asymmetries at the gross anatomical level. Advanced techniques have also allowed investigators to search for asymmetries at a more microscopic level, that of the distribution of brain-cell types. There are several variations in cell type and distribution that can be examined. The cerebral cortex, for example, is composed of several distinct layers consisting of specific types of neurons, each with a characteristic appearance. The number, thickness, and density of these layers within the cortex varies across regions of the brain, as illustrated in Figure 4.13. Anatomists have distinguished and labeled many areas across the cortical surface according to changes in the composition of cells and cell layers forming the cortex. Some have analyzed equivalent areas of the left and right hemispheres in search of any asymmetries. Postmortem evaluations of many brains have yielded several positive findings. Figure 4.14 shows the location of some of the areas involved. An area of the temporal lobe consisting of anatomically distinct cell layers, called *Tpt*, has been shown to be larger on the left side of the brain.[36] This area is part of what is called the auditory association cortex, a region involved in higher-level processing of auditory information, especially speech sounds. Another area defined by cell-layer types, called *PG*, lying mainly on the angular gyrus between the temporal and parietal lobes, was also found to be larger on the left side.[37] Lesions to this area have been implicated in speech disorders characterized by word-finding and naming difficulties.

It should be noted that enlargement of cell areas Tpt and PG in the left hemisphere is found most frequently in brains with larger

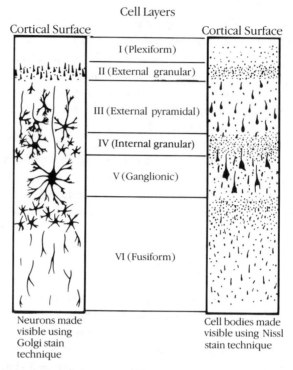

**Figure 4.13** Typical cell layer (laminar) structure of the cerebral cortex. The density of each layer varies across different regions of the cortex.

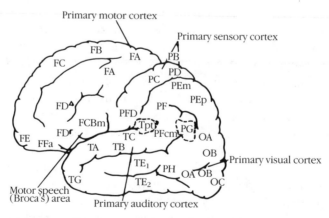

**Figure 4.14** The major "cytoarchitectonic" regions of the cortical surface. Differences in cellular arrangements and densities have been used as a basis for mapping the cortex. Areas Tpt and PG have been shown to be different in the left and right hemispheres.

left-temporal planes. Thus, there appears to be a link between the anatomical asymmetries, both gross and microscopic, that have been discovered so far in the hemispheres.

### What Do Anatomical Asymmetries Tell Us?

Much of the interest in techniques that can measure asymmetries in the living brain comes from a basic problem in interpreting anatomical asymmetries in general. Are the asymmetries that have been identified related in a meaningful way to functional asymmetries between the hemispheres?

At this point, we do not know. Most of the data on anatomical asymmetries have come from postmortem measurements of brains where nothing is known about the kinds of functional asymmetries that may have existed before death. In many cases, even the handedness of the individuals is not known. Clearly, this kind of information is necessary if we are to begin to answer questions like those posed in the preceding paragraph.

Procedures that permit measurements in the living brain offer us a way to get that crucial information. Batteries of behavioral and electrophysiological tests designed to study the distribution of functions between the hemispheres can be used with measurements of brain asymmetry in the same individuals to see whether there is a relationship. Some preliminary data indicate that, overall, left-handers show less anatomical asymmetry than right-handers—an observation that is promising.[38] It is clear, though, that investigators have only barely begun the process of studying how anatomical asymmetries and functional asymmetries are related.

## BIOCHEMISTRY OF THE HEMISPHERES

Neurons communicate through chemistry. Although electrical activity is associated with neuronal firing and interactions, the basic mechanisms generating this activity are chemical, and the mechanisms that transfer signals from one brain cell to another are also chemical. Neural pathways are established by groups of cells that utilize one specific chemical to transfer the discharges between them. Thus, brain cells communicate only with other brain cells using the same transmitter chemical, called a *neurotransmitter*. Many neurotransmitters have been discovered, and anatomists and chemists are busy mapping the cell groups and pathways defined by the neurons utilizing each particular transmitter chemical. Each neurotransmitter, in addition, has a host of biochemical processes associated with it, involving both its formation and breakdown.

A study conducted in 1965 with the hallucinogenic drug LSD suggested that the typical hallucinogenic perceptual responses associated with this drug were a result of its action on the right hemisphere.[39] LSD was administered pre- and postoperatively to patients undergoing right or left temporal lobe removals for alleviating epilepsy. It was found that the hallucinogenic responses to LSD disappeared after right, but not left, temporal lobectomy. One likely explanation of these findings is that there are some asymmetries in the biochemistry or the biochemical functions of the two hemispheres that make the right hemisphere more sensitive or vulnerable to the presence of LSD. One hypothesis was that LSD affects a certain neurotransmitter that may be used to a greater extent by the right hemisphere.

One of the first substantiations of true neurochemical asymmetries in the human brain came in 1978, when it was discovered that the neurotransmitter norepinephrine was distributed differently in the right and left halves of the thalamus, a subcortical structure that, among other things, serves as a main relay center for sensory impulses to the cortex.[40] Higher levels of norepinephrine were found on the right side. In 1981, a group of Italian scientists showed that there were neurochemical asymmetries at the cortical level as well. They found that an area of the left temporal lobe shows greater activity by the enzyme choline-acetyltransferase (CAT) than did the corresponding area of the right hemisphere.[41] CAT is involved in chemical processes associated with acetylcholine, a major neurotransmitter defining extensive neuronal networks in the brain. The area in which increased enzyme activity was found included the region Tpt, in which the cellular layer differences mentioned earlier were reported. Thus, a correspondence is seen between anatomic and physiologic asymmetries discovered through different techniques.

The list of neurotransmitter systems discovered in the brain continues to increase, and there is growing evidence that a number of transmitters are unequally represented in the left and right hemisphere. Dopamine, another major neurotransmitter may also define more extensive neuronal networks in the left hemisphere.[42] There is some speculation that the extra norepinephrine defined pathways of the right hemisphere complement the extra dopamine defined pathways of the left in terms of the kind of attentional mechanisms they subserve, which, in turn, lead to some of the well documented hemispheric asymmetries in function.[43] Dopamine has been implicated as playing a role in controlling fine movement, especially in the initiation of action sequences and, thus, may be a basis for the specialization of the left hemisphere for complex motor operations such as speech. Norepinephrine appears to facilitate arousal to novel stimuli and, thus, may be a basis for the specialization of the right hemisphere, for certain visuo-spatial–perceptual operations.[44]

A great deal of neurotransmitter research is conducted with laboratory animals. We review more biochemical findings pertaining to hemispheric asymmetry in Chapter 9.

## PHYSIOLOGY AND PSYCHOLOGY: BUILDING THE LINK

Anatomical measurements, recordings of electrical activity, blood-flow studies, and the scanning of metabolic processes offer investigators the opportunity to study relationships between mental processes, behavior, and brain activity. These techniques have at least partially validated some of the theoretical insights about brain function and hemispheric asymmetry developed in the brain-damage clinic and from psychological research with normal subjects.

Some researchers have claimed that physiological tools offer the ultimate resolution of questions that deal with relations between mind and brain; others argue against overreliance on such measures on both philosophical and practical grounds. Clearly, certain concerns must be confronted in the attempt to establish relationships between physiological processes and psychological functions. Although these concerns are important for the study of hemispheric asymmetries, their significance extends beyond any specific area of research and has applicability to the study of brain–behavior relationships in general.

One issue is the problem of selecting from among the various physiological measures available those that will prove most informative. Like all other tissues in the human body, the brain is dependent on complex metabolic processes for its functioning. Nutrients like glucose are converted for energy processes; other nutrients are used as cellular constituents; waste products are removed. A great deal of the brain's biochemistry, however, is unique and involves the communication of information between neurons. Biochemical processes operating in each cell generate electrical potentials, and biochemicals operating between cells effectively transmit electrical impulses between groups of neurons.

We do not know what aspects of this activity best reflect the behavioral or mental functions with which we are concerned. If, for example, we just want to know what areas of the brain are most active during particular human behaviors, we can look at cerebral blood flow, for it responds rapidly to changes in metabolic activity. Yet such measures may not be indicative of the true information-processing strategies or codes of the brain. Such codes could involve chemical pathways extending across many areas of the brain or could perhaps be reflected in patterns of electrical-wave activity. Neither would necessarily correlate with regional metabolic activity.

Even after deciding on a measure to study, we may be faced with further choices. The evoked potential, for example, may be broken down into several components and analyzed in different ways. In the absence of a comprehensive theory about the meaning of these components, investigators must decide how best to analyze their data to look for asymmetries or other effects. Anatomists, too, must decide what measurements of what regions of the brain will be most useful for the problem at hand.

Another issue involves the concept of localization of function in general. How much does attributing some psychological activity to a specific area of the brain contribute to insights about that activity? Certainly, findings on localization have been of tremendous clinical value. Furthermore, relationships between location and function may help establish the components of a complex behavior or task in terms of more basic processes. As a hypothetical example, it may be demonstrated that the memory of how to get somewhere involves linguistic processes in the left hemisphere as well as imagery processes in the right hemisphere. It is not clear, however, how far this kind of approach can take us. Ultimately, it is likely that dividing the brain in terms of "where" will not completely answer the question of "how."

Discovering brain–behavior and brain–mind relationships is not only an experimental problem and certainly not only one of localization of function. The problems are at least as much conceptual in nature: what are we trying to explain, how are we defining things, in what sense does some neurophysiological activity accompanying a mental event explain something about the event, what would constitute a satisfactory "explanation" of some mental or behavioral event?

Investigators have become more sophisticated, at least with respect to localization issues. They now talk of the "state of activity in the system," rather than "where." They realize most psychological functions should be associated with activity changes in multiple areas or defined pathways of the cerebrum. They also realize that these may be flexible and time varying, perhaps even probabilistic.[45]

More conceptual development will have to do with the nature of our questions and definitions, including a better appreciation of the levels of explanation involved. For the time being, it does seem that the interaction of psychology and physiology should be fruitful for the study of both mind and brain. Physiological injuries of the sort studied by neuropsychologists have had an impact on the way we break down mental functions. Physiological imaging of the sort described in this chapter has the potential to reorganize it further. Psychological questions are also guiding at least some investigations into anatomy and physiological processes. Although attempts at such interactions of the two disciplines often have led to premature simplistic conclusions, we are getting better.

A physiologist discovers that certain cells in the occipital lobe respond when very specific visual patterns, and only those patterns, are shown to subjects. A clinician in a hospital notices that a patient with a combination of lesions in both hemispheres can see clearly but seems to view objects in terms of parts and can't figure out what he is looking at. A psychologist suggests that visual perception involves both a pattern recognition system and some decision system to decide on what is relevant.

It is to be hoped that an interaction results from all these insights, both modifying what is meant by perception and identifying the processes that are involved. Similar interactions between psychology and physiology are possible in virtually every area of study dealing with brain–behavior relationships. It is our opinion that each component will be essential to achieving an understanding of such relationships.

# CHAPTER 5

# The Puzzle of the Left-Hander

An overwhelming majority of human beings use their right hands almost exclusively for writing and other skilled, unimanual activities. Cross-cultural studies put the incidence of right-handedness at around 90 percent. A variety of indirect evidence suggests that this has been the case as far back as prehistoric times.[1] Drawings of people found on cave walls and inside Egyptian tombs typically show the subjects engaged in activities involving the right hand, and an analysis of paleolithic tools and weapons suggests that they were made with, and for, the right hand.

A study of hand tracings believed to have been made by Cro-Magnon people showed over 80 percent to be of the left hand. If we assume the artists traced their own hands, these data also point to a very strong preference for the right hand in skilled activity. A study of 1,180 works of art spanning a 5,000-year period, from pre-3000 B.C. to 1950, showed that depiction of right- and left-hand use showed no significant change or trends over time, with left-hand use averaging 7 to 8 percent. Perhaps the most ingenious evidence of all for right-hand preference in early humans comes from an analysis of fossilized baboon skulls with fractures. On the basis of the locations of the fractures, the investigator concluded that the injuries were the result of blows inflicted by early humans wielding clubs with their right hands.

Animals may show preferences for one paw or the other in certain situations, but they divide up fairly evenly in terms of the numbers preferring the right paw and the left paw. Why, then, are most human beings right-handed? Conversely, why does a significant percentage of the population use the left hand, despite subtle and sometimes overt social pressure to conform to the handedness pattern characteristic of the majority?

We mentioned in earlier chapters that handedness is related in complex ways to the distribution of functions between the left brain and the right brain. Any analysis of brain asymmetry must deal with this problem if it is to be complete. What factors determine handedness? In what ways do left-handers and right-handers differ?

In this chapter, we consider modern theories proposed to account for variations in handedness and studies designed to examine possible differences between left-handers and right-handers. To provide a historical context for recent work, we turn first to a brief review of some of the older ideas about handedness.


## HISTORICAL NOTIONS OF LEFT-HANDEDNESS

### Is There Anything Sinister About Being Left-Handed?

*Webster's Third International Dictionary* lists several definitions of the adjective *left-handed*, including the following:

a: marked by clumsiness or ineptitude: awkward; b: exhibiting deviousness or indirection: oblique, unintended; c: obs.: given to malevolent scheming or contriving: sinister, underhand.

Left-handers are frequently referred to as "sinistrals," and *Roget's Thesaurus* lists *left-handed* as a synonym for *unskillfulness*. In other languages as well, the terms for *left* or *left-handed* have almost always contained at least one derogatory meaning, ranging from "clumsy" or "awkward" to "evil." The French word for *left, gauche,* also means "clumsy"; *mancino* is Italian for *left* as well as for *deceitful.* The Spanish idiom *no ser zurdo* means "to be very clever." Its literal translation is "not to be left-handed." Other examples abound.

Anthropologists have provided us with a number of examples of how symbolic associations with left and right are part of different cultures.[2] For example, the involuntary twitching of an eyelid is thought to be significant by the native people of Morocco. For them, twitching of the right eyelid signifies the return of a family member or other good news, whereas twitching of the left eyelid is a warning of an impending death in the family. In another part of the world, the Maoris of New Zealand at one time believed that a tremor during sleep meant that a spirit had seized the body. A right-sided tremor meant good fortune, whereas a left-sided tremor meant ill fortune and possibly death.

The Bible, too, reflects a bias against the left hand or side. One example from the New Testament that is especially striking is the Vision of Judgment in Matthew 25:31–34, 41, 46:

> When the Son of man shall come in his glory, and all the holy angels with him, then shall he sit upon the throne of his glory:
> And before him shall be gathered all nations, and he shall separate them one from another, as a shepherd divideth *his* sheep from the goats:
> And he shall set the sheep on his right hand, but the goats on the left.
> Then shall the King say unto them on his right hand, Come, ye blessed of my Father, inherit the kingdom prepared for you from the foundation of the world. . . .
> Then shall he say also unto them on the left hand, Depart from me, ye cursed, into everlasting fire, prepared for the devil and his angels. . . .
> And these shall go away into everlasting punishment: but the righteous into life eternal.

Michael Barsley, author of *Left Handed People*, has argued that the Vision of Judgment has been responsible for "fixing the prejudice against left handers [more] than any other pronouncement, and that this prejudice has come down through the ages, adopted by inquisitors, judges, soldiers, artists, teachers, nurses, and parents as the supreme example of the association of sinistral people with wickedness and the Devil."[3] Whether or not Barsley is correct, it is clear that the association of left with bad is of very long standing.

What is the origin of this bias? At this point we can only speculate. Carl Sagan, of Cornell University, has suggested one possibility in *The Dragons of Eden*, his book on the evolution of intelligence.[4] Sagan notes that in preindustrial societies, both now and in the past, the hand has been used for personal hygiene after defecation. This use of a hand is both unaesthetic and potentially harmful because it can spread disease, but these drawbacks can be reduced somewhat by using only the other hand to eat and to greet others. Right-handed individuals would perform activities like eating and throwing weapons with the right hand, leaving toilet hygiene to the left. Sagan suggests that the left-hand became associated with excretory activities, which have a long history of negative associations in human cultures. Thus the chain linking "left" with "bad" was forged.

Michael Corballis, of the University of Auckland (New Zealand), offers another explanation, which has two parts. First, the difference between the hands is not a structural one—the hands differ in function, but not in form. This, he argues, bestows on handedness a somewhat mysterious quality. Second, right-handedness, as we shall see in Chapter 9, appears to be a uniquely human trait, setting us apart from other animals. Corballis speculates, "Perhaps this is why virtually all cultures hold the right [hand] to be sacred and the left profane, as though right handedness, like human beings themselves, is a gift of the Gods."[5]

Both explanations assume that human beings begin with a preference to use the right hand for activities requiring fine control. We must still explain the basis for that preference. Speculation abounds on this issue, but we stand a good chance of bringing the tools of modern science to bear on and resolve the question in a satisfactory way.

## Nineteenth-Century Theories of Handedness

Let us first consider some of the ideas proposed in the nineteenth century to account for handedness. One popular theory was known as visceral distribution. Proponents argued that the asymmetrical placement of visceral organs, such as the liver, puts the center of gravity of the human body slightly to the right of the midline, and, as a consequence, human beings are better able to balance on the left foot. This leaves the right hand free, so that over time the muscles on the right side became better developed. This notion, however, does not explain why some people are left-handed, unless we assume a reversal in the orientation of their viscera.

Social-evolution explanations of handedness were also popular in the nineteenth century. There are several variations on this general theme, the most common being the sword-and-shield theory. According to this theory, attributed to English essayist and historian Thomas Carlyle and others, most soldiers hold their shields with their left hands to protect their hearts when they are engaged in battle and use their right hands to hold their weapons. As a consequence, during eons of armed conflict, the right hand gained in manipulative ability and came to be used for other unimanual activities as well. Again, there is no attempt to explain left-handedness or the apparently high incidence of right-handedness in humans before the invention of the shield.

The idea of cerebral dominance emerged in the last quarter of the nineteenth century, and with it came yet another theory of handedness. D. J. Cunningham, a Scottish anatomist, summarized this view in 1902 in a Huxley Memorial Lecture: "Right handedness is due to a transmitted functional preeminence of the left brain. Left brainedness is not the result but, through evolution, it has become the cause of right handedness." As it is stated, this view would not easily account for left-handers with left-hemisphere speech, who comprise about 70 percent of all left-handers. In addition, it fails to explain the reasons for the transmitted functional preeminence of the left brain.

## THE DIFFICULTY OF DETERMINING HANDEDNESS

Before we consider more modern theories of handedness, it is important to consider how handedness is actually assessed. We might assume that the best way to find out whether a given individual is a left- or a right-hander is simply to ask. Unfortunately, this direct approach does not always work. Few people use one hand exclusively for all unimanual activities, and simple self-classification does not indicate how someone weighed various activities when making the determination. Another approach is to ask people which hand they use for specific activities. The researcher can then compute a handedness preference based on the same weighting scheme for everyone.

A widely used questionnaire to measure hand preference was developed by Oldfield at Edinburgh University (see Figure 5.1). Sub-

Please indicate your preferences in the use of the hands in the following activities by *putting + in the appropriate column*. Where the preference is so strong that you would never try to use the other hand unless absolutely forced to, *put + +*. In any case where you are really indifferent, *put + in both columns*.

Some of these activities require both hands. In these cases the part of the task, or object, for which hand preference is wanted is indicated in parentheses.

Please try to answer all the questions, and only leave a blank if you have no experience at all of the object or task.

| | Left | Right |
|---|---|---|
| 1. Writing<br>2. Drawing<br>3. Throwing<br>4. Scissors<br>5. Toothbrush<br>6. Knife (without fork)<br>7. Spoon<br>8. Broom (upper hand)<br>9. Striking match (match)<br>10. Opening box (lid) | | |

**Figure 5.1** The Edinburgh Handedness Inventory, Short Form. To find the subject's laterality quotient, add the number of + signs in each column. Subtract the number in the LEFT column from the number in the RIGHT column, divide by the total of LEFT plus RIGHT, and multiply by 100.

jects are asked to indicate their preferred hand for writing, drawing, throwing, cutting with scissors, brushing teeth, cutting with a knife without a fork, using a spoon, holding a broom (upper hand), holding a match while striking, and holding a lid while removing it from a box. The questionnaire yields a laterality quotient that ranges from −100 for extreme left handedness, through zero for equal use of the two hands, to +100 for extreme right handedness.

In a study of over 1,000 undergraduates at the University of Edinburgh who completed the questionnaire, most showed a consistent preference for one hand; few showed no preference.[6] Those showing right preference, however, tended to show their preferences more strongly than those showing left preference. That is, the distribution of positive and negative scores was different. The positive scores were clustered toward the high end of the range, whereas the negative scores were more evenly distributed over the range of values. Findings like these have led some investigators to speak of right-handers and non-right-handers, rather than right-handers and left-handers.

The way in which subjects are classified into different handedness groups is critical for the outcome of research investigating handedness as a variable. Most studies using questionnaires attempt to classify subjects in terms of handedness based on their scores. Problems arise, however, because handedness is not a simple all-or-none dimension—a decision, most likely arbitrary, must be made about the placement of the boundaries between handedness group categories.

In an attempt to avoid this problem, other studies do not form groups based on test scores, but rather use the actual scores in the handedness measure. For either of these approaches, however, different types of questionnaires may yield different classifications for a group of subjects. In light of this, it should not be surprising that experiments investigating the effects of handedness sometimes yield conflicting results. Differences in the way subjects are classified may account for some or all of the conflict.

Keeping in mind this problem of handedness studies in general, we now consider the major theories of handedness currently receiving attention.

## IS HANDEDNESS HEREDITARY?

Is handedness, like eye color, blood type, and general body build, genetically determined? The probability of two right-handed parents having a left-handed child is 0.02. It rises to 0.17 if one parent is left-handed and to 0.46 if both are left-handed.[7] These figures are consistent with the hypothesis that genes play a role in determining handedness. The problem with interpreting the data, however, is that environmental factors can account for these differences as well.

Two left-handed parents could provide a child with different experiences relevant to the determination of handedness, just as they might provide specific genes. Nature (genes) and nurture (experience) are confounded in these figures, making it impossible to sort out the contribution of each.

### The Environmental View

Robert Collins has taken an extreme environmental position, arguing that handedness is transmitted from one generation to the next through cultural and environmental biases. Collins has based his conclusions in large part on his work with paw preference in mice. This work is discussed at greater length in Chapter 9 but can be summarized as showing that mice demonstrate consistent paw preferences in reaching for food in a glass tube. These preferences are not subject to genetic selection: it is not possible to breed right-pawed mice over several generations by mating mice that show a right-paw preference. The off-spring of such animals will show the same paw-preference distribution found among mice in general: 50 percent left preference, 50 percent right preference.[8] Collins has also shown that young mice that have not yet shown a preference for either paw become predominantly right-pawed if they are presented with the glass tube placed toward the right side of the case, making it easier to reach with the right paw than with the left paw.[9]

Collins's emphasis on the role of cultural and environmental biases in the determination of handedness is consistent with views expressed by another investigator who, after reviewing the evidence that existed up to 1946, concluded, "Preferred laterality is not an inherited trait. There is absolutely no evidence to support the contention that dominance, either in handedness or any other form, is a congenital, predetermined human capacity."[10]

The author argued that right-handedness is a learned response to a right-handed world and that left-handedness occurs when this response is not learned as a result of physical defect, faulty education, emotional problems, or the like. An environmental model of handedness determination must account, however, for the fact that right-hand preference has been found across all cultures studied and over all time periods for which evidence is available. It remains to be explained why environments biased in favor of the left hand do not occur.

## Genetic Models

Evidence for a genetic model of handedness, in contrast to environmental models, may be evaluated by formulating specific models of how handedness might be transmitted from generation to generation through the action of genes. Different models make different predictions of the actual figures. A good fit between the predictions of a specific model and actual data would suggest that genetic factors can account for most of the variations in handedness found among people.

One of the first genetic models of handedness proposed that handedness is a consequence of the action of a single gene that has two different forms, or *alleles*.[11] One allele, *R*, was dominant and coded for right-handedness. A second, *l*, was recessive and coded for left-handedness. An individual inheriting the *R* allele from each parent would be right-handed, as would someone with an *Rl* genotype (*R* from one parent, *l* from the other). Left-handers would be those individuals who inherited the *l* allele from each parent.

This model, however, cannot account for the fact that 54 percent of the offspring of two left-handed parents are right-handed. The model predicts that all offspring of such parents should be left-handed, because the *l* allele is the only one that left-handed parents can transmit to their offspring. There have been attempts to rescue this model by introducing the concept of *variable penetrance*. Variable penetrance means that all individuals with the same genotype may not express that genotype in the same way. In this case, it has been suggested that some individuals with the *Rl* genotype will be left-handed. These left-handers could transmit an *R* allele to their offspring, accounting for the nonzero incidence of right-handedness among the children of two left-handed parents. Even with variable penetrance built into the model, however, the model's "goodness of fit" to actual data is less than satisfactory.

A more sophisticated model has been proposed by Jerre Levy and Thomas Nagylaki,[12] who suggest that handedness is a function of two genes. One gene with two alleles determines the hemisphere that will control speech as well as the preferred hand. The allele *L* codes for left-hemisphere speech and is dominant, whereas the allele *r* codes for right-hemisphere speech and is recessive. The second gene determines whether the speech hemisphere controls the ipsilateral or the contralateral hand. Contralateral control is coded for by the dominant *C* allele, while ipsilateral control is coded for by the recessive *c* allele. Someone with an *LrCC* genotype, for example, would have left-hemisphere speech and be right-handed. Another individual with an *Lrcc* genotype would have left-hemisphere speech but would be left-handed.

This model assumes that an individual's handedness is a consequence of the pattern of hemispheric asymmetry as well as the type of motor control present in that individual. It does a better job of accounting for handedness patterns among relatives than do single-gene models, but it, too, is less than totally satisfactory. There is some question about whether ispilateral motor control of the sort postulated really exists. Nevertheless, the model is an ingenious attempt to account for variations both in brain organization and in handedness in terms of simple genetic mechanisms.

Marion Annett, of the University of Hull in England, has proposed a genetic model of handedness that is very different from those just considered.[13] She hypothesized that there is no gene for left- or right-handedness as such, but that there is a gene responsible for the development of speech in the left hemisphere, which, in turn, increases the chances of greater skill in the right hand. Annett refers to her theory as the "right shift" theory. In some individuals, however, the right-shift gene is presumed to be absent. When this occurs, Annett argues, there is an absence of systematic bias to one side, for either speech or handedness, with chance factors operating independently on the direction of lateralization for speech and handedness. Thus, an individual without the right-shift gene might have speech represented in either the left or right hemisphere, and be left- or right-handed, in any of the four possible combinations.

In one test of the right shift model, Annett examined the manual skills of parents and their children. Children of two left-handed parents, each of whom had a close left-handed relative, did not show a bias in ability when average performance for the two hands was compared. When neither parent had a left-handed relative, however, the children showed a bias to the right, even though they were raised by two left-handed parents.

These results can be predicted by the right-shift theory. Families with a number of left-handed relatives would be assumed to be lacking the right-shift factor. Handedness, then, would be randomly determined so that when the data of large numbers of offspring were averaged, there would be no difference between hands. Left-handers in families without other left-handed relatives are more likely to be left-handed as a result of pathological or other factors. They are presumed to possess the right-shift factor, although it is not expressed in them, and they can pass it on to their children. The children, then, would show the right shift itself, which is precisely what Annett found. Much more work needs to be done, however, to test the adequacy of this as well as other genetic models.

## Comparing Identical and Fraternal Twins

Assessing the fit of the predictions of specific genetic models to actual data is the approach most frequently taken by researchers testing the hypothesis that handedness is under genetic control. Another approach involves looking at the hand preferences of monozygotic (identical) and dizygotic (fraternal) twins. Monozygotic twins are genetically identical. They began life as a single fertilized egg that divided to form two individuals sometime within the first two weeks after conception. Dyzogotic twins, however, are no more similar genetically than ordinary siblings born at different times. They result from the simultaneous fertilization of two different eggs by two different sperm cells, and they have, on the average, 50 percent of their genes in common. Figure 5.2 shows the ways in which monozygotic and dizygotic twins are formed.

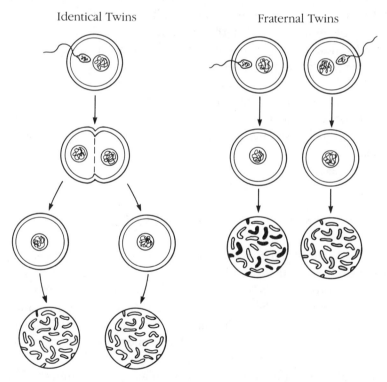

**Figure 5.2** The origin of identical and fraternal twins. Identical (monozygotic) twins are the product of a single sperm and egg. The resulting embryo divides at an early stage of development to form two individuals. Fraternal (dizygotic) twins develop from two different eggs fertilized by two different sperm cells. On the average they have half of their genes in common.

If a trait is under genetic control to some extent, monozygotic twins should be more similar in that trait than dizygotic twins. A number of studies have looked at handedness in twins. When the results of all these studies are combined, some interesting findings emerge. The percentage of concordance for handedness (both twins left-handed or both right-handed) is no higher in monozygotic twin pairs than in dizygotic pairs. Moreover, about 25 percent of the total number of pairs of each type are *discordant* for handedness—in other words, one of every four pairs of twins contains a left-handed twin and a right-handed twin.

The fact that monozygotic twins are no more similar in hand preference than dizygotic twins has been interpreted as evidence *against* genetic control of handedness. At first glance, the evidence from twins is a major setback for genetic models of any type. Regardless of the specific genetic mechanisms involved, genetic control of a trait means that individuals with all their genes in common should be more similar in that trait than individuals with fewer shared genes. This logic assumes, however, that the nongenetic factors that may affect handedness are the same in terms of their nature and incidence for both types of twins as well as for singletons (non-twins). As shown later, this assumption is probably incorrect. In addition, we consider how the factors that determine handedness in twins can help us understand the basis for hand preference in general.

## BRAIN DAMAGE AND LEFT-HANDEDNESS

The incidence of left-handedness in twins is about 20 percent, approximately twice that found in the singleton population. Twins also show a disproportionately high incidence of neurological and other disorders, which is believed to be a consequence of damage resulting from intrauterine crowding during fetal development.[14] It is a logical next step to suggest that the elevated incidence of left-handedness in twins is due, at least in part, to these factors.

The idea that minor brain damage may underlie much of the left-handedness in twins was first proposed in 1920.[15] Several pieces of evidence support that suggestion. First, the incidence of left-handedness is very high in populations that may have suffered minor brain injury before or during birth. In the mentally retarded, for example, the incidence is 20 percent. Left-handedness is also very common in children with learning disabilities, as well as in epileptics. Perhaps the minor brain damage that is the cause of the problem in many of these cases is also responsible for the shift in hand preference in individuals who otherwise would have been right-handed.

Second, clinical data from sodium amobarbital work suggest a relationship between handedness and early brain damage. In one study, the majority of left-handed patients with evidence of early damage to the left brain showed right-hemisphere language centers, whereas left-handers without signs of early damage had left-hemisphere language.[16] This suggests that damage to the left hemisphere early in life may result in a shift in the language hemisphere as well as in hand preference.

Paul Bakan and associates contend that all left-handedness is essentially pathological in origin and that trauma occurring at birth can account for most of it.[17] They believe that left-handedness is the result of left-hemisphere motor dysfunction following perinatal hypoxia, or reduced oxygen supply at birth. According to Bakan, sinistrality runs in families because of an inherited tendency for difficult births or abnormal pregnancies and not because handedness per se is genetically determined.

The data relevant to Bakan's hypothesis are mixed. Of the 25 studies reviewed that addressed the relationship between birth stress and left-handedness in the normal population, 9 were supportive of the relationship and 16 were not.

Less extreme views of the role of pathology have been taken by others. Paul Satz, for example, believes that pathological factors can account for a good deal of the elevated incidence of left-handedness among certain clinical populations, as well as some of the left-handedness in the population at large.[18] The remaining left-handers are, in his view, "natural" left-handers, whose left-handedness is genetic in origin.

Satz and his colleagues have become interested in other changes that may occur in individuals who are left-handed because of early brain injury. They view a shift in handedness as one of several alternatives in lateral development that form what they call the syndromes of *pathological left handedness* (PLH).[19] We have already mentioned one of these changes—a shift in hemispheric specialization for speech. Left-handers with a history of early brain damage are three times as likely to have speech controlled by the right hemisphere as left-handers without early brain damage.

Another component of PLH, according to Satz, is impaired visuo-spatial ability. He and his colleagues cite the earlier work of Herbert Lansdell with a group of left-brain-injured epileptics suggesting a link between early left-sided brain injury and impaired visuo-spatial ability.[20] Lansdell examined the association between the age at which neurological symptoms first appeared and the difference between verbal and nonverbal factors in the Wechsler–Bellvue intelligence scale. He noted that the verbal factors were affected less with early lesions, whereas the nonverbal factors suffered less with later lesions (5 years). Lansdell speculated that early injury to the left hemisphere may have shifted language functions to the right hemisphere, thereby disrupting and displacing the visuo-spatial functions that otherwise would have developed there. Later injury would not produce this shifting, resulting in impaired left-hemisphere function and intact right-hemisphere visuo-spatial ability.

A third component of the PLH syndrome is failure of the right side of the body to develop fully. Satz and colleagues cite studies in the 1930s and 1940s showing that decrease in the growth of all or part of half of the body can follow from early injury to the hemisphere on the opposite side. Their own research measuring foot size has shown that epileptic patients whose seizures began before age two had a shorter right foot if the lesion was located in the left hemisphere, whereas patients with early right-sided lesions had a shorter left foot.

Satz points out that much more work needs to be done before the existence of the PLH syndrome is established with certainty. Individuals with the syndrome would be relatively rare, and studies to test the hypothesis adequately would need to look for all the components at one time, not just one or two in isolation. This work is underway, although results may not be available for several years. Existing evidence, however, appears sufficient to support the more basic position that some left-handedness is pathological in origin, although few researchers would take the extreme view of Bakan, indicating that all left-handedness can be explained in this way.

The popularity of the pathological model of left-handedness has led investigators to compare the cognitive abilities of left- and right-handers. The rationale for such studies is simple. If left-handedness is a consequence of brain damage, however mild, then such damage may be reflected in lowered ability in various higher mental functions. We will review studies exploring this possibility in a later section. Before doing so, however, we will return to the issue of the elevated incidence of left-handedness in twins.

## TWINS AND HANDEDNESS: SOME FURTHER THOUGHTS

The evidence linking prenatal brain damage and left-handedness in singletons is sufficiently compelling for such damage to be considered a factor in producing the high rate of left-hand preference in twins, both monozygotic and dizygotic. As a result of their unusual prenatal conditions, twins are particularly susceptible to neurological damage, and left-handedness may be one of the results.

Another factor, operating only in monozygotic twins, may also contribute to the high incidence of left-handedness. About one-fourth of all monozygotic pairs are believed to demonstrate some aspect of a phenomenon known as *mirror imaging*. One twin may be left-handed, the other right-handed. One may have a clockwise hair whorl at the top of the head, the other a counterclockwise whorl. Fingerprints are also reported to show mirror-imaging effects. The print on the left index finger of one twin, for example, is more like the pattern on the same finger of the *right* hand of the other twin. Mirror imaging is typically limited to bodily tissues that derive from the ectodermal layer during development; it rarely extends to internal organs such as the heart and stomach.[21]

The embryological mechanism responsible for mirror imaging is not well understood, but there has been some speculation concerning how it might come about. At some point early in development, chemical gradients that establish an axis of bilateral symmetry are established in the embryo. If the division that forms two individuals occurs after that point (and in the proper plane), one embryo will develop from what was to be the left half of the original embryo, and one will develop from what was to be the right half.

This fortuitous division is believed responsible for the mirror imaging seen in certain monozygotic pairs. Relatively late division (around two weeks after conception) is generally incomplete, and the end result is so-called Siamese twins, joined together at some point along their bodies. Mirror imaging could operate only in monozygotic twins, for dizygotic twins begin life as two separate embryos, and division of the sort that occurs in monozygotic pairs does not take place. Thus, mirror imaging could help account for left-handedness only in monozygotic pairs.

We have seen that two factors—brain damage and mirror imaging—may contribute to handedness discordance in monozygotic pairs. Handedness discordance in dizygotic pairs may be the result of pathological factors and genetic differences because, on the average, the twins have only one-half of their genes in common.[22] The puzzle that remains is why the factors affecting monozygotic and dizygotic pairs operate in such away as to produce an incidence of discordance that is almost identical for both types of twin pairs. It may be a coincidence, or perhaps it is indicative of something more significant, possibly another factor associated with twinning in general that we have not accounted for. Nevertheless, this analysis suggests that twins are not a good population with which to test genetic models of handedness. They are subject to the influences of handedness-determining factors that affect singletons to a much lesser extent, if at all.

It is interesting to note that at least one investigator has suggested that all singleton left-handers are the surviving members of monozygotic twin pairs that divided at the time crucial for mirror imaging to occur.[23] We know of no evidence either to support or refute this, but it is an intriguing notion. In contrast, we have seen that some investigators are convinced that almost all left-handedness is genetic in origin; others argue that left-handedness is the result of early injury to the left hemisphere. At the present time, none of these extreme views has convincing evidence to support it, although each may contribute to understanding the incidence of left-handedness overall.

## HANDEDNESS AND FUNCTIONAL ASYMMETRY

In what ways does the brain organization of left-handers differ from that of right-handers? Both clinical and behavioral studies have helped answer this question.

The sodium amobarbital procedure discussed in an earlier chapter temporarily anesthetizes one hemisphere at a time, allowing the neurosurgeon to determine which half of the brain controls speech in a given patient about to undergo brain surgery. As we noted, a summary of sodium amobarbital testing at the Montreal Neurological Institute reported that over 95 percent of the right-handers had speech localized to the left hemisphere, and 70 percent of the left-handers showed the same pattern. Of the left-handers remaining, half showed right-hemisphere control of speech, and half had speech represented bilaterally.[24]

From these figures, one might conclude that the majority of left-handers are just like right-handers, whereas many of the others show a reversal of the pattern found in right-handers. Other clinical data, however, suggest that the picture is more complex.

Several studies have reported that the prognosis for recovery from aphasia following stroke is much better in left-handers than in right-handers.[25] Many investigators believe that recovery from massive damage to the speech hemisphere is a function of the extent to which the remaining, undamaged hemisphere can take over. If this is so, it suggests that language functions may be bilaterally represented in more than just the 15 percent of the left-handers identified by the sodium amobarbital data. Left-handers with speech controlled predominantly by one hemisphere may have the other hemisphere available "in reserve" to a much greater extent than right-handers.

Behavioral studies with normal subjects generally confirm this picture of complexity. Dichotic listening and lateralized tachistoscopic studies that compare the performance of left- and right-handers show less evidence of asymmetry in left-handers.[26] As a general rule, any asymmetry found in right-handers will be smaller and perhaps in the opposite direction when studied in left-handers.

By themselves, however, these summary statements do not allow us to differentiate between a situation where left-handers truly show no asymmetry in these tasks and a situation where approximately equal numbers show a right or left advantage. When data from individual subjects are examined, we find that left-handed subjects show smaller asymmetries than right-handed subjects, although there are some left-handers with strong left or strong right superiorities. These findings mesh nicely with the clinical evidence pointing to greater bilaterality in left-handers.

## The Role of Familial Sinistrality

The brain organization of left-handers appears to be more complex than the sodium amobarbital data would lead one to expect. Other clinical work has suggested that some of the variability between left-handers may be accounted for by determining whether a given left-hander has first-degree relatives (parents, siblings, or children) who are themselves left-handed.[27]

Left-handers with histories of *familial sinistrality* (left-handers in the immediate family) showed similar frequencies of language disturbances occurring after damage to either the left or the right side of the brain. In nonfamilial left-handers, language disturbances were almost nonexistent after right-hemisphere lesions. This difference suggests that there are at least two kinds of left-handers and that the patterns of brain organization in the two groups are different.

Studies with normal subjects have looked at the effect of familial sinistrality on performance. In one study using dichotic listening, left-handers without a history of familial sinistrality showed a right-ear superiority, and familial left-handers showed no left–right difference.[28] This difference has been found in several other studies, although some investigators have reported contradictory results.

In some studies, the left-handers with left-handed relatives showed the largest right-sided asymmetries, and the left-handers without left-handed relatives showed signs of bilateral or right-hemisphere speech.[29] Other researchers have reported no differences in asymmetry between familial and nonfamilial left-handers.[30] The bulk of the evidence, however, supports the idea that left-handers with left-handed relatives differ from those without. The conflict exists in showing how they differ.

The evidence pointing to differences in brain organization between persons with and without family histories of left-handedness has been taken by some to be a sign of a genetic component to handedness. The same relationship, however, may also be viewed as support for an environmental determinant of handedness.

## Inverted and Noninverted Writing Postures

The research of Jerre Levy and MaryLou Reid has identified another variable that may help sort left-handers into different groups on the basis of brain organization.[31] Some left-handers write in an inverted or hooked position, holding the pen or pencil above the line of writing. Other left-handers, as well as almost all right-handers, hold their writing instruments below the line of writing. These hand postures are shown in Figure 5.3.

Levy and Reid have argued that the position of the hand provides useful information about which hemisphere is controlling speech and language in an individual. Their view conflicts with conventional wisdom, which suggests that hand posture is due only to training. According to the conventional view, some left-handers, encouraged to position their writing paper in the same way as right-handers, have adopted the hooked posture out of necessity. Without it, their hand hides most of what they have just written.

In contrast, Levy and Reid argue that the inverted hand posture means that the speech hemisphere is ipsilateral to the preferred hand. Thus, the speech of a left-handed inverter would be controlled by

Left-handed Writers          Right-handed Writers

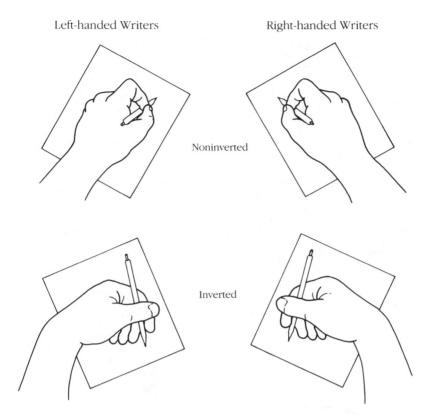

Noninverted

Inverted

**Figure 5.3** Noninverted and inverted writing postures of left-handers. [From Levy and Reid, "Variations on Writing Posture and Cerebral Organizations," Fig. 1, p. 337. *Science* (1976) 194, Oct. 1976. American Association for the Advancement of Science.].

the left hemisphere. The speech of a right-handed inverter (their study involved one subject in this category) would be controlled by the right hemisphere. The speech of noninverted writers would be controlled by the hemisphere opposite to the preferred hand.

The basis for Levy and Reid's conclusions is data from two tachistoscopic tests involving lateralized presentation of three-letter syllables or a dot randomly located in 1 of 20 possible locations within the left or the right visual field. These tests are shown in Figure 5.4. On verbal trials, subjects were asked to identify a syllable. On dot trials, they were to remember the position of a dot and locate it a few seconds later on a matrix of boxes displayed in free vision. Visual-field asymmetries in accuracy (measured as the number correct in the right field minus the number correct in the left field) were

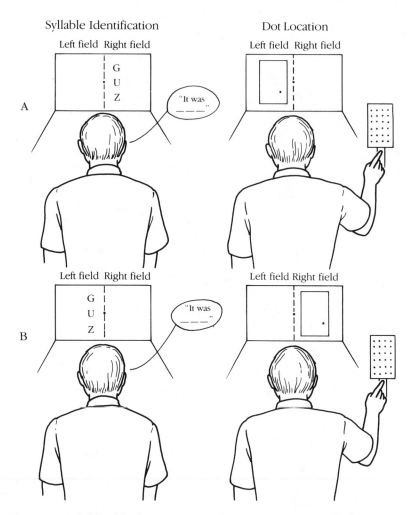

**Figure 5.4** Syllable identification ("What did you see?") and dot location tasks ("Point to the dot on the card that is in the same spot as the dot that appeared on the screen"). A. Noninverted right-handers and inverted left-handers were most accurate when the syllable task appeared in the right field and the dot task appeared in the left. B. Noninverted left-handers and inverted right-handers were most accurate when the syllable task appeared in the left field and the dot task appeared in the right.

computed for each type of stimulus to provide a measure of hemispheric asymmetry for verbal and spatial processing.

The results clearly indicate that right-handers who use the noninverted hand posture show a right visual field superiority for syllables and a left-visual field superiority for the spatial task. Left-handers who write with the noninverted posture show the reverse. In contrast, left-handers who write with an inverted posture perform like the right-handers with a noninverted posture. The sole right-hander who wrote with an inverted posture generated data comparable with those of left-handers writing in a noninverted fashion.

These results suggest that it is possible to tell a great deal about brain organization from an individual's handedness alone. Like most interesting findings, though, they raise more questions than they answer. What is the evidence for ipsilateral motor control of the sort postulated by Levy and Reid and, earlier, by Nagylaki and Levy? Assuming it exists, why should it result in an inverted hand posture?

Even more important are the questions raised by other studies that have attempted to test Levy and Reid's hypothesis in various ways. Using visual-field tasks with different kinds of verbal stimuli as a measure of hemispheric asymmetry, a number of studies have not confirmed the relationship predicted by Levy and Reid between language lateralization and hand posture.[32] Dichotic listening measures of language lateralization, in general, have failed to discriminate between left-handed subjects with normal hand posture and those with inverted posture.[33] However, additional support for some relationship between hand posture and lateralization has come from two other sources. In a study measuring the amount of alpha activity in each hemisphere, left-handers with normal posture showed more involvement of the right-hemisphere visual areas during reading and writing tasks than inverters did. No differences were found when subjects were asked to speak or to listen to verbal material.[34] In a study using elementary school children, it was found that the closer the child's writing posture was to an upright position, the better the child's reading ability.[35] Both of these studies point to the existence of a relationship between hand posture and asymmetry in the processing of printed language — rather than more general hemisphere asymmetries — and highlight the importance of not treating language as a unitary process.

What light do clinical data shed on the relationship between hand posture and asymmetry? The clinical data, unfortunately, present the same mixed picture. One set of investigators has stated that "the presence or absence of aphasia with a right or left hemiparesis has been appropriate as would have been predicted by hand posture utilized during writing."[36] These clinical data, however, have not been published. Other investigators have failed to find evidence for such a relationship in patients undergoing sodium amobarbital testing.[37]

At this point, the most prudent course of action is to defer judgment on the utility of hand posture as a predictor of brain asymmetry until some of these problems are resolved. It remains, however, a promising variable that may allow researchers to differentiate among individuals.

## HANDEDNESS AND HIGHER MENTAL FUNCTIONS

Do left-handers differ from right-handers in ways other than brain organization? The search for the relationship between handedness and brain asymmetry has led many investigators to consider the consequences of this relationship for other functions. Recall, for example, the pathological model of left-handedness. According to this view, some left-handers (one investigator believes all left-handers) have suffered from very early, minimal brain damage that resulted in a shift from what would have been a right-hand preference to a preference for the left hand. The pathological model leads readily to the prediction that minimal brain damage will result in lowered ability on various tests of higher mental functions.

### Evaluating the Case for Deficits in Left-Handers

Studies that compare the performance of left-handers and right-handers on tests of higher mental functions have yielded little in the way of data to support predictions of inferior performance by left-handers. A recent review of the literature cited 14 studies examining reading ability. Only one of them found a difference between left-handers and right-handers, and it reported that left-handers were superior.[38] Using measures of academic achievement, one study found no difference between groups, whereas another study reported that left-handers did more poorly on a college entrance exam. Three studies reported that left-handers did more poorly in perceptual tasks, although the sole study to be replicated failed to show a difference in subsequent work.

Despite this relatively meager collection of empirical evidence documenting performance differences between left-handers and right-handers, the association of left-handedness with deficit persists. This is most likely a result of the high incidence of left-handedness among the mentally retarded and reading disabled. This association suggests that some of the left-handedness in these groups selected for deficits is pathological in origin. The same damage that produces the impairment also may be responsible for the shift to left-hand usage. It does not follow, however, that a similar relationship holds for unselected groups of subjects obtained outside of the clinical setting.

The pathological model of left-handedness, then, has been responsible for much of the interest in the relationship between handedness and cognitive ability. Another theoretical approach to this question has been taken by Levy.[39] She noted that many left-handers show evidence of some language ability in the right hemisphere in addition to language ability in the left-hemisphere. What, she asked, are the consequences of this for the visuo-spatial functions typically controlled by the right hemisphere in the right-hander?

She proposed that language and visuo-spatial functions could compete for available neural tissue within a hemisphere and that language functions would predominate at the expense of the others. Thus, she predicted that left-handers should do more poorly than right-handers on visuo-spatial tasks but perform similarly on verbal tasks.

To test her hypothesis, she recruited 10 left-handed and 15 right-handed California Institute of Technology graduate students and administered the Wechsler Adult Intelligence Scale (WAIS) to them. The WAIS can be broken down into two parts, a verbal component and a performance component. The verbal subtests include general information, vocabulary, and similarities (simple abstraction). The performance subtests include block design (Koh's blocks), object assembly (puzzle assembly), and picture completion (noticing anomalies in drawings).*

Levy's study demonstrated that scores on the verbal component were the same for left-handers and right-handers. Left-handers scored significantly lower than right-handers on the performance score, however. Thus Levy's prediction of a deficit in visuo-spatial tasks was borne out.

It is important to remember, however, that this "deficit" is a relative one only. Levy's subjects, both left-handers and right-handers, showed markedly superior scores on both parts of the

---

*The verbal subtests seem most sensitive to damage to the left hemisphere, probably because they are so language dependent. The performance subtests are known to be quite sensitive to damage to either hemisphere, especially in the parietal region. In addition, the performance tests seem to be more sensitive than the verbal tests to brain damage in general, especially diffuse damage. They are first to show decline with increasing age and are the tests most affected by brain trauma and diffuse pathological processes.

WAIS compared with the overall population. The performance scores of the left-handers, though, were lower than their verbal scores, whereas there was no difference for the right-handers.

Levy's work has generated considerable interest as well as several attempts at replication.[40] One study, using a larger number of subjects from a college population, obtained similar results. Three other studies, with large samples from other subject populations, have failed to find any evidence of the differences expected.

Some have argued that Levy's results are an artifact of using a highly select sample of subjects. That objection, however, cannot explain the replication that was successful.

## Leonardo da Vinci Was a Lefty

Some investigators have suggested that the more bilateral distribution of language function that appears to characterize left-handers may result in superior abilities. The argument has been made that creativity might be enhanced in individuals whose brains permit a greater interplay between verbal and nonverbal abilities by virtue of their being housed within the same hemisphere. Occasional studies have reported superior performance by the left-hander, but these studies do not paint any more clear a picture than do those pointing to deficits in left-handers. Proponents, however, are eager to mention that Leonardo da Vinci, Benjamin Franklin, and Michelangelo were all left-handed.

It is interesting to note, however, that the incidence of left-handedness is considerably higher among artists than among the general population. For example, in one study comparing college undergraduates with less than two years of art training with students enrolled in an art-degree program, 20 percent of the artists were left-handed, compared with 7 percent of the nonartists. Mixed-handedness occurred in 27 percent of the artists and in only 15 percent of the non-artists.[41]

The meaning of these findings is uncertain. They clearly pose problems for Levy's cognitive deficit model of left-handedness, unless one argues that the deficit in visuo-spatial ability occurs in only a subset of left-handers. Another interpretation is that interest in and experience with art leads to greater utilization of the left hand, instead of the brain organization of left-handers directly predisposing them to greater artistic ability.

Despite the suggestion of deficits in left-handers and the amply justified reprisals mentioned, it is evident that any differences in the cognitive abilities of left- and right-handers in general are very small and of little practical importance. As in many such studies, it is clear that individual variation within a group is much greater than the statistical difference between groups. However, the issue of statistical differences in cognitive functioning and handedness will continue to be pursued because of its significance to theories of brain variability and organization.

## EYES, EARS, AND FEET

Handedness is clearly the most obvious human asymmetry. Most people, however, also have a preferred eye, ear, and foot. What is the nature of these preferences, and what, if any, relationship exists between them and brain asymmetry? In this section, we briefly review some of the evidence bearing on these questions.

### Eye Preference

Preference for one eye over the other can be measured in several ways, the most common being acuity dominance and sighting dominance. When acuity dominance is being measured, the dominant eye is the one that shows relatively better performance on standard tests of visual acuity (for example, the eye that can read letters further down on the Snellen eye chart). Strictly speaking, acuity dominance does not really reflect eye preference, because it assesses proficiency and does not require any choice on the part of the individual. Sighting dominance, in contrast, is a more direct reflection of eye preference.

The task used to measure sighting dominance is simple. The individual being tested stands about 10 feet from a wall with a small but clearly visible black circle placed at eye level. The observer is then asked to point to the circle quickly with an outstretched hand. Figure 5.5 shows two individuals performing the task. The male subject, a careful examination of the drawing will show, is aligning his hand with his left eye (left sighting dominance), while the female subject aligns her hand with her right eye (right sighting dominance).

Why don't subjects point straight ahead, aligning the hands with points between their eyes? The reason is that, because our eyes are

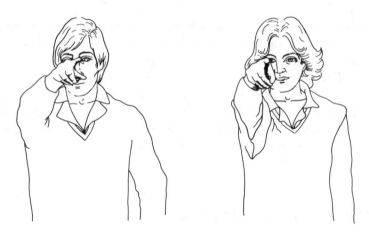

**Figure 5.5** The pointing test for sighting dominance. Note that the male is a left-sighter (his hand is aligned with the left eye), whereas the female is a right-sighter (her hand is aligned with the right eye).

slightly separated, each sees a slightly different image of the world. The average distance between the two eyes (measured from pupil to pupil) is about $2^1/_2$ inches. The closer the object, the greater the disparity or difference in the images formed in the two eyes. This does not pose a problem, because the brain is organized to receive these slightly different images and process them as cues for the perception of depth or three-dimensionality. When objects at different distances are viewed simultaneously, however, a double image will emerge. This can be easily demonstrated by looking at some point in the distance while holding a pencil directly in the line of sight a few inches from the nose. The image of the pencil will be double. When fixation is shifted to the pencil, the pencil will produce a single image, but the point at a distance will appear double. The double image problem is eliminated, however, if one eye is used. (Repeat the demonstration, but this time keep one eye open.)

In the sighting example illustrated in Figure 5.5, subjects kept both eyes open, yet they chose to align their sighting with one eye. In this process, in some ways not yet fully understood, the image from the other eye is suppressed so that it does not contribute to the double-image problem. Interestingly, subjects are typically unaware that they are making their alignments with one eye. There is, however, considerable consistency between the eye that is dominant in this task and the eye that is used in more conscious sighting tasks, such as looking through a microscope or sighting through a rifle.[42]

No relationship is found, however, between acuity dominance and sighting dominance for subjects within the range of normal vision.[43]

What relationship exists between eye preference and hemispheric asymmetry? Experimental evidence shows little relationship, a finding which, on further analysis, should not be surprising.[44] As shown in Chapters 2 and 3, the visual system is organized in such a way that each eye sends information to both hemispheres, from different halves of the retina. This differs from the way in which sensory and motor control of the limbs is arranged. Thus, although destruction of one hemisphere may affect only the opposite hand and foot, it will cause blindness in half the visual field of each eye. Because of these neuroanatomical arrangements, sighting preference for the left or right eye is not simply a reflection of preferential use of one hemisphere.

### Ear Preference

Ear preference can be measured in tasks that do not permit the subject to use the two ears simultaneously — pressing an ear against a watch to hear its ticking, for example. Sensitivity of the two ears relative to each other can also be assessed to give an auditory acuity dominance measure similar to that described under eye preference. Results have shown that within the normal range of hearing thresholds, there is no relationship between auditory acuity and ear preference in tasks requiring a choice between ears. In addition, there is little evidence for a relationship between handedness and ear preference. A weak relationship has been reported, however, between ear preference and ear asymmetry measured in dichotic listening, suggesting to some limited extent that both may be reflections of the same mechanisms.[45] The relationship is so weak, however, that it would be premature to view it as anything more than mildly suggestive.

### Footedness

Footedness refers to the preferred foot for such tasks as kicking a ball, grasping a small object with the toes, or stomping on a small object. Relatively few studies have looked at footedness, but those that have suggest that different measures of foot preference are highly correlated with each other. Claire Porac and Stanley Coren conducted a large-scale study of 5,147 subjects to obtain data on hand, foot, eye, and ear preference.[46] In their study, 46 percent of those participating were strongly right-footed, whereas 3.9 percent were strongly left-footed. This contrasted with figures of 72 percent and 5.3 percent, respectively, for hand preference. Correlations among the four kinds of preference were all positive and statistically significant, showing that the various preferences were related. The largest correlation was between hand preference and foot preference, although none of the relationships was exceptionally strong.

## NEW IDEAS ABOUT LATERAL PREFERENCES

This chapter has dealt with questions related to variations in lateral preferences—most notably handedness but to a lesser extent eye, ear, and foot preferences, as well. The basic issues explored have centered around their origins, their implications for human abilities, and their relation to hemispheric asymmetry of function. As we have seen, the evidence bearing on each one of these issues is considerably less than straightforward. In this section, we discuss two relatively new and very speculative ideas about the nature of lateral asymmetries.

### Left-Handedness and the Immune System

The possible relationship between handedness and the body's immune system is one of the newest and most exciting developments in the study of laterality. The idea emerged at a meeting in Boston in 1980, when neurologist Norman Geschwind commented that those interested in studying the genetics of dyslexia should not limit themselves to examining the frequency of dyslexia among the relatives of dyslexics—they should look for the presence of other conditions in these families as well.* In addition to psychologists and neurologists, the audience at his talk consisted of large numbers of parents of dyslexic children, who told Geschwind afterwards about their family histories of immune disorders and migraine. These observations led Geschwind to a series of studies with Peter Behan, which demonstrated an unexpected link between left-handedness and such disorders.

In the first two studies, a total of 500 strongly left-handed and 900 strongly right-handed subjects were compared.[47] The strong sinistrals had a rate of immune disorders 2½ times that of right-

---

*Dyslexia is the term applied to cases of reading disability unaccompanied by other problems such as sensory impairment. Dyslexia is discussed in greater detail in Chapter 10.

handers and a rate of learning disorders 10 times as high. In the most recent study, 652 strongly right-handed and 440 strongly left-handed control subjects were studied along with 304 patients with proven autoimmune diseases.[48] Among the control subjects, migraine, allergies, dyslexia, stuttering, skeletal malformations, and thyroid disorders were significantly higher in the left-handed group. Among the patients with proven autoimmune diseases, the rate of left-handedness was significantly higher than in the general population in five of the eight different autoimmune disorders included in this group.

These observations led Geschwind and neurologist Albert Galaburda to develop a far-reaching theory of lateralization that would account for these findings as well as many others.[49] A common factor, they speculated, may be responsible for both left-handedness and susceptibility to immune disorders. Such a factor most likely would be male related, they reasoned, because the incidence of left-handedness and the developmental disorders of language and cognition is higher in males. Because similar effects, although less marked, occur in females, however, the factor must also have the potential for affecting females. The male sex hormone testosterone met these criteria. Fetuses of both sexes are exposed to testosterone, although females are exposed to lower quantities.

They proposed that testosterone slows the growth of parts of the left hemisphere during fetal life, so that corresponding regions on the right develop relatively more rapidly. As a consequence, they argue, males will show a greater degree of shift to right-hemisphere participation in handedness and language and will more likely have augmented right-hemisphere skills. The delay in left-hemisphere development, in some cases, may result in a permanent developmental learning disorder, the incidence of which is higher in males.

At the same time testosterone is affecting the development of the left hemisphere, Geschwind and Galaburda believe that it may also affect the development of the immune system, thereby increasing susceptibility to subsequent immune disorders. Hence, testosterone could be responsible for both the apparent association between the incidence of left-handedness and the incidence of immune disorders.

Geschwind and Galaburda's ideas are intriguing and suggest a host of interesting possibilities. For example, they note that in some cases, the more rapid development of the right hemisphere mediated by testosterone may lead to special skills. Autistic individuals, for example, occasionally show very superior artistic ability (see Chapter 10 for further discussion). The effects of testosterone on the left hemisphere would account for the disabilities the person showed, while the accompanying enhanced development of the right hemisphere would account for the "island" of superior performance.

Such a mechanism could even account for certain types of superior performance in persons not showing cognitive deficits. In a study of a large, male predominant group of mathematically gifted children, the subjects had five times the rate of allergies and twice the rate of left-handedness as a less gifted group.[50] Could the testosterone hypothesis account for this as well? Geschwind and Galaburda tentatively suggest that it could—depending on the precise timing and levels of testosterone present in utero, the deleterious consequences of a slowing of left-hemisphere development might be avoided, while the advantages of right hemisphere enhancement might be realized.

It is clear that much more work needs to be done to test the testosterone hypothesis and its implications. For now, it presents researchers with a series of fascinating and, for the most part testable, hypotheses about lateralization and its correlates. Geschwind and Galaburda caution, however, that certain considerations should be kept in mind as work proceeds.

First, they note, it would be erroneous to conclude that left-handers are generally less healthy than right-handers: a group with an elevated incidence of certain conditions may have low incidence rates of other disorders. As an analogy, they point out that a number of diseases are limited to women although women overall have a lower mortality rate at all ages than males.

## Does a Gradient Determine Laterality?

An assumption implicit in the work just described is that the left hemisphere is normally dominant for speech. Psychologists Michael Morgan and Michael Corballis have suggested a way in which this might occur.[51] Corballis and Morgan propose that there is an underlying gradient operating during embryonic development that favors the left side of the body. This gradient, they claim, is responsible for physiological asymmetries in humans and animals which, in turn, are responsible for the functional asymmetries we see. According to this view, the leftward displacement of the heart in vertebrates, the left-sided control of song in certain birds (see Chapter 9), and the enlargement of the left temporal plane of the brain in chimpanzees, orangutans, and humans (see Chapters 4 and 9) are all examples of consequences of this developmental gradient. Both right-handedness and left-cerebral control of speech in humans are seen as further manifestations of this gradient.

Why are some people left-handed, and why do some have speech represented in the right or, perhaps, both hemispheres? Corballis and Morgan suggest that the hypothesized gradient is absent in some individuals and that in these cases, environmental factors play a major role in determining which pattern a given individual will show.

Corballis and Morgan's ideas are intriguing ones and are an attempt to place human hand preference and hemispheric asymmetry in a broader biological context. A gradient favoring faster development on the left side is a fundamental one shared by many species, they argue, and handedness and speech lateralization are simply a species-specific consequence of that gradient. Critics of their views, however, point to other examples, in both humans and other animals, in which the right side of the body appears to be favored.[52]

Corballis and Morgan[53] and Geschwind and Galaburda[54] offer new hypotheses regarding the basis for variation in lateral preference in human beings. They join the large number of investigators who are seeking to understand why about 10 percent of human beings prefer to use their left hands for different tasks, whereas the majority choose their right hands. It is likely that no single model of handedness will ultimately explain all the data and that many, if not all, of the theories we have considered will be shown to be true to some extent.

# 6

# Further Evidence from the Clinic: Neuropsychological Disorders

## CONTEMPORARY NEUROPSYCHOLOGY

In Chapter 1, we reviewed from a historical perspective how the concept of brain asymmetries developed from data on brain-injured patients. In this chapter, we further discuss the insights into brain function gleaned from evaluating the effects of various injuries to the cerebral hemispheres. This pursuit is the realm of clinical neuropsychology. Before the days of CT scans and other brain imaging methods, neuropsychologists emphasized the use of their clinical skills to predict the location of damage in patients showing various functional or behavioral disturbances. Modern neuropsychology still does this to an extent, with the emphasis on early diagnosis of the nature and location of lesions disrupting brain function, especially when neurological and physiological techniques seem insufficient.

In addition, modern neuropsychology attempts to extend our understanding of psychological processes by examining the ways in which they break down. Thus, the fact that visual impairments can take on a variety of forms leads to a theory or model of vision that incorporates many stages and takes into account the contribution of other psychological processes. In the same manner, investigators search for the ways in which memories break down and disorders of language, movement, and emotion occur. Sometimes, a behavior thought to be a unitary mental process turns out to be a complex interaction; other times, they discover that what were thought to be separate mental activities actually arise from the same brain mechanism.

Information obtained from the brain-damage clinic must be interpreted very carefully because of a variety of confounding problems. In Chapter 1, we mentioned some of these problems, including the brain's tendency to adjust its operations as best it can in the presence of damage. As neurologist John Hughlings Jackson pointed out a century ago, the abnormal behavior observed after a brain lesion reflects the functioning of the remaining brain tissue. This remaining tissue may compensate for the damage and thus minimize the deficit. However, it can also react adversely and operate more poorly, thus adding to the deficit—a concept called *diaschisis*.

The use of brain damage in studying brain–behavior relationships must rely on lesions occurring naturally or on lesions created by surgeons for medical reasons. These are usually less than ideal for answering specific questions an investigator may wish to ask. Natural lesions, such as those caused by stroke, do not respect anatomical boundaries. A lesion may destroy an area of the brain involved in some psychological process, it may disconnect areas contributing to this process, or it may do both.

These issues can explain why the interpretation of the effect of brain injury is difficult and usually confounded by a variety of plausible alternative explanations. In addition, however, the clinical investigator must also keep in mind that many of our current definitions and categories of mental function may not be suitable for interpreting the effects of brain damage or forming useful hypotheses about brain function.

Despite these and other difficulties, clinical neuropsychology has generated a substantial framework of data and theories that categorize and attempt to explain most brain-behavior dysfunctions. A discussion of neuropsychological disorders involves many concepts and definitions that have been developed over the years by notable investigators.[1] We do not attempt to trace this development but, rather, present certain concepts as fairly established while citing newer studies bearing on hemispheric asymmetries. The interested reader is referred to some of the excellent texts that review clinical neuropsychology in general.[2] We concentrate here on how newer neuropsychological data has furthered our understanding of functions within each cerebral hemisphere.

## DISORDERS OF SPEECH AND LANGUAGE

Language is a complex, multifaceted skill with many aspects, including the formation of sounds, sophisticated rule systems, and the existence of large memory stores containing meaning and significance information. Linguistics, the formal study of language, has developed many concepts dealing with the structure of language, which apply to all languages in general.

Linguists have defined four major components of language: *phonology*, dealing with producing and processing speech sounds; *syntax*, involving the rules of word order and form, or grammar; *semantics*, the processing of meaning; and *pragmatics*, involving intonation in speech, practical significance, and context.

The term *aphasia* has become the general heading for a broad class of speech and language dysfunctions caused by neurological damage. We review here the major categories of aphasia with respect to how they arise from damage to different areas of the brain and the extent to which they shed light on the organization of linguistic processes. The study of the aphasias also provides classic examples of the theoretical controversies that are often found when attempts are made to establish brain–behavior relationships by formulating psychological theories from clinical data.

### The Aphasias

There are many different types of aphasia, depending on the location and extent of damage to any of several regions of the brain. The two major categories are expressive (motor) aphasia and receptive (sensory) aphasia, although not all investigators adhere to this distinction.

*Expressive (or Broca's) aphasia* is a deficit involving primarily the patient's own speech; the patient's comprehension of the speech of others remains relatively intact. This type of aphasia is associated with damage to the frontal regions of the left hemisphere controlling speech output, particularly the region called Broca's area. Broca's area, as shown in Figure 6.1, is located just in front of the primary motor zone for speech musculature (lips, tongue, jaw, larynx, and so on). These speech motor areas, however, are spared in cases of classic Broca's aphasia; that is, there is no paralysis of the speech apparatus.*

A patient with Broca's aphasia speaks very little. When speech is attempted, it is halting—the patient has difficulty getting the words out. There is an absence of small grammatical parts of speech and proper inflection. Such speech is often called *telegraphic* or *agrammatic speech*. For example, in response to a picture showing a woman washing dishes, an overflowing sink, and some children tipping a stool as they attempt to get a cookie jar, a Broca's aphasia patient might say, "Sink . . . water . . . b . . . boy . . . boy fall . . . step . . . ." Severe cases will often be able to vocalize only one or two words over and over again in any attempt to speak or describe something.

When a patient does say a word, it is usually pronounced reasonably well. The ability to name objects is poor, but prompting helps significantly. These facts help justify the view that the deficit is not simply at the level of articulation. Most Broca's aphasics seem to understand spoken or written language, so the problem is considered to be at the motor output stage of language, rather than in comprehension. Patients also seem to be aware of most of their errors. Some investigators have argued, however, that the comprehension of Broca's aphasics is not as intact as many have believed. Edgar Zurif claims that many such patients understand a sentence only by inferring what makes sense from a sampling of its major nouns and verbs.[3] When the syntactic structure of a sentence is more complex, comprehension seriously falls off. Patients seem unable to properly utilize the information conveyed by complex grammatical structure.

*Receptive* (or *Wernicke's*) *aphasia* is a disturbance in which the patient has great difficulty comprehending speech. It is associated with damage to the posterior region of the first temporal gyrus, or Wernicke's area (see Figure 6.1). The speech of a patient with receptive aphasia is much more fluent than that of an expressive aphasic, but, depending on the extent of damage, it may vary from being

---

*Impairment of speech (such as slurring) due to partial paralysis of the speech musculature is called *dysarthria*.

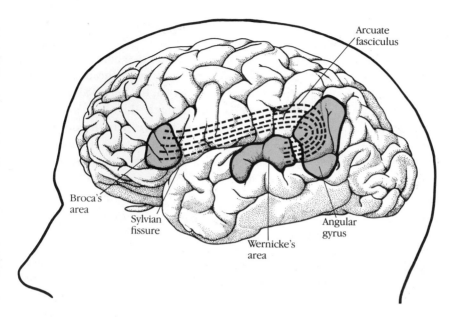

**Figure 6.1** The areas of the left hemisphere in humans associated with speech and language. The arcuate fasciculus is a nerve-fiber bundle beneath the cortex, connecting Broca's and Wernicker's areas. [Adapted from Geschwind, "Language and the Brain," Scientific American, Inc., 1972. All rights reserved.].

slightly odd to completely meaningless. Patients often use inappropriate words (paraphasias) or nonexistent words (neologisms). In some cases, the patient's output sounds like complete jargon or "word salad," although the rhythm and flow of speech seem preserved. One patient, when asked how he was, responded, "I felt worse because I can no longer keep in mind from the mind of the minds to keep me from mind and up to the ear which can be to find among ourselves."[4] In severe cases, the speech may not even have wordlike structures. It may consist mostly of meaningless utterances yet sound fluent, as in the following exchange [examiner's interjections in brackets]:

**Examiner:** How did you get sick?

**Patient:** Eeh, oh malaty? Eeeh, favility? Abelabla tay kare. Abelabl tay to po stay here. [stay here?] Aberdar yeste day. [yesterday?] and then abedeyes dee, aaah, yes dee, ye ship, yeste dey es dalababela. Abla desee, abla detoasy, abla ley e porephee, tee arabek. Abla get sik? [get sik?][5]

Such patients often seem unaware that their speech is defective or meaningless and continue to talk as if nothing is wrong.

Reading and writing are comparably impaired. There are aphasic patients who, when given a book, will go through the motions of reading it out loud but produce only gibberish, the length and timing of which bear little relationship to how quickly their eyes are scanning the text. A number of investigators believe that the deficit in Wernicke's aphasia is due to damage to verbal or semantic memory stores.[6] This is distinguished from the defect in syntactic and articulatory mechanisms involved in Broca's type of aphasia.

### Beyond the Receptive–Expressive Distinction

Although relatively pure forms of receptive and expressive aphasia do occur, the division of aphasia into these two categories implies a more clearcut distinction than is generally the case. Patients often show symptoms attributed to both types of aphasia, and some investigators feel the distinction is too artificial—not truly representing how language is organized in the brain. We deal with some of these criticisms later, but must first consider several other categories of aphasia. Beyond the expressive–receptive distinction, investigators have labeled other forms of aphasia, according to both patterns of brain damage and patterns of language deficits. Some of these categorizations are more controversial than the division of aphasia into expressive and receptive types, yet many neuropsychologists and speech pathologists argue that they truly represent distinct, recurring clinical syndromes.

Besides the receptive aphasia named after him, Wernicke predicted another type of aphasia that he claimed would arise from a lesion interrupting the neural pathways connecting the centers for speech production (Broca's area) and speech comprehension (Wernicke's area). This aphasia, now labeled *conduction aphasia*, is characterized by a patient's inability to repeat aloud what is heard. In addition, spontaneous speech may be meaningless, fluent jargon (as in Wernicke's aphasia), but unlike Wernicke's aphasia, comprehension of spoken and written material remains largely intact.

These symptoms can be explained as arising from a disconnection of the receptive and expressive language centers of the brain. In fact, damage to the neural tract called the arcuate fasciculus, connecting Broca's and Wernicke's areas (see Figure 6.1), has been implicated in such cases.[7] Stuart Dimond has claimed that the arcuate fasciculus, along with some subcortical structures (the thalamic region), is involved in integrating the input and output aspects of speech.[8] He also suggested that these neural tracts and associated structures form a store-house of linguistic information and may act as language generators.

The anatomical model for conduction aphasia was elaborated further by Norman Geschwind to explain several other combinations of symptoms observed in aphasic patients.[9] The *transcortical aphasias* involve lesions that spare the speech areas and their main interconnecting pathways but, in a variety of ways, isolate these areas from the rest of the brain. Depending on whether brain damage isolates Wernicke's area (transcortical sensory aphasia), Broca's area (transcortical motor aphasia), or both (transcortical mixed aphasia), there are varying degrees of comprehension and spontaneous speech problems. Such patients, however, are able to repeat quite well what is said to them. Transcortical aphasics, in extreme cases, may echo everything they hear, a condition known as *echolalia*. This sparing of repetition ability is what distinguishes transcortical aphasia from Broca's, Wernicke's, or conduction aphasia, where repetition is disturbed. Several additional aphasia types should also be mentioned:

*Word deafness* results from a lesion disconnecting Wernicke's area from auditory inputs. Comprehension is impaired for spoken language only; the ability to hear sounds in general is not affected. Comprehension of writing is normal, as is verbal and written expression, although the patient's speech may eventually also suffer because the patient lacks adequate feedback from his or her own speech.

*Anomic aphasia* involves difficulty in naming objects. Although this condition is present in most aphasics, a "purer" or isolated form results from damage limited to the cortical area at the junction of the temporal, parietal, and occipital lobes—the area called the angular gyrus (see Figure 6.1). A purely anomic patient will have normal comprehension and be able to speak almost normally in spontaneous casual conversation. When confronted with objects, however, or when trying to think of a word or name for something or somebody, the patient will falter badly. The difficulty is often severe and disheartening. It has been suggested that this impairment is a result of disruption of associations involving different sensory modalities (and, hence, different regions of the brain) that are part of the naming act.

*Global aphasia* refers to severe impairment of all language-related functions. Comprehension as well as production of speech are defective or absent in global aphasia. Communication may be attempted with a symbol system, as in learning to use plastic objects to stand for words, but even this is difficult and sometimes unsuccessful. Global aphasia results from widespread damage to the left hemisphere involving most of the areas thought to play a role in language.

## Theoretical Issues Arising from Aphasia Classification

In the preceding sections, we discussed how an anatomical model of language processes has been developed from an assessment of the language dysfunction associated with selective brain damage. The view that there are discrete cerebral centers performing specific aspects of language processing has been called the *localizationist-connectionist* view.* It has served to categorize the variety of language disorders seen in clinical settings and, to an extent, to predict the kind of disorder one may expect to see after specific types of brain damage. Evaluating a patient's language disorder in terms of the aphasia classifications can also do the reverse—that is, predict where the damage may be.

The localizationist approach has been criticized, however, by investigators who claim it is overly simplistic in its "flow diagram" view of the brain and the organization of language. Such criticisms can be traced back to the nineteenth-century holistic view of brain function, when neurologists such as Jackson argued that all aphasia is associated with defective comprehension—that is, that sensory aphasia underlies all others. Present-day investigators with more holistic views of brain function contend that the localizationist view places too much emphasis on independent components or depots interconnected by neural wiring.[10] The actual situation, they argue, is more dynamic, involving *simultaneous* interactions of many areas for any language function. The evidence mentioned for comprehension deficits in Broca's aphasia supports such criticisms to some extent.

Neurologist Jason Brown has proposed an alternative to the standard cortical localizationist view of the relationship between brain and language.[11] Synthesizing the work of several earlier theorists, he views the brain as organized in terms of evolutionary layers modified by maturational growth.[12] Broca's and Wernicke's areas are only the last stage "tips," not only in terms of the brain's evolution, but also in terms of brain function and language formation. Speech and

---

*This view is sometimes called *localizationist-associationist*, in the sense that most modern concepts that attribute functions to specific areas of the brain also place importance on the interactions between these areas in any complex mental activity.

language emerge at these cortical areas simultaneously from more primitive linguistic stages operating below. Thus, cortical lesions do not so much disconnect the cortical flow of information necessary for language as they force the language system to operate at a more primitive, incomplete level.

Some support for such a hierarchical view of language organization comes from evidence that certain subcortical structures, particularly the thalamus, play an important role in language.

*Subcortical Aphasia: The Role of the Thalamus* Our discussion of aphasia has dealt with lesions affecting mostly the cortex of the left hemisphere. Lesions to brain structures deeper within the brain, especially the thalamus, can also result in language disturbances. The thalamus, as shown in Figure A.1 in the Appendix, is also divided into a right and left half. Damage to the left thalamus has been reported to affect verbal fluency, creating word-finding hesitation as well as perseveration (repeating the same sound or word several times).[13] As mentioned in the discussion of conduction aphasia, it has been suggested that the thalamus is an integrating center between frontal and posterior cortical language areas, that is, Broca's and Wernicke's areas.

Neurosurgeon George Ojemann, who has conducted electrical-stimulation procedures during certain brain operations, has reported on the effects of thalamic stimulation. The procedure used was similar in principle to the cortical stimulation tests of Wilder Penfield in awake patients, described in Chapter 1. Stimulation of the left thalamus typically led to speech arrest or to problems with object naming coupled with perseveration of the initial syllable of the word a patient was attempting to say. Ojemann also reported that there was a general slowing, slurring, and distortion of speech. He has suggested that the thalamus has two general functions in speech: one, to serve as an alerting mechanism to direct attention to verbal information in the environment as well as to retrieve verbal information properly from verbal memory; the other, to control, at least in part, some of the physical substrates of speech, such as respiration and the speech musculature.[14]

## Left Hemispherectomy

Hemispherectomy, or removal of one half of the brain, is a rare operation and, despite the name, usually involves removing only the cortex of the hemisphere. It is sometimes performed in infants suffering from serious cerebral birth defects. Because of their age, such children often recover and develop remarkably well after the operation. We discuss childhood hemispherectomy in Chapter 8.

Hemispherectomy is performed very rarely in adults, usually for removal of malignant tumors. The operation is almost never performed on the dominant hemisphere, because of the very severe consequences. Left hemispherectomies offer investigators the opportunity to examine the functions of the right hemisphere in isolation. Neuropsychologist Aaron Smith and others have extensively studied such patients.[15] Smith reported that several of his patients made significant recoveries, although they initially showed markedly impaired language function. They were eventually able to produce short, relatively grammatically correct sentences. Most left-hemispherectomy patients show a surprising amount of verbal comprehension, although their voluntary speech, reading, and writing abilities remain severely impaired.

An important case for our understanding of how the two hemispheres may interact when one is damaged was described by Smith in 1969, when a patient underwent surgery to remove most of a damaged right hemisphere.[16] The patient *improved* after the surgery! This suggests that the damaged right hemisphere hindered the potential of the left hemisphere. It is very probable that normal communication between the hemispheres involves a substantial number of inhibitory signals, serving to coordinate function and prevent unnecessary duplication or competition. When one hemisphere is damaged, its inhibitory effects on the other may become pathological or, at least, inappropriate for recovery of function. The extent to which this is true makes interpretation of the effects of focal brain damage that much more difficult. It is also possible that understanding pathological inhibition eventually may allow surgeons to develop a rationale for when to remove damaged brain tissue for therapeutic reasons.

For the time being, cases such as the one described by Smith suggest why the general impression of right-hemisphere language function based on clinical data is more limited than some of the claims of right-hemisphere abilities in several split-brain patients (see Chapter 2).

## Reading and Writing

Disorders of reading and writing accompany some types of aphasia, especially aphasias resulting from posterior lesions. We mentioned, for example, how some Wernicke's asphasics go through the motions of reading aloud but produce only jargon. Reading and writing, however, can be selectively impaired; that is, a reading deficit or a writing deficit can be the primary problem after certain brain injuries, while speech production and comprehension remain relatively intact.*

Most reading and writing disorders involve either direct damage to the left angular gyrus or damage to adjacent regions. As mentioned in the discussion of anomic aphasia, the angular gyrus is located at the junction of the parietal, temporal, and occipital lobes and is thought to integrate the sensory, auditory, and visual information processed by these regions, respectively. This central position adjoining the major sensory and language-comprehension systems of the brain seems to make the left angular gyrus fundamentally important to reading and writing.

Disorders of reading and writing have been subdivided into two main categories: *alexia with agraphia* (inability to read and write) and *alexia without agraphia* (inability to read, but with writing spared). *Alexia with agraphia* almost always involves damage to the angular gyrus. In addition to deficits in reading and writing, it is often accompanied by some aphasic deficits, such as difficulties in word finding and naming. *Alexia without agraphia* is a rather astonishing condition to observe, for a patient with this disorder can write a sentence properly, either spontaneously or from dictation, but when this writing is shown to the patient, he or she cannot read it.

Alexia without agraphia has been explained as a "disconnection" between certain visual processing areas of the brain and the angular gyrus. It seems to arise when lesions damage the left occipital lobe and a part of the neural tracts forming the corpus callosum. The lesion to the corpus callosum disconnects the intact right occipital lobe from the left angular gyrus, leaving little, if any, visual information flow to the language processing areas.[17] Thus, a patient cannot read, although he or she can still see. Writing is preserved because the angular gyrus is intact and because writing can proceed with only minimal visual feedback.

A more controversial form of alexia, labeled *deep dyslexia*, has been described and is believed to demonstrate some right-hemisphere reading skills.[18] (The nature of right hemisphere language skills is discussed in the next section.) When asked, for example, to

---

*Our discussion of reading and writing disorders here concerns only those acquired following injury, *after* a person has developed the skills. Some developmental disorders in children are discussed in Chapter 10.

read aloud the printed word *table*, some alexic patients with left hemisphere damage will respond with "chair." This type of error is called *paralexic* and involves a wrong response that is nevertheless meaningfully related to the target word. It has been proposed that brain lesions have entirely inactivated the normal reading mechanisms of the left hemisphere in such patients. The right hemisphere, having some semantic (meaning) skills, understands the word and communicates some meaning information to the left hemisphere. The left hemisphere then forms the pronounciation of a word with a related meaning, because it does not "know" exactly what word the right hemisphere saw. The semantic information conveyed by the right hemisphere is not enough to distinguish among synonyms or closely related words, and thus the paralexic errors are made by the speaking left hemisphere.

As part of the evidence that supports this theory, patients who make paralexic responses in attempting to read do so to concrete words such as object nouns, whereas they show little or no response to abstract words. As we shall see, there is evidence that right-hemisphere comprehension abilities are limited to words that are more concrete in nature.

## THE ROLE OF THE RIGHT HEMISPHERE IN LANGUAGE

Semantic processing, the comprehension of word meanings, is severely disrupted in patients with damage to posterior regions of the left hemisphere, as in Wernicke's aphasia. No similar disruption can be demonstrated with right-hemisphere lesions. However, as mentioned in our discussion of split-brain patients in Chapter 2, investigators have demonstrated that the right hemisphere can show comprehension of certain words, especially object nouns. Some research with normal subjects suggests that the extent to which a word's meaning is understood by the right hemisphere depends on how concrete (as opposed to abstract) it is.[19] Thus, correct comprehension of words such as *justice, harmony,* and *hate* seems to depend more exclusively on left-hemisphere processing than does comprehension of *table, car,* and *hospital,* which the right hemisphere can also understand.

The right hemisphere's ability to understand certain words, however, probably does not contribute much to our speech and language skills, because the left can do the same and more. But does the right hemisphere make any unique contributions to our language communication skills? The answer, based on observing many patients and several studies with normal subjects, appears to be yes.

*Intonation* Communicating through speech and language involves many subtle nuances that are not an obvious part of the structure and content of sentences. Intonation patterns and emotional tone play an obvious, important part in speech communication. Intonation plays a major role in communicating the purpose of an utterance and can dramatically change its meaning—is it a declarative statement, a question, or a command?

Many left-hemisphere-damaged aphasic patients can discriminate the purpose of an utterance. Broca's aphasics, despite their problems with verbal output, attempt to use the correct pattern to produce a statement (as opposed to a question).[20] Patients with right-hemisphere damage, on the other hand, often speak with a flattened intonation; they also have difficulty judging the emotional tone of the speech produced by others.[21] Right-hemisphere-damaged patients have been known to add parenthetical phrases to their speech to emphasize their feelings—for example, "I am angry (and mean it)."[22] This is done after the patient realizes that his or her speech is not sufficiently forceful or emotional to evoke the desired response. Such handicaps, though not involving speech itself, point to the importance of other aspects of language communication in which the right hemisphere plays a major role.

*Melodic Intonation Therapy* The preservation of intonation and singing that often occurs in aphasic patients (see Chapter 1) has been exploited in therapy designed to teach such patients phrases through song. The program, called melodic intonation therapy, has been successful with certain patients who have reasonably good comprehension but poor speech production, such as Broca's aphasics. Word sequences are first incorporated in a song, and the melody is deemphasized gradually until the patient can speak the phrase without singing. It is presumed that the intact right hemisphere learns the phrases this way and, as a result, develops more language production skills that compensate, to a degree, for the left-hemisphere deficit. The program's developers claim that some aphasic patients, after not having had any meaningful speech for over a year following a stroke, are able to carry on short, meaningful conversations after a month or two of therapy.[23]

*Metaphor and Humor* There are several other language-related skills in which the right hemisphere appears to be involved. These are demonstrated by deficits found in right-hemisphere-injured, but not aphasic (left-hemisphere-injured), patients. These skills seem to involve more conceptual aspects of language communication. For example, right-hemisphere patients tend to be overly literal in their interpretation of words, stories, and cartoons. Given a choice, they often pick literal interpretations of metaphorical statements ("sour grapes") and popular sayings ("A penny saved is a penny earned").[24] They also very frequently pick totally inappropriate endings to cartoon strips, as if the humor is in a surprise ending.[25]

We see again that the right hemisphere contributes in important ways to language communication. In addition to possessing some comprehension abilities, as discussed earlier, it truly complements left-hemisphere speech and language processing through more subtle, but definitely important, communication skills. Emotional intonation, aspects of metaphor, and some qualities of humor seem to depend on right-hemisphere abilities. The extent to which the right hemisphere enriches other language skills remains to be determined.

## The Right Hemisphere in Recovery from Aphasia

Partial or complete recovery from initially severe deficits after stroke or head injury is not uncommon. Reports generally show that most improvement occurs during the first 6 to 12 months, depending on a number of factors such as age, cause, and severity of the original symptoms. The fact that recovery does take place raises a number of issues concerning the mechanisms responsible for it and the plasticity of the central nervous system.

One of the hypotheses offered to explain the recovery of language after left-hemisphere lesions is that structures of the intact right hemisphere become more involved in language processing. Wernicke was probably the first to propose this idea, which has continued to be entertained by investigators to this day. The hypothesis is supported by several lines of evidence. In the late 1800s it was observed that recovered aphasics who had sustained left-hemisphere injuries relapsed after new lesions developed in the right hemisphere.[26] Much more recently, Marcel Kinsbourne studied the effect of intracarotid injection of barbiturates (the Wada procedure) in three patients recovering from aphasia due to left-hemisphere lesions.[27] He found that although injection into the left carotid artery did not worsen speech, injection into the right carotid artery resulted in arrest of speech in two of the three patients. Other evidence for right-hemisphere involvement in recovery of language, although indirect, comes from the study of left hemidecortication or hemispherectomy in infants and very young children who develop apparently normal language (see discussion in Chapter 8), as well as from case studies such as that of a 54-year-old patient who recovered from global aphasia although he had sustained total destruction of the temporal–parietal regions of the left hemisphere.[28]

Several recent studies have examined such recovery using more direct physiological measures of brain activity. Using the probe evoked potential (EP) technique described in Chapter 4, one study examined four groups of subjects: patients who had recovered from aphasia after left-hemisphere injury, patients who had suffered left-hemisphere injury but were not aphasic, right-hemisphere stroke patients, and normal control subjects. Evoked potentials to a click stimulus were recorded during a control condition and during a verbal encoding task involving memorization of a list of common words. The normal control group, as well as the two patient groups who did not experience aphasia, displayed greater left-hemisphere attenuation of the probe EPs during the verbal task, indicating the expected greater involvement of the left hemisphere in that task. All recovered aphasics, however, showed the opposite pattern of greater right-hemisphere attenuation, suggesting much greater than normal involvement of the right hemisphere in that language task.[29]

Some cerebral blood flow data also supports increased participation of the right hemisphere in recovery from aphasia. Cerebral blood flow studies of regional cortical flow were conducted in 11 recovered aphasic patients during several conditions, including a phonological target detection task (picking out words with a "br" sound). Asymmetries in blood-flow activation, calculated as a change from resting baseline flow in each hemisphere, indicated a greater participation by the right hemisphere in a large percentage of patients during this task, compared with the normally greater activation seen in left-hemisphere regions in control subjects. Although the recovered aphasics showed larger than normal increases in blood flow in all cortical regions, including the undamaged areas of the left hemisphere, the asymmetry in activation was consistent with greater right-hemisphere involvement.[30]

Although the studies just described concentrated on recovery from aphasia and left-hemisphere damage, they have implications for the recovery of function in general, that is, from damage to either hemisphere. Although research to date is insufficient to reveal the precise nature of the hemispheric reorganization that occurs, there is little doubt that it does take place.

## PERCEPTUAL DISORDERS

Our interaction with the external world depends on intact sensory and perceptual processes in the two hemispheres. The ability to recognize external objects and events through vision, touch, hearing, and olfaction (smell) is acquired through this interaction and the subsequent formation of some sort of memory system.

We are all aware that damage to the peripheral organs of our senses, such as our eyes or ears, effectively destroys the use of a sensory modality. In a similar fashion, damage to areas of the brain receiving neural information directly from a sensory organ leads to simple blindness, deafness, and so on. However, there are many other more subtle injuries to our perceptual systems — injuries that result in such symptoms as not understanding what one is seeing. We review how some of these disorders have been categorized and what has been learned from them about the workings of the left brain and right brain.

### Agnosia

*Agnosia* is usually defined as failure of recognition that is neither due to impairment of the sensory input nor to a naming disorder of the kind seen in aphasia.* For example, a visually agnosic patient would not be able to tell what he or she is looking at, although one could demonstrate that the patient could see the object and have no trouble naming it if he or she held it. Definitions of agnosia suffer from an inability to carefully specify the difference between sensory loss and "higher-level" loss of recognition, because in fact there is no clear-cut distinction. For the most part, the distinction is based on some of the practical differences observed in patients with various kinds of perceptual problems.

---

*The patient's failure technically should also not be due to a general intellectual impairment, such as that seen in dementia.

Various agnosias have been classified according to the sensory modality that is affected, as well as according to the type of objects or sounds that cannot be recognized.

*Visual object agnosia*, as mentioned, is a failure to recognize objects for reasons that cannot be attributed to a defect of visual acuity or to intellectual or language impairment. Not all clinicians insist that good visual acuity has to be demonstrated, as is the case in the "purer" forms of visual agnosia. Certain cases of mixed sensory and perceptual loss have also been called agnosia. The decision as to whether a visual deficit is purely a sensory or a higher-level perceptual problem is often very difficult to make. Most cases fall somewhere in between. Most severe agnosias for objects occur with bilateral damage to parietal–occipital regions of the brain or with damage involving these areas in the left, dominant hemisphere coupled with damage to interhemispheric pathways. The latter situation is thought to mimic bilateral damage by disconnecting any remaining intact visual processing areas from the language centers of the left hemisphere. A patient with visual agnosia may still be able to recognize objects tactually, although extensive parietal damage often leads to problems in both modalities.

*Auditory agnosia* is a condition in which a patient with unimpaired hearing fails to recognize or distinguish what she or he hears. These sounds may include musical tones or familiar noises, such as a telephone ring or running water. They may also be limited to speech sounds, but such an auditory agnosia, known as word deafness, is usually considered a type of aphasia, as noted earlier in this chapter. Auditory agnosia is associated with damage to regions of the temporal lobe in the left, dominant hemisphere, although these disturbances are more severe when the injury is bilateral.

*Astereognosis* is a breakdown in tactile form perception (*stereognosis*). The patient cannot recognize familiar objects through touch or palpation, even though sensation in the hands appears to be normal. This condition usually results from damage to regions in the parietal lobe adjacent to the somatosensory projection areas (see Figure A.3 in the Appendix). It is thought that such damage interferes with tactile–kinesthetic memories that have been acquired and stored over the years and built up into perceptions of form, size, and texture. Evidence from clinical studies suggests that the right hemisphere plays a particularly important role in tactile form perception. Several studies have reported astereognostic conditions in patients with right-posterior lesions.[31]

## The Right Hemisphere in Perception

Of the three agnosias just discussed, only astereognosis results from right-hemisphere lesions alone. Our discussion of visual object agnosia did not implicate the right hemisphere in this disorder but, instead, pointed to damage to both hemispheres. This may be surprising to the reader, considering the general visuo-spatial nature attributed to the right hemisphere. In fact, one should not take visuo-spatial to refer to vision or visual perception. Both hemispheres are completely equipped to deal with most types of visual information. Although admittedly vague, the term visuo-spatial implies more complex operations on visual stimuli, such as those presented in Figure 1.4 in Chapter 1, or tasks involving judgments of spatial relationships. However, there are certain aspects of visual stimuli that the right hemisphere is truly superior at recognizing. Two relatively specific disorders involving visual perception point these out.

*Depth Perception* Normal human depth perception involves both the use of a variety of environmental cues (overlapping objects, figure-ground contours) and the three-dimensional stereoscopic effect (stereopsis) generated by the slightly different viewpoint of each eye. There is evidence that the right hemisphere plays the more significant role in stereoscopic vision. A technique developed by Bela Julesz allows the study of depth perception involving only stereopsis while eliminating all other cues to depth.[32] The technique involves random dot stereograms, computer-generated dot patterns in which an object can be seen only by viewing both members of a pair of dot patterns simultaneously, one presented to each eye. Figure 6.2 shows a pair of random dot stereograms. In two studies of patients with either left- or right-hemisphere lesions, left-hemisphere subjects showed no deficits when compared with normal controls. Those with right-hemisphere lesions, however, showed significantly more errors and longer response times than either of the other two groups.[33]

*Prosopagnosia: Agnosia for Faces* Our ability to distinguish between and recognize faces is truly amazing. We can recognize a familiar face almost instantly, despite the infinite number of expressions and orientations it can have; we can even distinguish it from hundreds of similar faces in a crowd. *Prosopagnosia*, an inability to recognize familiar faces, occurs following certain kinds of brain injury. A patient will not be able to recognize a previously known person's

Figure 6.2 Random dot stereograms generated by a computer. When the two images are viewed with a stereoscope, a geometric pattern is seen "floating" on a background of dots.

face and, in some cases, has difficulty recognizing his or her own face in a mirror. The patient has no trouble, however, recognizing that the face is in fact a face. There has been considerable controversy regarding whether this condition involves bilateral or right-hemisphere lesions. Originally thought to be a right-hemisphere deficit, prosopagnosic symptoms were later described as involving lesions to both hemispheres.

Neuropsychologist Arthur Benton has shed some light on the controversy by distinguishing between two forms of failure to recognize faces.[34] One is agnosia for familiar faces, or true prosopagnosia, and the other is a defect in discriminating between unfamiliar faces or in learning new faces. Benton claims that true prosopagnosia is largely due to right-hemisphere deficits but also involves the left hemisphere. The parietal–occipital regions of both hemispheres must sustain damage in order for the deficit to clearly manifest itself. On the other hand, defective discrimination of new (unfamiliar) faces, a much more common disorder, can result from just posterior-right-hemisphere damage.

These findings naturally raise the question of whether there are specialized mechanisms for facial discrimination and what their relationship to other right-hemisphere abilities might be. It is frequently speculated that facial recognition is accomplished so quickly because it involves some global or holistic analyses as opposed to feature-by-feature processing. This is, of course, exactly what many have speculated is the difference in processing strategies of the two hemispheres.

One may also wonder why the recognition of familiar faces seems harder to disrupt than simple discrimination between faces. It is likely that both hemispheres contain substantial, though perhaps different, kinds of information about a face they have seen many times.

## THE NEGLECT SYNDROME

A patient in a rehabilitation hospital wakes up in the morning and proceeds to shave his face. When he puts the shaver down to go eat breakfast, one notices that he shaved only the right side. While eating breakfast, the patient starts to look feverishly for his coffee cup until someone points out that it is just slightly to the left of his dish. At lunch or dinner, he may leave the food on the left half of his plate untouched while asking for more, only to be reminded that there is still food on the plate. If asked to draw a clock, the patient will draw a circle correctly but then crowd all the numbers into the right half. If asked to draw a person, he will draw only the right side of the body, leaving out the left arm and leg. If questioned about the drawings, the patient states that they look all right to him.

This phenomenon, known as the *neglect syndrome*, is observed in stroke or accident victims who have fairly extensive damage to the posterior (parietal or parieto-occipital) regions of the right hemisphere.[35] It sometimes occurs after similar damage to the left hemisphere, but much less frequently and in milder form. The impression one gets in observing such a patient is that he or she behaves as if the whole left side of space, and sometimes even the left side of his or her own body, does not exist. Figure 6.3 shows drawings made by a patient with neglect.

Several questions have long been asked about the syndrome. Why is there such blatant inattention to one half of space? To what extent is it related to damage in the visual system? Why are patients with damage to the right hemisphere much more likely to show long-lasting neglect symptoms than patients with equivalent damage to the left hemisphere? The answers are still not clear, but the phenomenon of neglect provides some valuable clues about the working relationship between the left brain and the right brain.

Although they may be initially unaware of it, many neglect patients are actually blind in their left visual fields. Because information from the left half of visual space is initially processed in the visual area of the right hemisphere, damage there can produce a *hemiano-*

Model                              Patient's Copy

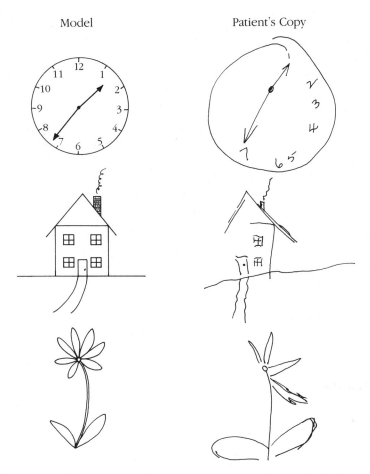

**Figure 6.3** Drawings by a neglect patient. A patient with a stroke in the posterior regions of the right hemisphere was asked to copy the model pictures.
Notice the profound neglect of the left side in each of his drawings. This
patient's pictures are quite representative of those of many such patients.

*pic* (literally, "half-blind") observer who cannot see any object to the
left of the point of fixation. This half-blindness, though, does not
solely explain the inattention of neglect patients.

Many examples can be found of patients who are blind to half of
the visual field but do not show neglect of that side of space.
Patients in whom damage is restricted to the optic-nerve pathways or
to the primary visual areas of either hemisphere typically compensate
for their half-field blindness through eye and head movements. Patients with damage to the left hemisphere who are blind in the right

visual field rarely display the kind of persistent functional neglect of one half of space shown by right-hemisphere patients.

Moreover, some neglect patients are not hemianopic at all. In testing situations, they can accurately report simple visual stimuli flashed alone in the left visual field. However, when stimuli are presented simultaneously in both visual fields, experimentally or in everyday situations, they will report only the items in the right half of visual space. Input from the right field reaching the undamaged left hemisphere appears to interfere with the brain's ability to process input from the left field coming into the damaged right hemisphere. The left half of the stimulus is "extinguished" by the right, but the patients see the left half of the pattern clearly if it is presented alone. Figure 6.4 shows typical stimulus presentations.

The extinction effects seen in these patients may explain at least part of the neglect patient's inattention to the left half of the world. Events in the right visual field may continuously extinguish information in the affected left field and consequently lead to orientation only to the right. This class of nonhemianopic neglect patients is particularly interesting to investigators of visual perception.

What happens to extinguished left-field information? Is it truly lost? Or is it present in the nervous system but unavailable to conscious experience? Several lines of research have studied this ques-

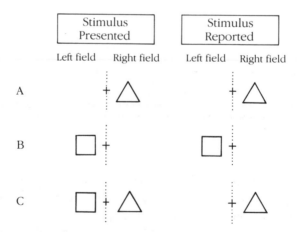

**Figure 6.4** Visual extinction. The left column shows three stimulus patterns as they were presented for a duration of 100 milliseconds each. The right column shows what the patient reported seeing. In stimulus conditions A. and B. the patient reports stimuli in either half of the visual field. In condition C., however, the patient does not see the item in the left field when another item is present in the right.

tion. Some investigators have found that under certain circumstances, the patients are able to report what appeared in the left field even when there was stimulation in the right. If forced to guess from among several choices, they perform much better than chance, although they may never acknowledge having actually seen the pattern in the left visual field.[36]

In a somewhat different line of research, patients who normally extinguished the left-field stimulus when two discrete patterns were presented did not do so when a single large pattern crossing the midline between the left and right fields was used. They were consistently able to identify meaningful drawings, such as of a key or a safety pin, presented on midline, even though relying only on the information in the right half of the drawing would not have provided them with enough information to recognize it.[37] Figure 6.5 illustrates stimuli of this type.

These findings can be interpreted in terms of a speculative but intriguing theory of why the neglect syndrome seems to arise from

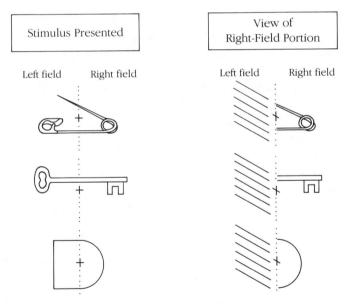

**Figure 6.5** The left column shows examples of continuous figures used to test bilateral processing in neglect patients. Neglect patients with true left-field cuts (partial blindness) were not able to report what these figures depicted after a 100-millisecond presentation. The right column shows how the stimuli would appear to a patient with a left-field cut. Neglect patients who normally exhibited the extinction phenomenon reported these figures accurately, thus showing bilateral processing ability under certain conditions.

damage to the right hemisphere. The left hemisphere normally possesses most of the speech and language skills of the brain. Furthermore, work with split-brain patients has shown that the left hemisphere often confabulates incorrect verbal responses based on that part of the visual information available to it. Perhaps after damage to the right hemisphere, the dominant, left hemisphere of the neglect patient acts in an egotistical fashion and assumes that what it sees encompasses everything there is. In other words, the left hemisphere, because it appears to be more self-sufficient than the right on account of its verbal capabilities, is more likely to act as if nothing is wrong in the presence of right-hemisphere damage than would the right hemisphere in the presence of left-hemisphere damage.

In the extinction patients just discussed, the left hemisphere seems very willing to report only information in its visual field as long as it can interpret that information in some comprehensible manner. If it cannot make sense out of what is presented to it, or if there is nothing at all in its field, only then does the left hemisphere make use of some of the information projected to the damaged right half of the brain.

Other explanations have been proposed for the asymmetrical nature of the neglect syndrome. One possibility is that mechanisms controlling selective attention or even arousal are lateralized to the right hemisphere. Another possibility is that the right hemisphere is more spatially adept in general and thus, in its absence, the left does a poor job of comprehending space.

These last two theories share the idea that neglect involves damage to centers responsible for proper orientation to the world, centers located in, or at least controlled by, the right cerebral hemisphere. This is in contrast to the notion of the egocentricity of the left hemisphere, an idea postulating that neglect is a result of the left hemisphere's inappropriate rationalizations in the face of impaired or inefficient input from the right.

We have stressed the visual problems and anomalies usually accompanying the neglect syndrome. Yet, many investigators believe that thinking about neglect in purely perceptual terms does not capture all its manifestations. A subtle aspect of the syndrome may be independent of any sensory processing problems. An anecdote about a neglect patient serves to illustrate this point.

An Italian neglect patient was asked to *imagine* entering a well-known plaza in Rome from the north end and to describe what he saw. The patient had been very familiar with the plaza before his stroke. He proceeded to describe all the buildings to the west — that is, to the right—of where he would have entered, but he failed to mention any of the buildings to the east. He was then asked to imagine entering the plaza from the south and to describe what he saw. The patient proceeded to describe all the buildings in the eastern half of the plaza.

This story suggests that neglect can be independent of visual processing, because it even affects the recall of images from memory. If neglect truly is a visual deficit, it must be a high-level one involving complex aspects of perception. The fact that some neglect patients even deny their illness further attests to this point. An understanding of this unusual, lateralized deficit may add in important ways to our knowledge of how the left brain and the right brain contribute to awareness and perception.

## DISORDERS OF PURPOSEFUL MOVEMENT

Our daily activities involve many movements that have become almost automatic. We perform many complicated acts without having to think about how to do them, from picking up a pen to drinking from a cup, to putting on perfume. Patterns of complex learned movements are organized in terms of both position and timing and follow intricate sequences established through experience. *Apraxia* is the inability to perform certain learned or purposeful movements despite the absence of paralysis or sensory loss. This breakdown in movement can occur in a number of ways.

*Kinetic (or motor) apraxia* is most frequently associated with lesions of the premotor area of the frontal lobe on the side opposite to the affected side of the body. This form of apraxia affects the finer movements of one upper extremity, such as properly holding a pen or placing a letter in an envelope. Reaching out and properly grasping an object consists of a largely unconscious series of movements that depend on a built-up memory of acts similarly performed. Kinetic apraxia may be regarded as a breakdown in the program or "memory" of the motor sequences necessary to perform some basic act.

*Ideomotor apraxia* is usually due to damage in the parietal lobe of the left (dominant) hemisphere, but it seems to have bilateral effects behaviorally. A patient is unable to perform many complex acts on command, although he or she may perform them spontaneously in appropriate situations. The difficulty is especially noticeable when the patient is asked to use pantomime—for example, when asked to "pretend you are brushing your teeth" or when asked "How do you strike a match?" or "How do you wave goodbye?" The patient seems to know what he or she has been told to do but is unable to do it. Given the actual objects and appropriate context, the patient will usually perform much better. The main disturbance seems to be in voluntary recall of some action, not in its actual execution. Therefore, the motor memory of the action is not believed to be disturbed, as in kinetic, or motor, apraxia. Ideomotor apraxia is considered to be a result of the interruption of pathways between the center for verbal formulation of a motor act and the motor areas of the frontal lobe necessary for its execution.

*Ideational apraxia* involves an inability to formulate an appropriate sequence of acts or to use objects properly. A patient seems to know how to perform isolated movements, such as striking a match, but will do them inappropriately. For instance, given a candle and a book of matches, she or he may strike the candle up against the matchbook cover. A patient may pick up a perfume bottle and bring it up to her mouth instead of to her nose. Sometimes complex sequences are done out of order, such as when a patient starts the hand motions involved in writing before picking up a pen.

The patient's appreciation of what she or he is doing often seems to be defective, so it has been suggested that such apraxia is a form of agnosia. The locus of damage in such disorders has been controversial. A classic view was that ideational apraxia arose from lesions in the parietal lobe of the left (dominant) hemisphere or in the corpus callosum. It is most frequently found, however, in cases of diffuse bilateral damage, such as that following disruption of the oxygen supply to the brain (anoxia).

*Constructional apraxia* involves a loss in the ability to reproduce or construct figures by drawing or assembling. There seems to be a loss of visual guidance or an impairment in visualizing a manipulative output, although basic visual and motor functions appear intact. It is seen in certain cases of damage to the occipital and parietal cortex, perhaps to pathways between them.

The incidence of deficits called constructional apraxia by various investigators seems to be the same for either left- or right-hemisphere lesions. This is due, in part, to the rather broad class of disorders labeled as constructional in nature. More recent reviews show that there are characteristic differences in the quality of performance on constructional tasks between left- and right-hemisphere patients.[38] The nature of the errors made is different. For example, when the left hemisphere is damaged, patients draw pictures that preserve the overall configuration of objects but tend to lose detail; this supports the view of the right hemisphere as better at perceiving overall spatial relationships. When the right hemisphere is damaged, patients draw pictures that include much detail but lack an overall coherence. Proportion and spatial relationships are often quite poor.

## The Role of the Hemispheres in Apraxic Disorders

As noted above, ideomotor apraxia and, possibly, ideational apraxia much more often involve lesions of the left hemisphere than of the right. The anatomical model for ideomotor apraxia explains it as a disconnection between posterior brain areas for verbal formulation of an act and those areas of the frontal lobes that generate the motor output.

There is some question as to the extent of verbal involvement in apraxic disorders in general, in the sense that "internalized speech" may mediate many kinds of movement. There is a high incidence of apraxia in aphasic patients, but the fact that the two disorders can occur relatively independently suggests that apraxic disturbances involve motor memories that in some case can be separated from the speech system. It is intriguing to speculate, nevertheless, that there is a similarity in the mechanisms required to produce speech and those required to produce fine motor movements of the limbs. We return to this topic and its relationship to handedness in Chapter 12.

Constructional apraxia, as we have seen, appears to be not one but many different disorders involving either or both hemispheres. Arthur Benton has provided some perspective on constructional apraxia in the context of distinguishing among various kinds of visual deficits.[39] He separates *visuo-constructive, visuo-perceptive, and visuo-spatial deficits* and argues that the right hemisphere is most involved in the latter two disorders. At the visuo-constructive level, involving block designs and construction and figure drawing, both hemispheres are usually involved, although in different ways, as demonstrated in our brief discussion of constructional apraxia. At the visuo-perceptive level, involving separating a figure from complex ground, recognizing deformed objects, discriminating between faces, the right hemisphere plays a greater role than the left. Finally, at the visuo-spatial level, involving judgments of depth, line orientation, and matching simple patterns, the right hemisphere plays an almost exclusive role.

## AMNESIA AND LOCALIZATION OF MEMORY

Concepts of localization in the brain have long included the idea that specific storage sites exist for human memories. The search for the *engram*, the storage unit of memory, has continued for decades. Karl Lashley, following extensive experiments with rats whose brains were lesioned in a systematic fashion with respect to location and size, formulated the *principles of mass action and equipotentiality*.[40] He concluded that memory was critically affected by the amount of cortex removed (principle of mass action) but did not depend on the area removed; that is, all areas of the cortex were equally important for memory (principle of equipotentiality). He arrived at these conclusions because he was unable to reduce significantly a rat's performance on a learned task following removal of small areas of brain tissue from any of a great many regions of the brain. However, in destroying a rather large portion anywhere in the brain, he significantly affected the rat's memory of what it had learned.

Human clinical data over the years has provided evidence that aspects of what we loosely term *memory* are organized in both diffuse and focal ways in the brain. Memory complaints are common in both neurological and psychiatric clinics and seem to accompany a variety of neurological and mental disorders. Most neurological disorders affecting higher mental function have some impact on memory. Diffuse neurological damage, such as that often observed in accidental head injury, typically results in prominent memory disorders. Fortunately, many head-trauma patients make substantial recoveries, including a gradual decrease in their amnesia. Memory loss in these and many other kinds of patients involves amnesia for events prior to the accident (*retrograde amnesia*) and loss of new learning capacity (*anterograde amnesia*). Retrograde amnesia usually diminishes in an orderly fashion, with oldest memories coming back first. Both types of memory loss typically diminish simultaneously during recovery. Ultimately, it is only the recall of certain events after the accident that may seem to be lost; that is, learning, immediately after the accident, is most permanently affected.

*Alzheimer's dementia*, a disease that most frequently affects the elderly and in which there is diffuse degeneration of cerebral tissue, also results in a very prominent memory disorder. Although the "senile" symptoms of this disease involve most intellectual functions, deficits in orientation and memory are the most obvious impairments. Dementia patients usually retain older memories—that is, memories of people and events they encountered earlier in their lives—until the later stages of their disease. The ability to learn and remember new events fails first. Unfortunately, the cause of the neural degeneration is not known or curable, and all such patients continue to deteriorate until they die.

## Isolated Memory Disorders

In addition to the memory loss that can frequently occur in neurological disorders affecting other functions, striking disorders of memory can occur in isolation, that is, out of proportion to any other deficit of higher function. Such isolated disorders of memory are associated with damage to relatively specific areas of the brain, notably the temporal lobes, the hippocampus (an older part of the cortex deep within the temporal lobes), and several other structures deeper within the brain. Figure 6.6 shows some of the regions that have been implicated in memory disorders. Patients with some damage to these structures can appear normal under casual observation and may have normal intellectual capacity. Their defect is primarily in acquiring and retaining new memories. Many remember their past histories and earlier events very well, although the extent of this preservation varies substantially.

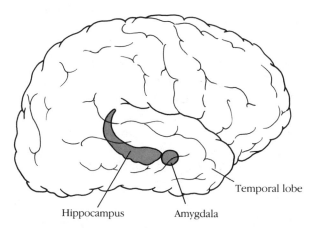

Temporal lobe

Hippocampus          Amygdala

**Figure 6.6** Areas of the human brain involved in memory disorders. Certain memory processes appear to be associated with structures on the inner surface of the temporal lobes, such as the hippocampus and amygdala. Unilateral lesions of these structures have been reported to impair memory selectively, depending on which hemisphere is involved. Bilateral lesions have been known to cause severe memory disorders.

## Episodic Versus Semantic Memory; Cortical Versus Hippocampal Lesions

Investigators have defined two types of long-term memory. *Episodic memory* records information about specific events within the context of other events in a person's lifetime. *Semantic memory* concerns our permanent knowledge of the world; that is, it primarily concerns facts, concepts, rules, and meanings.* It is thought to contain the information necessary for perceptual recognition and complex motor skills, including speech (for all of us) and playing the piano or typing (for some of us).

The cerebral cortex is thought to subserve semantic memory. The loss of meaning information in certain aphasias and the loss of object recognition in certain agnosias can be viewed as loss of semantic memories resulting from damage to the language regions and the perceptual regions of the brain, respectively. Thus, the memory loss associated with damage to cortical regions can be relatively specific, as in Wernicke's aphasia, where left temporal-lobe damage appears to interfere with language knowledge.

In contrast to the role of the cortex in semantic memory, the hippocampus (and associated structures) is thought to be primarily involved in episodic memory because bilateral hippocampal lesions (which occur in conjunction with deep damage to the middle of the temporal lobes) produce a severe loss for new episodic information.[41] Patients with such damage quickly forget events in their daily lives: where they are, what they had for lunch, where they put their checkbooks, or if in fact they wrote a check. Their verbal skills, however, may remain intact, and they are able to have normal conversations, at least about events that occurred before their injuries. It has been shown that where damage is restricted more or less to the hippocampus, patients can learn to perform new tasks, such as playing a new card game. They will be able to use their knowledge of the rules and play correctly when tested at a later time, without remembering how or when they learned the game.

## Hemispheric Differences in Memory

Hemispheric differences have been reported in the kinds of memories lost after either left or right temporal-lobe lesions. The most

---

*In this context, *semantic* has a broader definition than it does in linguistics, where it refers to word meanings. Semantic memory refers to a more general kind of knowledge, encompassing perceptual codes, motoric skills, and other "how" and "what" information.

striking asymmetries related to memory function have been observed in cases involving surgical removal of one temporal lobe. These unilateral temporal lobectomies were performed to remove tissue responsible for epileptic seizures or tumors. Left, or dominant, temporal lobectomy led to difficulty in the learning and retention of verbal material. This deficit was evident independent of whether the material was presented visually or through auditory means, and occurred when memory was tested by either straight recall or recognition procedures.[42]

Right temporal lobectomy led to difficulties with nonverbal material, whether visually or auditorily presented.[43] ("Nonverbal material" involves stimuli that are difficult to name or encode verbally, such as abstract patterns.) In addition, Brenda Milner showed that patients with right temporal-lobe removals have difficulty with maze learning, whether by visual or proprioceptive (exploratory touching) means.[44]

Thus, memory deficits resulting from lateralized lesions, such as unilateral temporal-lobe removals, seem to involve loss in specific semantic memory skills. They are often coupled with some impairment of the contextual (episodic) information involving the hippocampus, however, because this structure deep in the temporal lobe may also be damaged.

Analysis of split-brain patients has supported the evidence from lesion studies of some differences in the memory processes of the two hemispheres. As mentioned in Chapter 2, cutting the corpus callosum seems to have negligible effects on a patient's memory when tested in a conventional manner. However, investigators have shown that when the hemispheres are tested separately, there is a clear difference in the kinds of information each hemisphere can learn and remember.[45] When techniques such as those described in Chapter 2 are used to present information to only one hemisphere at a time, it is primarily language information that is retained best by the left hemisphere and primarily visuo-spatial information that is retained by the right hemisphere. These differences, of course, are expected based on the data concerning what types of information each hemisphere is best equipped to deal with.

## Some Final Observations About Memory

Most amnestic syndromes do not convincingly show a true obliteration of long-term memories. Memory disorders typically affect recent events and new learning. When older memories are affected, there is evidence that the defect is in accessing the memories, for most do, indeed, "come back" when patients recover. Prompting or cuing an amnesic patient can also bring back many memories.

Electrical stimulation studies by Wilder Penfield and his associates, some of which are described in Chapter 1, have been seen as providing evidence bearing on the localization of long-term memories.[46] As part of the procedure to remove diseased brain tissue, Penfield electrically stimulated the brain in certain awake patients at various points in the vicinity of the diseased region. He reported interesting responses from stimulation of points in the temporal lobes, the hippocampus, and the amygdala. Patients at times reported experiencing visual or auditory memories and claimed that these experiences were very vivid, as though they were being lived over again. However, excision of the whole area did not seem to erase any memories. It is likely that most memory impairment after brain damage to a particular region is not so much a removal of localizable engrams as an interference with *part* of the mechanisms or steps involved in forming or retrieving memories.

Finally, it must be kept in mind that our concepts of memory are very vague and ill-defined. A useful understanding of the brain processes behind memory functions will require, at the least, some conceptual clarification of the many psychological functions we refer to loosely as memory. It is hoped that some clarification will come from further analysis of memory disorders.


## MUSIC AND THE HEMISPHERES

In Chapter 1 we presented some evidence for the role of the right hemisphere in music. Patients who had suffered left-hemisphere strokes that affected their speech were often unaffected in their ability to sing. Conversely, right-hemisphere strokes often resulted in the loss of musical abilities while leaving speech unimpaired.

Early research was consistent with the idea that most aspects of musical perception are right-hemisphere functions. Pre- and postoperative testing of musical skills was performed on patients undergoing excision of either the left or the right temporal lobe to remove epileptic tissue.[47] It was found that the operation significantly increased errors on tests of melodic pattern, loudness, sound duration, and timbre when the right hemisphere was removed. Left-hemisphere removal did not result in a change in performance. The ability to sing was also investigated in patients undergoing temporary anesthetization of the right hemisphere using the Wada procedure. Singing was grossly disturbed, and, although rhythmic elements were preserved, melody was reduced to a monotone.[48]

Evidence from other clinical cases, however, has suggested that the right-hemisphere predominance in music is not always complete, especially when music skills are highly developed. Musicians who have sustained left-hemisphere stroke have shown documented impairment of at least some of their skills. Composer Maurice Ravel (1875–1937) suffered a stroke (presumed to be in the left hemisphere) and developed a Wernicke's type of aphasia while at the peak of his career. Many of Ravel's musical skills remained intact. He could recognize melodies and notice the smallest mistakes in performed music. He maintained the keenest awareness of how well a piano was tuned. In contrast to these preserved skills, however, Ravel experienced a substantial loss in ability to identify (label) notes and recognize written music. He also could not play the piano or write music, even by dictation. His career as a composer had come to an end.[49]

Although one could argue that most of Ravel's musical deficits seem related to his language disorder (as in his loss of writing and dictating skills) and to some motor output problems (as in his inability to play the piano), research with normal subjects points to left-hemisphere involvement in certain aspects of musical processing. In a dichotic listening study looking at the detection of pitch and rhythm changes, the right ear proved more accurate in detecting changes in rhythm as well as in pitch in five-note sequences.[50] Thomas Bever and Robert Chiarello have reported findings suggesting that laterality differences in music perception are a function of training.[51] In a memory recognition task, nonmusicians showed a left-ear advantage. Listeners with musical training, however, showed a right-ear superiority. The investigators explained their results as reflecting differences in the way melodies are processed by trained and untrained listeners. Naive listeners focus on overall melodic contour, they suggest, whereas experienced listeners perceive a melody as an articulated set of component elements.

Although the Bever and Chiarello findings remain controversial because different results have been found by some investigators, overall the data on music and the hemispheres suggests that, just as all of the components of language do not appear to be equally lateralized to the left hemisphere, all aspects of musical skill do not reside exclusively in the right hemisphere. Those aspects of musical processing that require judgments about duration, temporal order, sequencing, and rhythm differentially involve the left hemisphere, whereas the right hemisphere is differentially involved when judgments about tonal memory, timbre, melody recognition, and intensity are required.

## EMOTION

Emotion is not an easily definable phenomenon. It involves many kinds of human mental states, reactions, and attitudes. Some of these may be highly related in terms of the brain mechanisms involved, whereas others may not be. There are also many ways in which emotion is conveyed. Emotional information is reflected in our facial expressions, as well as in less noticeable physiological signs. Emotional information may be conveyed directly in speech, or it may be superimposed in the tone by which other information is conveyed in speech. As in other studies of brain–behavior relationships, the answers to where and how emotional processes take place in the brain depend, to a great extent, on what aspects of emotional behavior one is investigating.

### Emotional Responses to Hemispheric Injuries

A number of investigations have focused on the emotional behavior of patients with unilateral brain lesions. Left-hemisphere patients have been reported to display feelings of despair, hopelessness, or anger (often referred to as a catastrophic–dysphoric reaction), whereas right-hemisphere damage produces what is known as an indifference–euphoric reaction, in which minimization of symptoms, emotional placidity, and elation are common. A frequently cited study, for example, compared the frequency of the catastrophic and indifference reactions in 150 patients with unilateral brain lesions. Of the patients with left-hemisphere lesions, 62 percent showed a catastrophic reaction, whereas that response was observed in only 10 percent of right-lesion patients. The incidence of indifference reactions, however, was 38 percent among those with right lesions and only 11 percent among those with left lesions.[52]

Extreme emotional reactions have also been reported after unilateral injection of sodium amobarbital into the carotid artery (the Wada test). Several investigators have observed dysphoric reactions, frequently accompanied by crying, after left-side injections.[53] Indifference–euphoric reactions were found in significantly fewer patients. One researcher described the catastrophic reaction in the following way:

> . . . the patient especially when spoken to despairs and expresses a sense of guilt, of nothingness, of indignity and worries about his own future or that of his relatives. . . . [54]

After right-side injection, however, indifference–euphoric reactions were more common than dysphoric reactions, with patients sometimes breaking out into peals of laughter as the effects of the sodium amobarbital wore off. The same investigator describes the indifference reaction that occurs as:

> a complete opposite emotional reaction, a euphoric reaction that in some cases may reach the intensity of a maniacal reaction. The patient appears without apprehension, smiles and laughs and both with mimicry and words expresses considerable liveliness and sense of well being.[55]

Although not all investigators have reported results that are this consistent,[56] the findings we have just reviewed strongly suggest that the two sides of the brain differ in the emotional states they subserve. However, there are two problems with this interpretation that need to be addressed. First, the reported emotional changes accompanying insults to either half of the brain may not result from disruption of brain mechanisms underlying emotion but, instead, may be a consequence of the patient's reaction to the deficits resulting from the brain insult. Thus, the catastrophic reaction following left-hemisphere injury or inactivation would be seen as a reaction to the inability to speak and does not represent lateralization of emotion per se. Although an analogous explanation to account for a euphoric reaction after right-hemisphere injury is not as intuitively obvious, it is possible, nevertheless, that both the dysphoric and euphoric reactions are secondary manifestations of other deficits and not the direct result of alterations to the lateralized mechanisms subserving emotion.

The second problem deals with the relationship of the two sides of the brain to the emotional states under discussion. If we assume for the moment that the emotional changes are a direct consequence of changes in brain function, we still need to determine how those changes operate. For example, damage to one side of the brain may produce emotional reactions through its effects on the same hemisphere, or it may exert its influence on the side contralateral to the damage, e.g., through the destruction of regions that normally inhibit certain activities of the other hemisphere. To understand the nature of hemispheric asymmetry for emotion, it is important to determine which of these two actually occurs.

Psychologist Harold Sackheim and his colleagues have reviewed some relevant clinical literature in an effort to address these issues.[57] Initially, they looked at cases of pathological laughing and crying in which patients show spontaneous uncontrollable displays of emotion that are uncorrelated with objective events. Their review showed that patients with pathological laughing were three times more likely to have right- as opposed to left-sided lesions, whereas pathological crying was more than twice as likely to occur in cases of left- than right-side damage. Sackheim argues that pathological laughing and crying are unlikely to be secondary results of other deficits because the symptoms often preceed the appearance of other deficits and are often the first sign of a lesion and that, hence, these data support the hypothesis that the two sides of the brain do differ in subserving positive and negative emotional states.

Sackheim then looked at cases of uncontrollable emotional outbursts of laughing and crying that sometimes accompany epileptic seizures. Of the 91 patients showing outbursts of laughing, a left-sided focus was twice as likely as a right-sided focus. Many fewer cases of crying were found. In the six cases of crying that were reported, however, a different pattern was observed. Four patients were judged to be right sided, with one left sided, and one indeterminate.

It is interesting to compare these findings with those obtained through the study of pathological laughing and crying resulting from brain lesions. In the latter case, pathological laughing was strongly associated with predominantly right-sided lesions. In the case of epilepsy-induced uncontrollable laughing, however, the epileptic focus was more often left-sided than right-sided. Similarly, results were reversed in the few cases of pathological crying and epilepsy induced crying that were studied. Pathological crying was associated with left-hemisphere lesions, whereas a right-sided focus tended to accompany seizure-associated crying. Although the results may appear to conflict, they are actually quite consistent if one keeps in mind the fact that seizures are associated with hyperexcitability in the regions comprising the focus, whereas lesions involve destruction of tissue. The data suggest that uncontrollable outbursts of laughter may result from excitation within the left half of the brain (as in epilepsy) or disinhibition of the left side resulting from damage to the right (as in the case of brain injury). The conclusions regarding uncontrollable crying must be more tentative because of the small number of cases. However, the data that exist are consistent with the idea that uncontrollable crying results from excitation within the right half of the brain, or disinhibition of the right hemisphere following left-hemisphere injury.

The notion of disinhibition, as used here, implies that ordinarily the two halves of the brain exert inhibitory effects on each other in the area of emotional expression, resulting in a normal balance that is free of uncontrollable outbursts of any kind. In the event of damage to one side, however, this mutual inhibition is disrupted and the damaged side no longer exerts the same degree of inhibition on its partner; hence, the other hemisphere is disinhibited.

The model of hemispheric control of emotional experience that emerges from this review, thus, is one in which the left side of the brain typically subserves positive emotions, whereas the right side typically subserves negative emotions. Normally the two sides exert inhibitory influences on one another. In the case of lesions or epileptic seizures, however, this pattern of inhibition is disrupted, producing the effects we have just discussed. The model is a useful working hypothesis that helps explain a good deal of the data just reviewed, although it is far from being a complete and universally accepted explanation of the relationship between emotion and the hemispheres. Let us turn now to some other evidence bearing on hemispheric asymmetry and emotion that illustrates how complex an area this is.

## The Perception of Emotion

*Clinical Data* As mentioned in the discussion of language disorders, some clinical evidence has suggested a role for the right hemisphere in the processing of emotional information. Kenneth Heilman and his colleagues, for example, report that patients with damage in the right hemisphere have greater difficulty picking up on the emotional messages conveyed by speech intonations than do patients with damage in the left hemisphere.[58] Patients sat in front of pictures of four faces—one happy, one sad, one angry, and one indifferent— and listened to sentences read in different tones of voice. The sentences were neutral and not emotional in content; emotional information was conveyed only by the way in which the examiner read the sentences. The patients' task was to point to the face that best illustrated the emotional tone that the examiner was expressing on each trial. Aphasic patients, even one global aphasic, did quite well — often flawlessly — on the task. In contrast, patients with right-hemisphere lesions had great difficulty with this task; their overall performance was much poorer than that of the aphasics.

Another study was designed to address the question of whether this failure on the part of right-hemisphere patients was due to an inability to identify emotional expression — that is, a perceptual loss — or to a loss in the concepts of what different emotions mean — that is, a cognitive loss. The investigators required patients with right-hemisphere lesions to discriminate between pairs of sentences that had the same words but were spoken with either the same or different intonations. The patients did not have to identify the emotion but merely tell if the sentences sounded the same or different.

The right-hemisphere patients performed more poorly on this task than did aphasic controls, as they had in the Heilman study. On the other hand, when right-hemisphere patients were tested on whether they could identify the emotion conveyed by the *contents* of a story, they performed as well as controls. These results have been interpreted as showing that right-hemisphere patients have not lost the concept or comprehension of different emotions but, rather, that they exhibit difficulty with standard perceptual cues to emotion.[59]

*Behavioral Tests in Normals* Studies with normal subjects also support a major role for the right hemisphere in the perception of emotion. In a study looking at possible asymmetries in the expression of emotion, full-face photographs and their mirror reversals were split down the midline.[60] Composites were put together from two left sides or two right sides. Subjects were asked to rate the intensities of emotional expression evident in a series of such pictures depicting different emotions. Figure 6.7 shows one such face and the composites formed from it.

Left-side composites were judged to express emotion more intensely than right-side composites. The researchers noted the preponderance of contralateral projections controlling facial muscles and argue that these results point to greater involvement by the right hemisphere in the production of emotional expression. A number of subsequent investigations have produced basically similar results overall. Findings are conflicting, however, when the expressions are divided into positive and negative categories. Some investigators

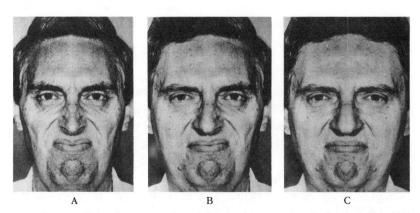

A            B            C

**Figure 6.7** Comparison of the intensity of emotional expression in composite faces. A. Left-side composite. B. Original face. C. Right-side composite. [From Sackheim, "Emotions Are Expressed More Intensely on the Left Side of the Face," Fig. 1, p. 434. *Science* 1978, 202, Oct. 1978. American Association for the Advancement of Science]

have reported differences in the pattern of asymmetry for positive and negative expressions. Joan Borod and her colleagues, for example, found that negative expressions were consistently and significantly left-sided, whereas positive expressions were not systematically lateralized.[61] Other studies, however, have shown left-side effects for both positive and negative stimuli under certain conditions.[62]

Other tests of neurologically normal subjects have also shown a pattern of results in which it is the right hemisphere alone that appears to be specifically involved in the recognition of emotional states, while the left hemisphere plays no special role. In a dichotic listening study using nonverbal human sounds, such as laughing and coughing, a small left-ear advantage was found, and a study asking subjects to identify both the emotional intonation and the verbal content of dichotically presented sentences found a slight left-ear advantage in identifying the emotional tone of the sentences.[63] A study using visual stimuli presented to the left and right visual fields also showed evidence of differential hemispheric involvement. The stimuli were five cartoon characters, each with five emotional expressions — extremely positive, mildly positive, neutral, mildly negative, and extremely negative — presented briefly one at a time in the left or the right visual field. The subjects' task was to judge whether the emotional expression was the same as that of a second cartoon presented in the center of the visual field. Results showed a left-visual-field superiority, consistent with right-hemisphere superiority for the task.[64]

Thus, there appears to be a good case for believing that the right hemisphere is involved in both the processing of emotional information and in the production of emotional expressions to a greater degree than is the left. It is important to keep in mind, however, the data reviewed earlier pointing to a specialized role for the left hemisphere in the expression of positive emotions. To speak of the right hemisphere as the one specialized for emotion clearly oversimplifies what we know about hemispheric asymmetry. Adding even more to this picture of complexity are the data reviewed in Chapter 10, dealing with a possible role of hemispheric differences in psychopathology. We look to future research to provide additional clues about how it all fits together.

# 7

# Sex and Asymmetry

Consider the following simple experiment. In one condition, subjects are asked to run mentally through the alphabet and count the
number of letters, including the letter *e*, that when pronounced
contain the sound "ee." In a second condition, subjects are asked to
count the number of letters that contain curves when they are
printed as capitals. In both conditions, the subjects must perform the
task "in their heads." Writing or speaking out loud is not permitted.
Participants are told to do each count as quickly as possible because
the results are scored for speed as well as for accuracy.

Which task is harder — counting sounds or counting curves? The
outcome of this study depends on whether male or female subjects

are being tested. Males are more accurate and slightly faster in the shape task; females do better in the sound task.[1]

This study is one of many pointing to sex differences in certain human abilities — in this case, verbal and spatial skills. Considerable evidence suggests that females are superior to males in a wide range of skills that require the use of language, such as fluency, speed of articulation and grammar.[2] Extensive evidence shows males to be superior in tasks that are spatial in nature, including maze performance, picture assembly and block design tests, mental rotation, and mechanical skills.[3]

Identifying sex differences such as these, however, does not necessarily reveal anything about the origin of the difference. Biological factors may play an important role, as may sex differences in child-rearing practices. Recent research into the left brain and right brain has suggested that sex differences in verbal and spatial abilities may be related to differences in the way those functions are distributed between the cerebral hemispheres in males and females.

In this chapter, we review the evidence on this question and consider its theoretical and practical significance. The picture we have of sex differences in the brain comes from both clinical and behavioral studies.

## EVIDENCE FROM THE BRAIN-DAMAGE CLINIC

### Sex Differences in the Effects of Brain Damage

Herbert Lansdell, working at the National Institutes of Health, was among the first investigators to note that the consequences of damage to one half of the brain appeared to differ for males and females.[4] Lansdell was interested in studying the effects of the removal of part of the temporal lobe on one side of the head in patients operated on to alleviate epileptic seizures. A wealth of earlier research had led him to predict greater deficits in visuo-spatial tasks after operation on the right hemisphere and greater deficits in verbal tasks following left-hemisphere surgery. His predictions were borne out, but only for male patients. These unexpected findings led Lansdell to speculate that some physiological mechanisms underlying visuo-spatial and verbal ability may overlap in the female but may be located in opposite hemispheres in the male brain.

Later work has pointed to the same conclusions. For example, psychologist Jeannette McGlone reported data from 85 right-handed adults with damage to the left or the right side of the brain.[5] Most had suffered a stroke, although some were tumor cases. Each patient was given a battery of psychological tests, including the Wechsler Adult Intelligence Scale (WAIS) and an aphasia test, to determine if the pattern of verbal and nonverbal deficits that emerged was a function of both sex and side of damage.

The results for language impairments were striking. Aphasia after damage to the left hemisphere occurred three times more frequently in males than in females. Even when patients showing signs of aphasia were excluded from the analysis, deficits in higher verbal tasks in the remaining patients continued to be more common and more severe in males.

In contrast, performance on the nonverbal subtests of the WAIS did not show any overall significant effects due to sex or side of damage. When performance on the nonverbal tests was compared with performance on the verbal tests, however, differences by sex and side of lesion again appeared. The relevant measure is the difference between the score on the nonverbal IQ items and the verbal IQ score. For men, left-hemisphere damage impaired verbal IQ more than nonverbal IQ, and right-hemisphere damage lowered nonverbal performance relative to verbal. Women showed no effect of side of lesion. Their verbal and nonverbal IQ scores were not significantly different for damage to the left or the right side. These data also support Lansdell's speculation that both language abilities and spatial abilities are represented more bilaterally in females than in males.

## Have Sex Differences Always Been Present?

How can these findings be reconciled with almost 100 years of clinical investigations of hemispheric asymmetry that did not report sex differences? One explanation is that many of the older studies included patient populations that were predominantly male. Patients in Veterans Administration hospitals have been extensively studied, and they are almost exclusively male. Patients suffering from war-related brain damage have also been the object of much research; they too are overwhelmingly male. Populations having surgery on the temporal lobe are biased as well. Most surgery of this type is done to alleviate epilepsy, a disease that is much more common among males.

Another important factor in explaining the failure of early work to notice sex differences is simply that no one looked for them. There is tremendous variation from patient to patient (even within one sex) in the effects of unilateral brain damage. Damage to the left hemisphere of some right-handed people can produce a massive disruption of language-skills, whereas comparable damage in other individuals has minimal effect. This variability in the effects of brain damage within groups of males and females makes it difficult to find differences between males and females unless the investigator is working with a large subject population and is specifically looking for differences.

With these ideas in mind, James Inglis and J. S. Lawson have performed an interesting reanalysis of a number of older studies that investigated the effects of unilateral brain damage on verbal and spatial abilities without looking for sex differences.[6] Inglis and Lawson predicted that those studies reporting significant verbal and spatial deficits in groups with left- and right-brain damage, respectively, would be found to contain many more male than female patients. Those studies that failed to find this pattern of deficits would be expected to contain more female patients, they argued, because reduced laterality effects in women would mask the stronger effects found in men. The reanalysis strongly supported these hypotheses and has provided additional evidence for the importance of sex differences in the study of brain injury and brain lateralization.


## EVIDENCE FROM BEHAVIORAL TESTS

### Auditory and Visual Studies

Many researchers doing behavioral studies of laterality have begun to look for sex differences. Several verbal dichotic listening studies have reported greater right-ear advantages among males than among females. Philip Bryden, a psychologist who has conducted numerous dichotic listening studies to assess brain asymmetry, has combined the data from several of his studies using dichotically presented digit pairs to look for possible sex differences.[7] Of the 98 subjects he tested, 73.6 percent of the males (11 left-handers and 42 right-handers) showed a right-ear advantage, and 62.2 percent of the females (3 left-handers and 42 right-handers) showed right-ear superiority. Sex differences in ear asymmetries have also been found in studies using spoken syllables as dichotic stimuli.

Not all attempts to look for sex differences in verbal dichotic listening performance have found them, however. Overall, about half of the verbal dichotic listening studies that look for sex differences do not find them; the remaining half report greater lateralization for males.

Much less attention has been paid to possible sex differences in the processing of nonverbal auditory stimuli. Two studies that have measured ear asymmetry for melodies and familiar sounds reported a significant left-ear advantage for women and a small, but statistically insignificant, left-ear advantage for men.[8] These findings suggest that lateralization for certain nonverbal auditory stimuli may be greater in women than in men, in contrast with the trend found in studies using verbal stimuli.

Visual-field studies have also been employed to address the possibility of sex differences in brain organization. For the most part, the results show greater lateralization in males when tasks involve the processing of words, and there is also a weak trend toward greater lateralization in males when subjects are asked to indicate the location of a dot or to judge the number of dots represented in a display. A number of visual-field studies, however, have also failed to find sex differences.[9]

The failure of many studies to find reliable sex differences have led some investigators to question the reality of sex differences in laterality in the first place. Some have argued that this area of research is plagued by the *type I error.*

Type I is the name given to the kind of error made when an investigator concludes that the differences observed in a study are real when in fact they are due to chance. Investigators are much more willing to report differences between groups (and journal editors are much more eager to accept such studies) than they are to publish negative or "no-difference" results. Critics have suggested that journals contain only the tip of the sex-differences-in-laterality-research iceberg and that the majority of studies with negative results are never published.

Those who believe that sex differences in laterality are real counter this argument with one that challenges the sensitivity of studies that fail to find evidence of sex differences. They note the tremendous variability in lateralization within a given sex and point out that this variability makes it quite difficult to detect real, but small, differences between the sexes. Small studies with 10 or 15 subjects per group (the size of many studies) will especially suffer from this problem.

### Studying Sex Differences in Children

Significant sex differences in the lateralization of spatial functions have been found in children. Standard behavioral techniques for studying the right hemisphere's role in spatial processing proved difficult for young children. Thus, Sandra Witelson devised a test of tactual perception that could be used over a wide range of ages.[10]

The test, known as the dichaptic stimulation test, requires that the subject simultaneously feel two different objects held out of view, one in each hand. After holding the meaningless shapes for 10 seconds, the subject chooses the two shapes from among a group of six that are displayed visually. The data are then scored for the number of objects correctly selected by each hand. Figure 7.1 shows this test.

Witelson tested 200 strongly right-handed children ages 6 to 13. The results showed a significant interaction of hand and sex. The left-hand scores of the boys were significantly better than their right-hand scores, but there was no difference between hands for the girls. A dichotic digits test administered to the same subjects did not show any sex difference in the proportion of children showing a right- or a left-ear advantage.

The results of the Witelson study suggest that sex differences in lateralization of spatial abilities may have their origins quite early in life. Later in this chapter, we consider mechanisms that may underlie these differences. In the next section, we summarize some of the remaining data that provide additional evidence for the existence of sex differences.

## ACTIVITY AND ANATOMY: ADDITIONAL PIECES OF THE SEX DIFFERENCES PUZZLE

### Differences in Brain Anatomy

In Chapter 4, some of the evidence pointing to anatomical differences between the hemispheres was reviewed. Mounting interest in sex differences in lateralization has encouraged investigators to see

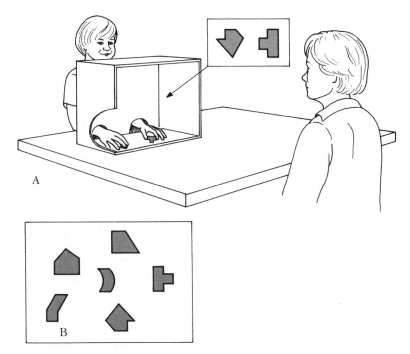

**Figure 7.1** Dichaptic stimulation test. A. The subject is given two objects with meaningless shapes, such as those shown in the inset. Without being able to see the objects, he or she simultaneously feels both of them, one with each hand, for 10 seconds. B. The subject is asked to identify the two shapes from among a group of six displayed visually.

whether sex is a factor in these asymmetries, and findings have begun to appear suggesting that it is.

Although data on sex have not been reported in some studies, one large investigation obtained gender information for most of the brains that were examined postmortem.[11] Results were reported as ratios of the length of the right temporal plane to the length of the left temporal plane for each brain. Overall, this ratio was less than 1, reflecting a longer plane on the left side. Of those individuals showing a reversal of this pattern, however, most were female. If a reversal is assumed to reflect greater bilaterality of function, the findings with human subjects are consistent with the other data reviewed so far. Females seem to be less lateralized.

Sex differences in brain asymmetry have also been reported for a species of white rat.[12] A more detailed discussion of brain asymmetries in the rat is presented in Chapter 9; we confine discussion here to the evidence on sex differences. Marian Diamond and her colleagues found that male rats showed significantly thicker right hemispheres at all ages except very old. Female rats, in contrast, showed somewhat thicker left hemispheres, although the differences for females were not significant statistically.

In studies unrelated to hemispheric differences, investigators observed that pregnancy could induce increases in cortical thickness in female rats. The finding that male and female rats differ in their pattern of cortical asymmetries led the investigators to consider that ovarian hormones might play a role in these asymmetries. To test this hypothesis, a group of female rats who had undergone ovarectomy (removal of the ovaries) at birth was compared with a control group at 90 days of age. Nine areas of the brain were measured. The control rats revealed thicker left cortices in seven of the nine regions, with none of the differences reaching statistical significance. In the ovarectomized rats, however, the *right* cortex was thicker in seven of the nine regions, with statistically significant differences in three regions.

The effects of testosterone on brain asymmetry was examined in male rats whose testes were removed at birth. At 90 days of age, the intact control group had a thicker right cortex in all of the regions measured, with the differences in three regions reaching significance. The rats whose testes were removed at birth, however, showed a strikingly different pattern — all regions but one were thicker on the left side than on the right, a pattern similar to that of intact females.

The evidence from asymmetries in the rat brain point to a powerful role for sex hormones in establishing and maintaining asymmetries. We must re-emphasize, though, that the link between anatomical asymmetries and functional asymmetries is, at present, an untested assumption. That link must be firmly established before anatomical data can be used to infer function. In addition, in the study of human brains, relatively few specimens showed a reversal — that is, a right temporal plane longer than the left — thus, this effect may hold true for only a small percentage of females, overall.

## Electrical Activity and Sex Differences

Some other evidence pointing to sex differences in lateralization has come from electrophysiological studies. One study correlated the degree of EEG alpha asymmetry (left-alpha power minus right-alpha power) with the speed of performance on different tasks thought to engage the left and right hemispheres differentially.[13] For males, a significant correlation was found between the magnitude of the asymmetry and performance in the right-hemisphere task. The correlation for the left-hemisphere "vocabulary" condition approached, but did not quite reach, statistical significance. A task believed to involve both hemispheres did not show any correlation with performance. In females, however, none of these correlations was significantly different from zero. These results suggest some differences in laterality as a function of sex, but a direct analysis of alpha power did not show evidence of the sex by type of task by hemisphere interaction that was originally predicted.

Another study looked for sex differences in a situation where subjects were trained to use biofeedback techniques to generate symmetrical or asymmetrical EEG patterns.[14] In a task where the subject can control the onset or offset of a tone by generating a particular EEG pattern (such as greater left-hemisphere alpha, greater right-hemisphere alpha, or low or high alpha in both hemispheres), subjects quickly acquire the ability to produce the required distribution of activity. Results showed that females were better able to maintain asymmetric patterns of alpha activity than males, but there were no sex differences in the ability to maintain *symmetrical* patterns in the two hemispheres.

Although this last study points to a sex difference in brain asymmetry, the difference is the reverse of what would have been predicted on the assumption that females are less lateralized. The investigators proposed that the apparent conflict may arise from other studies' use of perceptual tasks to measure asymmetry, whereas the investigators employed a task involving production (the production of the alpha asymmetry). They suggest that sex differences in asymmetry may depend heavily on whether perception or production is studied.

Electrophysiological studies, then, contribute to the idea that the lateralization patterns of males and females differ. This area of research, however, confronts the same difficulties as the electrophysiological work reviewed in Chapter 4. Studies are often difficult to repeat, and even seemingly successful studies are not always clear-cut in their results or their interpretation.

## Cerebral Blood Flow

A study comparing hemispheric blood flow during a verbal analogies task with that seen during a task involving judgment of line orientation showed significant differences in the extent of the hemispheric asymmetry of flows, depending on the sex of the subject.[15] Both female and male right-handed subjects showed comparable increases (relative to resting state flow) in left-hemisphere flow during the verbal task. Females, however, showed a greater increase in right-hemisphere flow during the spatial task than did the males. The most surprising aspect of these findings is the stronger lateralization of blood flow in right-handed females, which seems to run counter to the bulk of evidence showing weaker lateralization in females. These results are intriguing but need to be studied further and interpreted with great care as we improve our knowledge of the many factors contributing to metabolic changes during task performance (see Chapter 4).

## ARE SEX DIFFERENCES IN LATERALITY REAL?

Are there sex differences in the distribution of verbal and spatial functions between the hemispheres? Much of the data reviewed in the preceding sections suggest that there are. A variety of evidence suggests that males tend to be more lateralized for verbal and spatial abilities, whereas women show greater bilateral representation for both types of functions. But what about type I error? Are there studies (some of which we do not know about because they are unpublished) that fail to find these purported sex differences?

Our review of the lateralization literature in general has given us a healthy respect for the type I error and the scientific chaos it can create. The frequency as well as the consistency of reports of sex differences in cerebral organization, however, lead us to accept their reality, at least as a working hypothesis. The strength of the case, in our opinion, rests on the diversity of methodologies (clinical studies, dichotic listening, tachistoscopic presentation, and electrophysiology) that point to the same conclusion: females are less lateralized than males.

A review of the studies that do not support this conclusion shows that most report no differences between the sexes. It is a rare study that reports sex differences in the direction of greater lateralization in females. This consistency suggests that there are true differences that are small in magnitude and easily masked by individual variability or other factors that may not be controlled.

# THE ORIGIN OF SEX DIFFERENCES

Assuming for the moment that sex differences are real, how can they be accounted for? Several intriguing proposals have been offered. Deborah Waber has suggested that sex differences of the sort reviewed here are attributable not to sex per se but, rather, to differences in the rates at which males and females develop.[16] Waber noted that females generally gain physical maturity at an earlier age than males. She hypothesized that maturational rate might be systemically related to sex differences in verbal and spatial abilities. Specifically, she predicted the following relationships that would be independent of sex: first, early maturers have better verbal than spatial abilities, whereas late maturers perform better on spatial tasks than on verbal ones; second, early maturers show less speech lateralization than late maturers.

Waber tested her predictions with a sample of 80 children, divided into eight groups on the basis of age (10 and 13 for girls; 13 and 16 for boys), sex, and maturational level (early or late, based on a medical examination for secondary sexual characteristics). Individuals were classified as early maturers if their chronological ages were at least one standard deviation below mean age for their stages of sexual development and as late maturers if their chronological ages were one standard deviation above the norms used.

Several standard tests of verbal and spatial ability were administered to each subject, as well as a consonant–vowel dichotic listening test to assess speech lateralization. In general, the results confirmed Waber's predictions. Within individuals and independent of sex, late maturers scored better on spatial tasks, and early maturers scored better on verbal tasks. Further analysis showed that only the spatial scores were related to maturational rate. The verbal scores did not differ as a function of maturation. Among the older subjects, late maturers also showed larger ear advantages than early maturers. The younger children did not show a difference in ear advantage as a function of maturational rate. Differences due to sex alone were not significant in the study.

Waber's data lead to the proposal that sex differences in verbal and spatial ability and the lateralization of these functions may be due not to sex but to a variable that is *correlated* with sex— maturational rate.

Jerre Levy has suggested an evolutionary basis for sex differences in lateralization.[17] She argues that males have been the hunters and

leaders of migrations throughout hominid evolution, and those with
good visuo-spatial skills have had a selective advantage. At the same
time, females were likely to have had selective pressures for skills
involved in child rearing, such as use of language as a tool for
communication, development of social sensitivity, and facility with
nonverbal communication. Levy proposes that greater bilateraliza-
tion of function may facilitate the skills needed by females, whereas
stricter separation of function is necessary to ensure a high level of
visuo-spatial skills in males.

## THE SIGNIFICANCE OF SEX DIFFERENCES

From a theoretical standpoint, the significance of sex differences in
brain organization is considerable. If sex differences are real, what is
(or was) their adaptive advantage? How does brain organization
relate to patterns of higher mental function? Do sex differences in
child-rearing practices affect brain asymmetries? These are a few
important questions that remain unanswered.

Particularly interesting is the issue of how ability is related to
extent of lateralization. Does greater lateralization for a given function imply superior performance for that function? Is the spatial
ability of males better than that of females because males seem to
rely more on one hemisphere to process spatial information? There
is, of course, no logical reason to expect that greater lateralization
necessarily leads to superior ability. In fact, we have to assume the
opposite to explain the superior verbal ability of females. According
to behavioral tests and clinical data, women appear to be less lateralized for language functions, yet as a group they are superior to men
in language skills.

There may be a relationship between lateralization and ability that
is different for different tasks. If this is the case, it would be fascinating to know why the brain organizes itself so differently for the
optimal functioning of different abilities. At this point, we can only
speculate about the relationship of lateralization and ability. For
example, assume that complex visuo-spatial capability preceeded the
evolution of language in humans (which is a reasonable assumption).
One can then postulate that in men only the left hemisphere became
involved in language, leaving visuo-spatial functions intact in the
right, whereas in women language was established in both hemispheres, crowding most specialized visuo-spatial capability. If this in

fact occurred, "more lateralized" would be better for visuo-spatial function, whereas "less lateralized" would be better for language.

Although most investigators would probably agree that theoretical questions of this sort are significant, undoubtedly there would be less agreement concerning the practical meaning of sex differences in brain organization and their possible correlates in cognitive function. Sex differences in higher mental functions are typically on the order of one-fourth of a standard deviation. This means that there is a great deal of overlap in the distribution of ability across men and women. Some women have better spatial abilities than most men, whereas some men have better verbal skills than most women. On the average, though, the groups do differ in these abilities to a limited degree.

Awareness of the extent of the overlap in ability tends to temper any suggestion that sex be used as a major criterion, by itself, for determining career options and educational opportunities. Witelson has proposed that data on sex differences in brain organization be the basis for devising educational programs (at the elementary school level) that are best suited to the abilities of each sex. This approach, though, denies the importance of individual differences within groups of males and females. The need for curricula better geared to the abilities of specific groups is clear. It is perhaps wiser, however, to determine the composition of those groups through individual testing rather than to determine it only on the basis of gender.

# 8

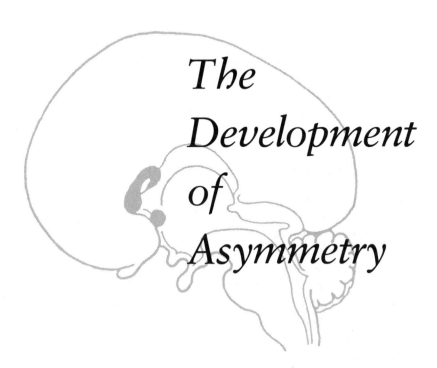

# The Development of Asymmetry

At birth, the brain of a human infant is one-fourth the weight of an adult brain. By the time a child is 2 years of age the brain will have more than tripled its mass and come close to its full size. Accompanying this dramatic change in physical size are equally dramatic changes in the child's capabilities. By the age of 2, the average child has begun to talk and to show the beginnings of many of the higher mental functions that characterize human beings.

In this chapter, we discuss how and at what point the basic differences between the left brain and the right brain found in adults fit into this picture of physical and functional change in childhood. Do these asymmetries emerge over time as the child develops, or are they present at birth or even before? What roles do genetic and environmental factors play in the establishment of asymmetry? Can the pattern of asymmetry be changed and, if so, what are the limiting factors?

These fundamental questions are the focus of considerable research using many different methodologies. The answers have the potential for contributing in important ways to our understanding of language disorders, both in children and in adults. They may also help investigators better understand other problems that have been linked to the division of functions between the hemispheres.

## WHEN IS LATERALIZATION COMPLETE?

### The Case for Lateralization by Puberty

The person perhaps most responsible for current interest in the development of lateralization was Eric Lenneberg, a psychologist at Cornell University. In the mid 1960s, Lenneberg reviewed a variety of evidence and concluded that lateralization of function in the brain develops over time but is complete by puberty.[1] His research also indicated that puberty marks a crucial turning point in the ability to learn new languages, without signs of a foreign accent, through mere exposure. Lenneberg believed it was not merely coincidence that both lateralization and language-learning ability appear fixed at puberty. He saw one as the biological basis of the other.

In drawing his conclusions about the time course of lateralization, Lenneberg relied heavily on clinical data collected by the neurologist L. S. Basser.[2] Basser reported that about half of a group of 72 children with brain injury occurring before the age of 2 began to speak at the usual time, whereas the other half showed some delay. The results were the same for children with damage to the left or the right hemisphere, suggesting that hemispheric asymmetry for language is not well established by age 2. Results from a group of children with injuries occurring between the onset of speech and age 20, however, showed the emergence of hemispheric differences. In this group, injury to the left side resulted in speech disturbances in 85 percent of the cases, but injury to the right side produced disturbances in only 45 percent of the cases.

Despite these differential left–right effects, this pattern of impairment is still different from that found in right-handed teenagers and adults who sustain brain injury. Here, aphasia very rarely follows damage to the right hemisphere but occurs even more often after damage to the left half of the brain. On the basis of this evidence, Lenneberg concluded that lateralization begins at the time of language acquisition but is not complete until puberty.

## Lateralization by Puberty Reconsidered

Lenneberg's interpretation of these data has not gone unchallenged. A careful re-examination of Basser's findings has shown that each of the cases where damage to the right hemisphere resulted in speech disturbances involved injury occurring before the age of 5. In the sole case where right-hemisphere injury occurred after that age, no speech loss was noted. Thus, Basser's findings are consistent with the hypothesis that lateralization is complete by age 5 rather than by puberty. They do not, however, provide an adequate number of patients to test the hypothesis that lateralization is completed later.[3]

Another investigator has argued that the data are consistent with the hypothesis that lateralization is complete at birth, not by age 5 or at puberty. Kinsbourne has reviewed the neurological records in Basser's cases and argues that most of the cases in which right-hemisphere damage in infancy resulted in aphasia were really cases of injury to the left as well as the right hemisphere.[4] If this is so, the early childhood data look no different from adult data in terms of the incidence of aphasia after damage to the left or the right side of the brain.

In 1978, Bryan Woods and Hans Lucas Teuber reported 65 cases of children with unilateral hemispheric injury occurring after the onset of speech.[5] They found that 25 of the 34 children with left-hemisphere lesions were initially aphasic, whereas only four of the 31 children with right-hemisphere lesions (including two left-handers) were aphasic. In reviewing earlier literature, the authors concluded that there had been a striking change in the incidence of aphasia after right-hemisphere injury in children, with a sharp drop seen in studies begun after 1941.

They attribute this in part to the use of antibiotics, which resulted in the virtual elimination of aphasia and hemiplegia in children as a consequence of complications from scarlet fever, measles, diphtheria, and other diseases. Studies had shown that these infections, if severe and untreated, could produce localized brain lesions as well as diffuse damage to both hemispheres. A child who showed both left hemiplegia and aphasia after such an infection probably would have been classified as a right-hemisphere case, when, in fact, the left hemisphere was most likely also affected. The investigators concluded that the incidence of aphasia after right-hemisphere lesions in children had been greatly overestimated and that the data as a whole supported the idea that the pattern of language functions seen in adults is essentially complete soon after birth.

Thus, recent clinical evidence suggests that hemispheric specialization for language is present at birth and does not develop over time. This conclusion, however, does not question in any way what we know about the ability of the right hemisphere to take over language functions after very early lesions of the left hemisphere. We know that there are dramatic differences in recovery from aphasia in children and in adults, and we will consider the theoretical implications of this finding later in this chapter. What is called into question is the postulation of an initial active role of the right hemisphere in speech production in normal children.

## AGE AND ASYMMETRY: THE SEARCH FOR THE BEGINNINGS OF LATERALIZATION

Clinical evidence dealing with the effects of early brain damage on language functions has played a central role in shaping current thinking about the development of asymmetry. Several other sources of evidence bearing on this issue are also available, and we turn now to consider them.

### Dichotic Listening in the Crib

Many dichotic listening studies have sought to determine the earliest age at which the right-ear advantage may be found. This technique, discussed at length in Chapter 3, involves the presentation of two different speech messages simultaneously, one to each ear. Subjects are typically asked to report what was heard, a procedure that obviously places a lower limit on the age of the children who can be tested. The standard dichotic listening test has been used with children as young as 3, though, and a right-ear superiority has been found.[6]

More recently, ingenious methods have been used to take the dichotic technique to the crib to determine if infants show a right-ear advantage. In one study, infants averaging 50 days of age first learned to suck on a nipple in order to receive dichotic presentations of a pair of words. Each time the infant sucked with a previously specified force, the same words were presented to them. This procedure continued until the infant habituated to the dichotic pair, as evidenced by a sustained reduction in the sucking rate. At this point, either the left-ear stimulus or the right-ear stimulus was changed, and the investigator monitored the infant for changes in sucking rate. The results of this study showed that the infant noticed a change in either ear (the sucking rate increased), but a change in the right ear produced a larger increase in sucking.[7]

Work by other investigators has shown that infants typically increase their rate of sucking when a novel stimulus is presented. The results with the dichotic speech stimuli, then, suggest that the difference between old and new stimuli is easier to detect in the right ear — a right-ear advantage. A similar study by the same investigator found a greater increase following left-ear change when nonspeech stimuli were used. This is further evidence that the "ear difference" in the dichotic task reflects brain asymmetry.

Although this modification of the dichotic paradigm is ingenious and encouraging to those who believe lateralization of function is present at birth, other investigators have had difficulty replicating the findings. One study repeated the work with speech stimuli modifying the procedures slightly to prevent inadvertent experimenter bias.* That study failed to obtain evidence of differences in the sucking rate in response to stimuli changed in either ear.[8] Further work is needed to determine whether ear asymmetries can be found in newborns.

Attempts have also been made to see whether the magnitude of the ear advantage in the standard dichotic task changes with age. Perhaps the beginnings of lateralization of function are present at birth, and the degree of asymmetry increases as the child matures. Results on this issue are not clear-cut. Some investigators have reported that the asymmetry does not change between 5 and 12 years of age; others have noted differences over that period.[9]

---

*Experimenter bias is a potential problem in all behavioral research that does not strictly control for it. In the study just discussed, the experimenter working with the infant was not "blind" to the order of stimulus conditions; that is, the investigator knew which ear received a change in sound stimuli on a particular trial. Thus, the experimenter may have inadvertently influenced the infant to respond in the predicted direction. In the attempted replication of this work, the interaction of experimenter and infant was reduced to a minimum, and the experimenter present in the room with the infant had no knowledge of the particular condition being tested at any given time.

## Evoked Potentials In Infants

Because electrophysiological recording techniques do not require a deliberate response of any sort from the subject, they are ideally suited to the study of hemispheric asymmetries in infants. Psychologist Dennis Molfese was one of the first investigators to find evidence of asymmetries in the electrical recordings of the left brain and the right brain in neonates. In one study, he and his collaborators presented speech sounds, such as "ba," to infants ranging in age from 1 week to 10 months while they recorded evoked potential (EP) activity from both hemispheres.[10] They found responses of greater amplitude, presumably reflecting greater involvement in the processing of the sounds, on the left side in 9 of the 10 infants tested. The effect held for the youngest infants as well as for the older ones. The one infant showing a reversal was 8 months of age. When Molfese presented the infants with certain nonspeech sounds, such as a noise burst or a piano chord, the opposite results were obtained: all 10 infants showed EPs of greater amplitude in the right hemisphere.

These findings are exciting because they suggest that although a newborn may not "understand" what is being presented, the brain is already equipped with specialized centers that will be responsible for processing the sounds at deeper levels later in life.

Wada and Davis have taken another approach to the study of EP asymmetries in infants. "If fundamental asymmetry of the neurocircuit exists before the development of language and speech function," they note, "then we ought to be able to disclose such a difference without using verbal stimuli."[11] Wada and Davis recorded the EP to clicks and flashes of light and measured the *coherence*, or similarity of the forms, of the EP in the temporal and occipital regions of the brain in infants.

In earlier work with adult patients tested with sodium amobarbital, they had observed that coherence was largest for clicks in the speech-dominant hemisphere and for flashes in the non-speech-dominant hemisphere. Similar results were found in their study of 50 infants ranging in age from 1 day to 5 weeks. Findings indicated that the forms of the occipital and temporal responses to clicks were more similar within the left half of the brain than the right half; the similarity shifted toward the right hemisphere when flashes were presented. The investigators argued that their findings reflect the specialization of the two hemispheres for processing different kinds of information and that this specialization is present at birth.

## Head-Turning in Infants

Newborns are very limited in the range of behavior they demonstrate, leaving little opportunity to observe any lateral preferences such as hand usage. However, infants do turn their heads to the left and right, and thus the frequency of left-side turns and right-side turns becomes a measure of potential interest. Several studies have shown that infants just a few days old show a marked preference for right-side head turns.[12] Although the meaning of this preference has not been firmly established, there is some preliminary suggestion that it may be related to hand preference later in life.

One group of investigators has reported a statistically significant correlation between direction of head turning in infancy and lateral preference at age 7, although the correlation is not large.[13] There are at least two possible explanations for this relationship. The first holds that head-turning preference in infancy affects the subsequent development of hand preference. For example, those infants who prefer to turn their heads to the right would see their right hands more often than their left hands. This might result in better eye–hand coordination with the right hand, leading to a preference for the right hand in visually guided reaching. A second possibility is that both head-turning preference and later hand preference are related because they are determined by the same set of brain mechanisms.

## Anatomical Asymmetries in Infants

Other evidence to support the idea that brain asymmetry has its origin early in life comes from anatomical studies in fetuses and infants. In the largest study, 207 brains were measured. Ages ranged from 10 to 44 weeks after conception. A longer left temporal plane was present in 54 percent of the brains; the relationship was reversed in 18 percent of the cases. In 28 percent no significant difference in the size of the temporal plane was observed between the two sides.[14]

In another large study of 100 brains, comparable results were found. The mean age in this study was 48 weeks, including the gestational period. The left-temporal plane was 77 percent larger, on the average, than the right-temporal plane. There were 12 infants with the right side larger than the left side and 32 with approximately equal measurements on the left and the right.[15]

In an interesting twist, anatomists have shown that parts of the right hemisphere develop more rapidly than corresponding parts of the left during the fetal stage of human life. The folding of the cortex into the characteristic convoluted shape of the brain's surface takes place earlier and proceeds faster in the right temporal lobe than in the left. Right-sided folding may occur as much as two weeks ahead of folding on the left. Although the left-hemisphere language regions may develop more slowly than equivalent right-hemisphere regions, they ultimately reach a greater size and complexity of organization.[16] Investigators have speculated that the relative slowness of development of the left hemisphere may be an example of the principle that slowly developing structures in the brain ultimately become larger and better.[17] (See Chapter 4 for a discussion of related issues.)

Once again, however, there is a major difficulty in interpreting such anatomical studies. We do not know the precise nature of the relationship between anatomical asymmetry and functional asymmetry. Is the former the structural basis of the latter? If so, are functional differences between the hemispheres operative whenever we find anatomical differences? Only when additional information is available to help answer these questions will we be able to interpret the asymmetry data with confidence. Until then, the evidence will remain suggestive and intriguing but by no means a complete answer to the issue of whether lateralization of function is present at birth.

## HEMISPHERECTOMY IN INFANCY: REMOVING HALF A BRAIN

Occasionally, it is medically necessary to remove most of one cerebral hemisphere. We discussed in Chapter 6 some of the consequences of hemispherectomy in adults. The operation is also done early in infancy when extensive damage to one hemisphere threatens to impair the function of the undamaged side as well.

Reports of several dozen hemispherectomy cases have appeared in the literature and serve as a source of information on the development of hemispheric asymmetry of function. The consequences of the operation are a function of the age of the patient at the time of the surgery and of which hemisphere is removed. As we discussed, adult patients with the right hemisphere removed typically show little or no language impairment, but the removal of the left hemisphere generally results in marked aphasia that improves only slightly with time. Similar lateralized effects occur in children. The severity of impairment is directly related, and the prognosis for recovery of language is inversely related, to the age of the child at the time of surgery.[18]

Several reports have noted that if surgery is performed early enough in infancy, no signs of lateralized deficits in higher mental functions remain in adulthood. This finding suggests that the remaining hemisphere, whether it is the left or the right, is able to take over for the hemisphere that is removed and to perform those functions that ordinarily would be lateralized to the other half of the brain.

It is possible to draw at least two different theoretical conclusions from these data. One is that no shift of functions has taken place in early hemispherectomy cases because lateralization of function is not present in early infancy. A second interpretation is that hemispheric differences are present early in infancy, but the young brain has a tremendous ability to reorganize itself in the face of damage to specific regions.

Some recent, in-depth studies of the abilities of patients with left and right hemispherectomies suggest that of the two possibilities, the latter "plasticity" explanation is more likely to be correct. Maureen Dennis and Harry Whitaker tested early hemispherectomy patients on various language tests and found very subtle signs of lateralized effects.[19] Standard measures of verbal intelligence do not seem to differentiate between early left and early right hemispherectomy. This does not mean, though, that other tests might not reveal a difference.

Dennis and Whitaker studied three 9- to 10-year-olds who had undergone hemispherectomy by the age of 5 months. One was a right-hemispherectomy patient; the other two had had the left hemisphere removed. Results showed that both discrimination and articulation of the sounds of speech were normal in all three children. The three were also equally good at producing and discriminating words. Important differences between the hemispheres, though, appeared in tests of the patients' ability to deal with syntax — the rules for combining words into grammatically correct sentences. For example, each child was asked to judge the acceptability of the following sentences:

1. I paid the money by the man.
2. I was paid the money to the lady.
3. I was paid the money by the boy.

The right-hemispherectomy patient correctly indicated that sentences 1 and 2 are grammatically incorrect and that sentence 3 is acceptable. The two left-hemispherectomy patients did not make these distinctions.

The researchers concluded that the right hemisphere in the left-hemispherectomy cases does not accurately comprehend the meaning of passive sentences. Other tests led them to conclude that the right-hemisphere defect is an organizational, analytical, and syntactical problem, rather than one rooted in the conceptual or semantic aspects of language. The results suggest that there are limits to the plasticity of the infant brain and, more importantly for our purposes, that the asymmetries between the hemispheres are present very early in life.

Dennis and Whitaker's conclusions, however, have been criticized as premature considering the evidence presented in support of them. Dorothy Bishop has noted problems with the statistical analysis used, as well as with the absence of appropriate control groups against which to compare patients' performance.[20] Bishop notes that later studies showed that the sole right-hemispherectomy patient studied by Dennis and Whitaker did better than most other right-hemispherectomy patients in a variety of linguistic tasks, and that it is unsound to use one patient as the sole standard against which to evaluate the linguistic abilities of the left-hemispherectomy patients. Bishop argues for caution in accepting Dennis and Whitaker's conclusions until stronger data are presented.

It may well be the case that data definitively showing the limits of plasticity eventually will be provided. These limits, however, whatever they may be, do not detract from the very important role plasticity plays in much of the dramatic recovery from aphasia that is found after left-hemisphere damage in children. The ability of a brain to readjust its function relatively quickly makes it hard to distinguish between a system in which lateralization does not exist or exists only in rudimentary form and one in which lateralization is extensive but rapid compensation for unilateral damage is possible. Only through the use of very sensitive tests designed to measure subtle differences in performance can we begin to tease apart these alternatives.

## DOES LATERALIZATION CHANGE OVER TIME?

A good deal of the evidence just reviewed suggests that hemispheric differences, both functional and anatomical, are present at birth.

What changes in this early lateralization take place as the infant matures? How, if at all, does asymmetry change over the life span of a human being?

The brain of most mammals, including humans, is largely under-developed at birth and undergoes a major portion of its structural and functional maturation during infancy and early childhood. In addition to its obvious growth, the brain undergoes dramatic changes at the microscopic level. The connections between neurons multiply tremendously in the first few years and are thought to continue changing throughout a person's lifetime. In addition, insu-lating fatty layers called myelin are laid down around nerve fibers, making them more efficient conductors of electrical impulses.

The corpus callosum is present at birth but appears disproportion-ately small in cross section when the brain of a newborn is compared with the brain of an adult. Figure 8.1 shows the growth of the cerebral commissures during three stages of human development. Some investigators feel that the slow maturation of the neocortex and the interhemispheric fibers leads to differential development of the two sides of the brain during the postnatal period.[21]

The fact that the effects of unilateral brain damage occurring early in life contrast with the effects of later damage certainly suggests that important changes in the brain occur with time. Language impair-ments after damage to the left hemisphere generally are less severe and of shorter duration the younger the individual at the time of the injury. Does this imply that lateralization becomes more extensive or complete with age? Not necessarily. Another interpretation of these brain-damage findings is that the plasticity of the brain decreases with age — that is, as the individual grows older, the right hemi-sphere loses the ability to take over the control of language.

To answer the question of whether lateralization itself changes with age, we must obtain measures of lateralization in subjects of different ages and compare the degree of asymmetry present in each age group. This approach has been used most extensively in investi-gations of dichotic listening. The pattern of findings, unfortunately, is not consistent. For example, one large study using 30 children at each of five ages (5, 7, 9, 11, and 13) in a dichotic consonant–vowel task found a right-ear advantage across all age groups, with the magnitude of the ear asymmetry consistent at all age levels.[22] In contrast, another study using 24 subjects in each of five age groups (6, 7, 10, 12, and 14) found an increase in the magnitude of the ear asymmetry over this age range. The right-ear advantage was signifi-

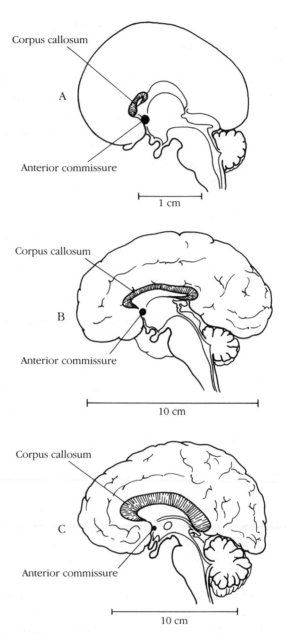

**Figure 8.1** The corpus callosum and anterior commissure at three stages of human development. A. Fetal (16 weeks). B. At birth (40 weeks). C. Adult. [From Trevarthen, "Cerebral Embryology and the Split Brain," Fig. XI-7, pp. 228–229 in *Hemisphere Disconnection and Cerebral Function*, ed. M. Kinsbourne and L. Smith, Springfield, IL: Charles C. Thomas, 1974]

cantly different from zero, in fact, in the 12- and 14-year-old groups only.[23] The stimuli employed were syllables, as in the previous experiment. In a review paper dealing with the issue of developmental change, the authors tallied four dichotic listening studies showing an increase in asymmetry over this time period and five showing either a mild decrease or a plateau after 3 to 5 years of age.[24]

Other measures have also been used to address the question of change in lateralization with age. Molfese's study of EPs to speech and nonspeech stimuli mentioned earlier in this chapter also involved children between 4 and 11 years of age and adults 23 to 29 years old.[25] Analyses showed that the asymmetry in the size of the EP to the nonspeech stimuli was proportionately greater in the infants than in the children and adults. The speech stimuli resulted in a comparable asymmetry in the infants and children, whereas both groups showed greater asymmetry in response to these stimuli than did the adults. The authors suggest that the EP asymmetry may decline with age because of the maturation of the cerebral commissures that connect the hemispheres. To support their argument, they cite anatomical studies showing that the corpus callosum is incompletely developed at birth.

We noted earlier that anatomical asymmetries have been found in infant brains. One study used both infant and adult brains measured in a manner permitting comparison of the degree of asymmetry in the two groups. By expressing the size of the right temporal plane as a percentage of the size of the left-temporal plane, a measure independent of absolute size is derived. The investigators could then directly compare the infant and adult series. The average R/L ratio was 67 percent for infants and 55 percent for adults, indicating a greater degree of asymmetry in the adults.[26] These findings suggest that the asymmetry in the size of the temporal plane in the two hemispheres increases with age.

Given the variability in outcome of studies using different methodologies, as well as the variability found in studies using the same measure of lateralization, it is clearly premature to draw conclusions regarding change in asymmetry with age. Further research using more refined measures of lateralization should provide the answers. It would also be valuable to investigate hemispheric asymmetries over the entire life span to see if the aging process differentially affects the hemispheres. This is an area in which very little work has been done.

## A MODEL OF BRAIN LATERALIZATION

Sandra Witelson has presented an interesting model of brain lateralization that bears on the issues we have been considering.[27] She takes
the position that hemispheric specialization is present from birth for
both hemispheres, and that the essential processing difference between the two hemispheres does not change over development.
Although there may be an increase in the number and nature of
cognitive skills that appear to be lateralized, she argues, what is
actually occurring is an increase in the amount and nature of cognitive processes that are available to be mediated asymmetrically by the
brain.

Witelson suggests that some fundamental differences in information processing may characterize the basic differences between the
hemispheres at birth, and that later asymmetries may be reflections
of this earliest one as newly acquired cognitive skills draw on it. She
notes that both behavioral and anatomical evidence for hemispheric
asymmetry is present before the onset of speech production and
language comprehension; thus, processes more basic than language
must be the essence of hemispheric differences.

In Chapter 12 we present a more detailed discussion of specific
ideas about the underlying nature of hemispheric differences.

## THE ROLES OF NATURE AND NURTURE IN THE
## ESTABLISHMENT OF ASYMMETRIES

### Nature

Much of the evidence reviewed in this chapter suggests that
hemispheric asymmetries in some form are present at or near birth.
The earlier the age at which asymmetries are detected, the more
confident we may be that they are part of the biological makeup of
the organism and independent of experience.*

Several genetic models have been proposed to account for hemispheric asymmetries. We reviewed some of them in Chapter 5 in the
context of our discussion of handedness. One model, for example,
postulates separate genes coding for left-hemisphere and right-hemi-

---

*Asymmetries occurring later may also be part of an organism's biological makeup.
Genetic factors may determine the emergence of asymmetries in later stages of
development.

sphere dominance; another holds that only left-hemisphere dominance is controlled genetically.

More recently, some investigators have begun to consider other
ways, not genetic in the strict sense, in which patterns of lateralization may be inherited. Research has shown that cytoplasm, the fluid
contained in all cells, including the maternal egg, can transmit certain
traits from parent to offspring in some species. Such "cytoplasmic
inheritance" has been proposed as a possible basis for the transmission of asymmetry from parent to offspring in human beings.[28] This
is the mechanism that Corballis and Morgan proposed to account
for the gradient underlying differential development of the left side
of the embryo in different species (see Chapter 5).

Because brain asymmetry is not easily observable, it is difficult to
evaluate these various models. Different measures of hemispheric
asymmetry are available, yet the measures do not always agree in
terms of the direction and degree of asymmetry they reveal in a given
subject. Philip Bryden has conducted a family study of dichotic
listening performance in which he obtained ear-advantage scores for
parents and offspring in 49 families. Results showed significantly
positive correlations between parents and offspring in ear asymmetry
but negative correlations between siblings.

Both genetic and cytoplasmic models of inheritance would predict positive correlations between siblings as well as parents and
offspring. Bryden notes, however, that the ear-asymmetry score is far
from an ideal index of hemispheric differences and that until better
measures are developed it will be difficult to rigorously test models
of the inheritance of lateralization of function.[29]

Some additional evidence suggestive of the role of heredity has
come from a recent study looking at a different measure of asymmetry, head-turning preference in newborns. The investigators
found that the direction of infants' head-turning response to stimuli
presented simultaneously to the left and to the right of the infant
was biased to the right in infants with two right-handed parents but
not in those with a non–right-handed parent.[30] Because the infants
were only a few days old, it is presumed that learning could not have
played a role in determining preference.

### Nurture

What can be said about the role of experience or environmental
factors in determining hemispheric asymmetries? At one extreme, we
have seen that early damage to one hemisphere of the brain can

result in a dramatic reorganization of lateralized functions. The fact that persons with the left hemisphere removed in infancy develop language skills in the right hemisphere is but one piece of evidence pointing to the tremendous plasticity of the brain. The compensation for early removal of one hemisphere, however, is not total. Sensitive tests reveal language deficits, suggesting that the basic blueprint for asymmetry is present very early in life and that its traces remain despite damage-induced reorganization. In our discussions of left-handedness, we noted that some investigators believe all left-handedness (and presumably all right-hemisphere control of speech) is a result of brain injury, however subtle. Other evidence, however, has suggested that the quality and quantity of exposure to language itself may affect the development of lateralization.

*Socioeconomic Factors* Several studies have looked at the effect of socioeconomic class (SEC) on hemispheric asymmetries as measured by behavioral tests. In one experiment, 104 right-handed children, ranging in age from 4 to 7 years and from low-SEC backgrounds were matched for age and sex with 104 right-handed children from middle-SEC homes. All were given a dichotic digits test. Results revealed a significant right-ear superiority in the 4-, 5-, 6-, and 7-year-old children from the middle-SEC group, whereas only the 7-year-olds from the low-SEC group showed a right-ear advantage.[31]

In another study, a right-ear advantage was found in both low-SEC and middle-SEC children, but the middle-SEC children showed right-ear advantages of significantly greater magnitude.[32] SEC differences in the ear asymmetry have not been found in all studies that have looked for them.[33] If the differences are real, they suggest that environmental factors correlated with SEC affect lateralization of function.

*Exposure to Language* A very different type of finding that also points to early environment as a factor in asymmetry is based on the study of Genie, an adolescent girl who endured 11$^1$/$_2$ years of extreme social and experiential deprivation. Genie was discovered at the age of 13$^1$/$_2$, after having spent most of her life in almost complete isolation, during which time she was punished for making any noise whatsoever. Two years after she was found, she was reported to have made slow but steady progress in language learning. This fact is of considerable significance for the theoretical issue of whether a first language may be acquired after puberty.

Of particular interest to us here, though, is Genie's performance on dichotic listening tests. Two special tests were prepared for her. One was composed of familiar words, the other of familiar environmental sounds. Genie was able to identify correctly each of these stimuli when she was tested one ear at a time. This finding is typical. When the words were presented dichotically, however, her performance departed markedly from what was expected. Instead of the moderate right-ear advantage that is generally found in right-handed subjects, Genie showed an extreme left-ear advantage. Her left ear performed perfectly, while the performance of her right ear was at chance level. For the environmental sounds, Genie showed a small left-ear advantage, in keeping with the prediction that such sounds are processed more efficiently in the right hemisphere.[34]

On the basis of dichotic listening performance, then, it appears that the processing of both language and nonlanguage stimuli is taking place in Genie's right hemisphere. The investigators working with her have argued that her left hemisphere may have begun language acquisition before her confinement but through disuse was no longer able to fulfill its original function. As Genie began to learn language a second time, the right hemisphere assumed control because its functions presumably had been exercised (by visuo-spatial processes) in spite of her confinement.

The problem with a single subject study such as this is that there is no way of knowing the pattern of asymmetry that would have developed in Genie's brain had she had a normal childhood. Perhaps she would have shown right-hemisphere specialization for language and nonlanguage stimuli anyway. Nevertheless, the results are intriguing, especially in light of work looking at hemispheric asymmetry in the congenitally deaf.

Walter McKeever and his colleagues at Bowling Green State University in Ohio have used tachistoscopic presentation to compare the degree of lateral asymmetry in normal subjects and in congenitally deaf persons.[35] They argued that if experience with auditory stimuli plays a major causal role in the lateralization of language, congenitally deaf persons should show smaller visual-field differences for linguistic stimuli than hearing subjects. In several different tasks with words and letters as stimuli, they found that both groups showed a right-visual-field superiority in identification, but the differences were considerably smaller for the congenitally deaf subjects. This finding has been replicated by others.[36] They concluded that auditory experience is a major determinant of lateralization of visual language processing in humans.

Using pictures of the manual signs used by the deaf, several studies have found a left-visual-field superiority in the congenitally deaf.[37] Before concluding that the pattern of hemispheric asymmetry is reversed in the deaf, however, it is important to note that manual signs have a considerable spatial component and that this may be responsible for the right-visual-field advantage.

This hypothesis was tested in a study using congenitally deaf subjects born to deaf parents.[38] These subjects showed a right-visual-field superiority for signs that were alphabetical and a left-visual-field superiority for meaningless signs. Hearing subjects, in contrast, showed a left-visual-field superiority for both. The investigators concluded that auditory experience is unnecessary for normal development of left-hemisphere language specialization.

We are still left, however, with the finding that deaf subjects show a reduced right-visual-field advantage for letters and words. At this point, the conflicting evidence points to the need for further research to clarify the role of auditory experience in language lateralization.

*The Bilingual Brain* Our discussions of hemispheric asymmetry, to this point, have been limited to patterns of brain organization in monolinguals, or individuals fluent in one language. Does the experience of acquiring two languages change those patterns? This question is currently the subject of considerable controversy. Evidence has come from case studies of bilingual persons who have become aphasic as well as from experimental studies using such measures as tachistoscopic presentation, dichotic listening, and electrophysiological recording. A number of studies have concluded that the left hemisphere is dominant for processing the native language as well as the non-native language of the bilingual speaker. Other studies, however, have reported weaker left lateralization for language among bilinguals; still others have reported differential hemispheric asymmetry for language in the bilingual speaker. A recent review by Loraine Obler and her colleagues has identified some important factors that must be considered in conducting or evaluating research in this area.[39]

Subject-selection factors are critical. Obler notes that a great number of studies have not specified the criteria used to screen subjects for proficiency in their two languages. According to one hypothesis, bilinguals will rely on the right hemisphere to a greater extent in second-language processing in the early stages of learning, but as proficiency increases, the left hemisphere will be engaged to a greater extent. Linguistic analysis of beginning second-language learning forms the basis for this hypothesis. Beginning learners, for example, rely more on content than on function words and more on prosodic (rhythmic) features than on phonetic features in speech comprehension—components believed to be within the competence of the right hemisphere. To ideally test this hypothesis, a study would trace the relative participation of the two hemispheres of a group of learners at various levels of proficiency in their second language. Because of the difficulties in conducting such research, investigators have relied on a cross sectional approach looking at different groups of subjects differing in proficiency. In a review of the dichotic listening and tachistoscopic studies that have looked at proficiency, Jyotsna Vaid and Fred Genesee, of McGill University, note that three experimental studies have provided evidence for what has become known as the stage hypothesis, whereas six have reported an equivalent pattern of hemispheric asymmetry in both first and second languages of nonproficient bilinguals.[40]

Another factor identified by Obler is the age at second-language acquisition. She notes that proficiency is often confounded with age; proficient bilinguals typically acquire both languages during infancy, whereas nonproficient bilinguals typically begin second-language acquisition during adolescence or later. If the two languages of a bilingual are acquired successively, the maturational state of the brain will be different during first- and second-language acquisition. In addition, there may be differences in the processing strategies used during first- and second-language acquisition. Together, these two factors lead to the prediction that hemispheric asymmetry in bilinguals will more closely resemble that of monolinguals the earlier the acquisition of a second language takes place. Vaid and Genesee cite seven experimental studies relevant to this hypothesis, with five supporting the hypothesis that hemispheric processing of language in early bilinguals resembles the pattern found in monolinguals, while late second-language acquisition engages the hemispheres differently. In one study, EPs were recorded from the left and the right hemispheres of French–English bilingual adults during a language recognition task. The latency of components of the EPs was shorter in the left hemispheres of bilinguals who had acquired their second language in infancy or early childhood but shorter in the right hemispheres of bilinguals who had acquired the second language after age 12.[41]

The manner of second-language acquisition also has been identified as a factor that may affect the pattern of hemispheric asymmetry for a second language. One hypothesis holds that there will be less left-hemisphere participation if second-language acquisition is informal (attention to content rather than form) and greater left-hemisphere involvement if acquisition is formal (emphasis on rule isolation and error correction). Vaid and Genesee cite several experimental studies consistent with this hypothesis, although the effect of manner of acquisition varied with age and proficiency in these studies.

The nature of the relationship between hemispheric asymmetry and bilingualism is clearly complex. As a result, the controversy surrounding this issue is likely to continue until reasons for the variation from study to study are identified and explained.


## IN SUMMARY

Although investigators are far from having definite answers to the questions posed in this chapter, a pattern of findings is emerging.

Of great theoretical significance are the observations suggesting that hemispheric differences are present at birth. In apparent conflict with the lateralization-at-birth view is clinical evidence showing that the effects of very early unilateral brain damage do not vary as a function of the side of injury. The latter data, though, are compatible with the lateralization-at-birth position if we take into account the plasticity that allows the young brain to compensate for the effects of damage. In this context, we pointed to the importance of tests that are very sensitive to subtle impairment and could perhaps differentiate between the results of damage-induced reorganization and the absence of lateralization in the first place (presuming damage-induced reorganization is in some way less than optimal).

Research investigating the time course of lateralization and the factors that affect it is difficult for several reasons. First, our measures of laterality are far from perfect. Does failing to find differences between the hemispheres mean such differences do not exist? Can we be sure that we have not simply failed to set up conditions that would allow us to detect a real difference?

A related issue is that many tests apparently are sensitive to factors other than brain lateralization. In Chapter 3, we discussed how differences in the way a task is approached can dramatically affect the type of asymmetry observed in behavioral tests. Perhaps any differences found in hemispheric asymmetry as a function of age reflect different strategies adopted by the subjects rather than differences in lateralization per se.

A second major problem in studying factors involved in lateralization is related to the difficulty of answering nature–nurture questions with human beings in general. We are severely limited in the kinds of environmental effects that can be studied, and genetic models frequently cannot be adequately tested.

The state of affairs is a challenging one for which there are no simple solutions. As more and more investigators appreciate the significance of developmental issues and the care with which they have to be investigated, we can expect progress toward some answers.

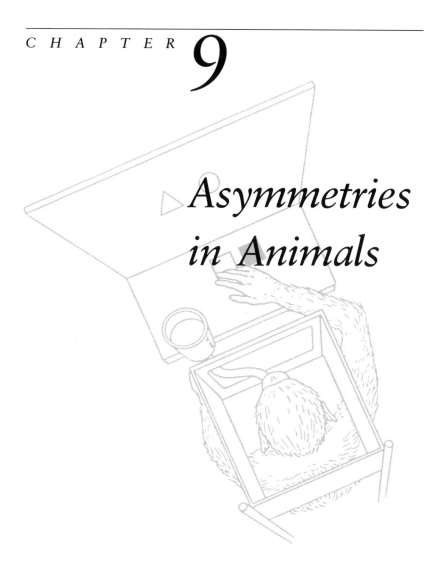

# CHAPTER 9

# Asymmetries in Animals

Do animals show any evidence of lateral asymmetries similar to those found in humans? Do differences exist between the left brain and the right brain in creatures other than human beings? These questions bear on some issues critical to our understanding of hemispheric differences. At the core of questions about asymmetries in animals is the assumption that laterality is a true biological trait that can be studied in much the same way as other biological phenomena, such as color vision and digestion, and that precursors of human laterality will be found by studying other species.

Although most research in laterality during the past 100 years has tacitly assumed that laterality is a biological characteristic, only within the last 20 have active efforts been made to study its biological foundations. Research on anatomical asymmetries in the brain (see Chapter 4) and Geschwind and Galaburda's immunological theory of left-handedness (see Chapter 5) are examples of this new biological approach. So are the studies of laterality in animals that are presented in this chapter.

Research demonstrating the existence of hemispheric asymmetries in animals would have important implications for our understanding of the origin and significance of asymmetry in humans. Some investigators have argued that brain asymmetry is intimately related to higher linguistic abilities. The presence of hemispheric differences in nonlinguistic animals would suggest that this view is not correct. The asymmetries found may then provide clues to the actual evolutionary basis for brain asymmetry. On the other hand, convincing evidence pointing to the absence of asymmetries, even in the closest evolutionary relatives of human beings, would argue that brain asymmetry is unique to *Homo sapiens* and may be fundamentally related to language ability.

On a practical level, research on hemispheric differences in human beings would progress more rapidly if it were possible to study similar asymmetries in animals. Experiments on brain asymmetry involving surgical and environmental manipulations that are not possible with people could be conducted with animals showing hemispheric specialization.

In this chapter, we review evidence that has emerged from the search for asymmetries in animals. The data, although often conflicting or inconclusive, are often tantalizing and inspire speculation about the origin of brain asymmetries.

## WHICH PAW DOES YOUR DOG SHAKE HANDS WITH?

The most obvious sign of lateralization in humans is handedness. Thus, investigators have looked for paw or limb preferences in animals as evidence of brain lateralization, and they have found that many species do show such preferences.[1] Cats typically use one paw in tasks that involve reaching for an object. Monkeys too use one limb predominantly in unimanual tasks. Even mice show consistent preferences in a task in which they must use one paw at a time to reach for food.

Although the pattern of limb preference in a given animal bears some resemblance to hand preference shown by human beings, there is an important difference. Approximately 50 percent of cats, monkeys, and mice show a preference for the right paw, and 50 percent show a preference for the left paw. This is strikingly different from the breakdown found in human beings — 90 percent right-hand preference, ten percent left-hand preference.

The 50–50 split in animals has led some investigators to propose that paw preferences are the result of chance factors. According to this hypothesis, the limb first used by an animal is determined by chance. The additional dexterity gained as a result of the experience increases the probability that the same limb will be used again. This kind of use–dexterity loop rapidly produces preference for that limb in the animal under consideration. Some support for such a mechanism has come from geneticist Robert Collins' work with paw preference in mice, which was discussed briefly in Chapter 5 when we considered the factors that determine handedness.

Collins compared the predictions of the chance, environmental model of paw preference with predictions that follow from the assumption that paw preference has a genetic basis. If a trait is under genetic control, it should be possible to select for it. That is, if individuals with the trait are selectively mated, each successive generation should show a higher incidence of the trait. If the trait is determined by chance, however, no such increase across generations should occur.

Collins began his study by mating mice that shared the same paw preference. In the next generation, he mated those offspring who showed the same paw preference as the parents. After repeating this selective inbreeding three times, Collins looked at the proportion of left-pawed and right-pawed offspring in the last generation. He found a 50–50 split, the same proportion he had started with in generation 1.[2]

Collins interpreted his data as evidence against genetic control of lateral preference in mice and argued that chance is the determining factor in such preferences. His data, of course, address only the question of the basis for paw preference in mice. Selective inbreeding studies have not been reported for other animals. However, we can say with some assurance that the favored paw in animals showing a preference is equally likely to be the left or the right. Human beings appear to be the only animals with lateral preferences strongly biased in one direction.

Although the paw-preference data are not particularly encouraging for those seeking evidence of fundamental hemispheric asymmetries in animals, it is important to remember that the relationship between hand preference and hemispheric specialization in human beings is also less than clear-cut. With this in mind, investigators have turned to more direct tests of hemispheric asymmetry of function in animals. They frequently employ the same approaches that have proved useful in studying brain asymmetries in human beings.

## DAMAGE TO ONE HEMISPHERE: ARE THE EFFECTS ASYMMETRICAL?

Many studies have focused on the kinds of deficits in behavior that follow surgical lesions in specific brain structures. In general, deficits following lesions on one side only (unilateral lesions) are less serious than those that follow bilateral brain damage, regardless of which side the lesion is on. In monkeys, for example, studies have shown that visual discriminations involving color, shape, and orientation are disturbed equally by lesions in a particular region of the left or the right hemisphere and that the deficits are independent of the monkey's limb preferences.[3] Figure 9.1 shows a typical visual discrimination test. Deficits in the discrimination of complex sequences of

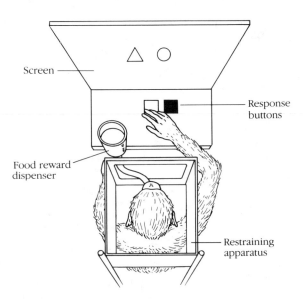

**Figure 9.1** Visual discrimination training. A monkey is positioned in front of a screen and a panel containing several buttons. The animal receives a reward, such as a raisin, if it presses the black button when a pair of similarly shaped figures appear on the screen. It is also rewarded for pressing the white button if the figures are dissimilar.

auditory stimuli after damage to the auditory region also have been shown to be independent of the side of the lesion.[4]

More recently, however, James Dewson of Stanford University has reported some evidence for hemispheric asymmetry in monkeys in a complex, cross-modal matching task.[5] In this task, monkeys are taught to push a red light after hearing a tone and a green light after hearing a brief noise. The test is conducted with varying delays between the presentation of the noise or tone and the appearance of the lights. The task is a difficult one for monkeys, particularly at delay intervals of as long as 15 seconds.

Dewson taught the task to six monkeys and then removed part of the temporal lobe on one side of the brain in each of the six. After surgery, the four monkeys with lesions on the left side could no longer do the task when the delays were longer than 2 seconds. The two monkeys with right-side lesions continued to perform normally, even at the longest delays.

Dewson's data suggest that animals, or at least monkeys, do show some evidence of hemispheric specialization. Why is it that other lesion studies have not produced similar results?

Charles Hamilton of the California Institute of Technology reviewed the evidence on asymmetries in animals and makes two important points.[6] First, the Dewson study and some other studies that have reported asymmetries are based on a very small number of animals. The results are suggestive but cannot be considered definitive until they are replicated on larger numbers of animal subjects.*

Hamilton's second point is the importance of the tasks used to study hemispheric asymmetry in animals. He notes that many experiments, particularly those involving visual discrimination of simple patterns and objects, would probably fail to reveal evidence of hemispheric asymmetry in human beings. What is needed are tasks that are sufficiently complex to tap the brain asymmetries that may exist in animals. Dewson's delayed cross-modal matching task certainly meets the criterion of complexity, but it is a difficult one for monkeys to learn.

## SPLIT-BRAIN RESEARCH WITH ANIMALS

Split-brain studies are also used to test for hemispheric specialization in animals. We have already considered at some length what has been

---

*Type I errors are a problem in animal studies as well as in laterality research with humans; the best safeguard against such errors is successful replication.

learned about brain asymmetry from split-brain studies with human beings. We noted that findings from animal research played an important role in the decision to try split-brain surgery with epileptic patients. More recently, the dramatic results of human split-brain research have led to a renewed interest in the work of investigators searching for brain asymmetries in other species.

In principle, split-brain research is ideal for this purpose. Cutting the fiber bands that connect the two hemispheres allows the investigator to study separately the abilities of each half of the same brain. Except for possible hemispheric differences, which are the object of the research in the first place, both hemispheres are genetically identical and have been exposed to the same environmental influences.

In contrast to research with human patients, limited by necessity to persons with epilepsy (generally of long standing), animal studies may be done with healthy animals with two intact hemispheres. Interpretation of any differences that might be found is therefore much more clear-cut. In addition, split-brain research avoids the problem of inferring the function of specific regions of the brain from the effects of lesions in those areas. Lastly, in lesion studies, investigators must have some idea in advance about which parts of the brain control specific functions. In split-brain work, it is not necessary to localize a function to a specific region; the performance of the whole hemisphere is studied.

What are the results of studies with monkeys and cats investigating the relative abilities of the two hemispheres to learn and perform different types of problems? Results from tests of simple pattern discrimination suggest that the two hemispheres possess similar learning capabilities.[7] A few studies have reported quantitative differences between the hemispheres in learning and performance. However, there are no consistent differences favoring one hemisphere in these studies.[8] The absence of consistency within a study suggests that the differences found may be a consequence of asymmetrical damage resulting from the surgical procedure.

Like the lesion work, however, most of the tasks used to study asymmetries in split-brain animals are simple and bear little resemblance to the stimuli and tasks that reveal asymmetries in humans. An exception is several studies by Hamilton that have tested the surgically separated hemispheres of rhesus monkeys with stimuli similar to those that show evidence of asymmetry in humans.[9] Hamilton's studies are models of how research in this area should be done, and we will consider them in some detail.

The work used 18 rhesus monkeys, with equal numbers of left-handed and right-handed, male and female individuals trained in each task wherever possible. The surgery for all animals involved midline division of the optic chiasm, the corpus callosum, and the anterior and hippocampal commissures. This procedure allows the experimenter to present stimuli to just one hemisphere by presenting it to the ipsilateral eye. For each task, comparisons were made between the left and right hemispheres and between the hemispheres contralateral and ipsilateral to the preferred hand. The experimental design also eliminated possible biases from asymmetrical surgical procedures or the order in which the two sides of the brain were tested.

Stimuli were projected on a screen located in front of the monkey. The compartment in which the animal sat allowed the experimenter to determine which eye and hand would be used on a particular trial. Hamilton first ran control experiments to determine the ability of each hemisphere to learn simple visual discriminations. Twelve two-choice discriminations were taught to each animal. Animals were taught to press the screen after seeing one member of each pair and to refrain from pressing after seeing the other. The number of trials needed for the animal to reach a criterion of 90 percent was then calculated for each half of the brain.

The results showed no overall difference between hemispheres in the speed of learning these discriminations, nor was there any systematic relationship between sex, hand preference, or hemisphere retracted during surgery. These control tasks demonstrated that Hamilton had been successful in eliminating some of the biasing factors that may have affected other studies, and they provided further evidence that the two hemispheres of the monkey brain are equally capable of learning a simple pattern discrimination.

The purpose of the experiment, though, was to test tasks that would have a high likelihood of showing hemispheric differences. Two tasks that would be considered right-hemisphere tasks in human terms were used. The first was a facial recognition task in which monkeys were taught to discriminate colored pictures of two monkeys with each hemisphere. Five different pictures of each of the two monkeys were used to reduce the probability that the monkeys would perform the task on the basis of some incidental feature and not the face itself.

The second task was a series of spatial discrimination tests involving (1) two-dimensional drawings of horizontal surfaces that receded toward the horizon from either above or below eye level; (2) lines of different orientation, 0 versus 135 degrees and 45 versus 90 degrees; and (3) a spiral form rotating clockwise or counterclockwise. Again, the monkeys were taught to press the screen in the presence of one member of each pair of stimuli and to refrain from pressing it in the presence of the other.

These are difficult tasks for monkeys, but with many weeks of training they can learn to perform them. Results from these tests did not provide evidence for hemispheric asymmetry of function in rhesus monkeys of the sort that favors the right hemisphere in humans.

Hamilton also employed a more analytic, left-hemisphere task with his animals to determine if asymmetry would be observed. In this task, the monkey was rewarded for a response to two successively presented stimuli that were the same. If the two stimuli were different, the animal was rewarded for withholding a response. The task can be made more difficult by increasing the time between stimuli; the data, however, showed no hemispheric asymmetries even at the longer delays.

Despite the absence of hemispheric asymmetries in these experiments, Hamilton has found evidence for differences in what each hemisphere likes to see. In this study, the monkey holds down a lever for a specified period of time to obtain food. Independent of its relationship to the food, the lever also controls the presentation of a picture projected on a screen in front of the monkey. If the lever is released and then pressed again, the picture changes. Because the lever may be released and pressed again without affecting the food reward, this procedure provides a way to measure a monkey's preference for various pictures.

Hamilton's data using this task suggest that there may be consistent differences between the hemispheres of the same monkey in preferences for pictures. This work is preliminary but promising and suggests that the left hemisphere has a greater preference than the right for viewing colored pictures, especially photos of other monkeys and people, over viewing a plain white screen.

## ANATOMICAL ASYMMETRIES IN ANIMALS

Anatomical studies have suggested that in the temporal-lobe region of some non-human primates there may be structural asymmetries between the hemispheres similar to the asymmetries found in human brains. In one study, comparable measurements were made in the brains of 25 humans, 25 chimpanzees, and 25 rhesus monkeys. Results showed asymmetries favoring the left hemisphere in humans and, to a lesser extent, in chimpanzees, but no significant differences between sides in the rhesus brain.[10]

Another study examining the brains of a variety of monkeys and apes reached a similar conclusion. Sixteen of 28 great apes (orangutans, chimpanzees, and gorillas) showed an asymmetry favoring the left hemisphere. One showed the opposite. In contrast, only 3 cases among 41 monkeys and lesser apes (gibbons and siamangs) showed a sizable asymmetry.[11] Skull size, rather than brain size, has been studied by another investigator. In this study examining skull length in three species of gorilla, only the mountain gorilla showed evidence of gross asymmetry. The other species did not.[12]

It is tempting to speculate that these asymmetries are related to the ability of the apes, particularly chimpanzees, to learn language. Chimpanzees have shown an ability to learn words, some grammar, and even some abstract concepts through the use of sign language or the manipulation of plastic symbols. Some investigators believe the anatomical asymmetries in the great apes are a reflection of their having reached a "prelinguistic" evolutionary stage in which their thought patterns are similar to those of humans but much more primitive.

Evidence for anatomical asymmetries in the brain has not been limited to primates, however. For almost 20 years, Marian Diamond and her colleagues had studied how the cerebral cortex in the rat could be altered by environmental experience. They had pooled the data from the two hemispheres assuming they would be similar, but renewed interest in hemispheric differences led Diamond to begin to examine the hemispheres separately, revealing an intriguing pattern of asymmetries.[13]

Measuring cortical thickness in seven regions of the brain in a species of rat known as the Long Evans, she found asymmetries that were a function of both age and sex. For young, adult, and aged male rats, the right cortex was thicker than the left in six of the seven regions measured. For very aged male rats (900 days old), however, the asymmetry was considerably reduced and did not attain statistical significance in any region. For females, the results were less clear-cut: overall, the left cortex was thicker than the right, but the results were not statistically significant in any region, and no consistent age-related trends were observed in the females.

Asymmetries in subcortical structures were also observed in this series of studies. Measurements of the hippocampus, a structure that plays an important role in memory, show laterality effects as well. The male rate has large, significant differences favoring the right hippocampus early in life: these differences decrease considerably with age. The female rat shows the reverse asymmetry: left hippocampus thicker than right, with the differences reaching statistical significance only at 21 and 90 days of age.

Diamond's results are exciting because they suggest it may be possible to study factors influencing hemispheric asymmetries in simple experimental animals. In Chapter 7, for example, we discussed the implications this work might have for understanding sex differences in brain asymmetry. The white rat is an easy organism to work with, and a wide range of experiments looking at the effects of age or different environments, for example, which would be impractical with primates, can be conducted on it.

Of course, it is still important to keep in mind that we do not yet have evidence linking anatomical asymmetries in animals to actual asymmetries in function, such as those for speech and language in human beings. In fact, there is little convincing evidence of a link between anatomical asymmetries and functional asymmetries in human beings. It is possible that asymmetries in the brain of primates and rats are not related to behavioral asymmetries, just as it is possible that the asymmetries in the human brain may be unrelated to behavioral differences. Underlying much of the interest in anatomical asymmetries, however, is the as yet unproven assumption that such a relationship will ultimately be established.

## PHARMACOLOGICAL ASYMMETRIES

Further evidence suggesting that the rat may be a useful animal in which to study brain asymmetries comes from the work of Stanley Glick and his colleagues at the Mt. Sinai School of Medicine.[14] They found that rats rotate or move in circles at night, and that individual rats show a preference in the direction in which they run. Some prefer to run to the left, and others consistently prefer to run to the right. This preference seems to be established very early — the direction in which newborn rats turn their tails predicts their turning preferences later in life.

Glick has shown that a rat's characteristic turning preference is related to a chemical imbalance in the region of the brain called the *nigrostriatal pathway*, an area that helps regulate movement. They found that the concentration of dopamine, a chemical transmitter released by the neurons in the nigrostriatal pathway, is higher by about 15 percent in the side of the brain opposite to the direction of the animal's turning preference. Thus, animals with a higher concentration of dopamine in the left side of the brain prefer to turn right, and those with a higher concentration on the right prefer to turn left. The relationship is not coincidental—other studies have shown that dopamine is in fact the neurotransmitter responsible for the circling behavior.

Studies with humans have also revealed asymmetries in the concentration of neurotransmitters in the brain. In reanalyzing data collected by others, Glick and colleagues found higher concentrations of some chemicals in the left hemisphere, and higher concentrations of others in the right hemisphere. A particularly intriguing piece of data was the observation that dopamine concentrations were higher in the left side of the brain. Because most of the patients whose brains were studied at postmortem may be assumed to have been right-handed, this finding suggests that dopamine concentration apparently is higher on the side contralateral to the preferred hand, a finding consistent with the rat data they obtained.

This work suggests that studies in the rat may reveal functions and mechanisms of brain asymmetry that apply to humans, as well. Although research to test this began only recently. Ernst Mach considered the possibility more than a century ago.

> The idea that the distinction between right and left depends upon an asymmetry, and possibly in the last resort upon a chemical difference, is one which has been present to me from my earliest years. . . . Human beings and animals that have lost their direction move, almost without exception, nearly in a circle . . . we have here a teleological device to help parents to find their hungry young again when they have been lost.[15]

## BEHAVIORAL TESTS

We have reviewed lesion, split-brain, and anatomical studies of hemispheric asymmetries in animals. In many respects the search for asymmetries in animals has followed a progression similar to that of laterality research with human beings. A major difference between the human and animal research, however, lies in the role played by behavioral studies. Behavioral work forms a large part of the literature on human laterality but, with the exception of research on paw preference, there have been very few studies involving behavioral approaches to hemispheric differences in animals.

One recent study, however, fits nicely into this category, and we will present it here because of its relevance to the issue of asymmetry in animals as well as the cleverness of its methodology. The study involved teaching Japanese macaque monkeys to discriminate two different types of vocalizations made by members of their own species. The sounds were prerecorded and presented to the left or the right ear in a random sequence. The investigators found that all five of the monkeys tested performed more accurately when the sounds were presented to the right ear. Only one of five monkeys of other species showed ear asymmetry when presented with the Japanese macaque vocalizations.[16]

If we assume that sounds presented to the right ear are preferentially delivered to the left hemisphere, these results suggest a hemispheric asymmetry in Japanese macaques for the processing of vocalizations produced by members of their own species.* This, of course, is precisely what we find with human subjects. If these results can be replicated, they open up the exciting possibility that at least one hemispheric asymmetry exists in primates, which has striking parallels to hemispheric asymmetry for speech in human beings.

## AVIAN ASYMMETRIES: WHAT THE BIRD'S BRAIN CAN TELL US

Up to this point, our review of asymmetries in animals has been confined to studies using mammals, particularly the non-human primates. There is some evidence to suggest the existence of asymmetries in these species, but the evidence is far from clear-cut. Given this background, it is especially interesting to note that researchers working at Rockefeller University have discovered a striking asymmetry between the halves of the brain in an unexpected source: songbirds. To appreciate their findings, we must make a brief digression to consider how bird song is produced.

The vocal system of birds consists essentially of a set of bellows that act on an air-driven structure called the syrinx. The position and

---

*It is commonly assumed that dichotic presentation involving simultaneous presentation of material to the two ears is necessary to lateralize auditory inputs. As discussed in Chapter 3, however, some studies have reported monaural ear differences in human subjects.

tension of tissue folds and membranes in the syrinx determine the frequency and amplitude of the sounds produced. The syrinx is divided into a left half and a right half, which are controlled independently by the left and the right hypoglossus nerve, respectively.† Song birds typically develop song during the first year of life. They require auditory feedback both to acquire and to maintain normal song.

Fernando Nottebohm and his colleagues demonstrated that sectioning the left hypoglossus in adult chaffinches and canaries results in a dramatic change in song. Most of the song components disappear and are replaced either by silence or by poorly modulated sounds. Sectioning of the right hypoglossus, in contrast, has minimal effects on song; for the most part, song remains intact.[17]

Further investigation has shown that the right hypoglossus may come to control song to varying degrees, depending on the age at which the left hypoglossus is cut. Canaries with the left hypoglossus cut within two weeks after hatching develop song of normal complexity that is completely controlled by the right hypoglossus. Birds operated on as adults also show some plasticity in that they can learn new song under control of the right hypoglossus; the end result, though, is less accomplished than that produced by intact canaries and canaries with damage occurring earlier in life.

The asymmetries in control of bird song appear to extend to the highest vocal-control stations in the brain. Results show that lesions of the left hemisphere produce a song almost completely lacking in structure, without any of the components that were present preoperatively. In contrast, the song in right-lesioned birds retains its structure, although some components are lost. With time, canaries with damaged left hemispheres recover their ability to sing; the right hypoglossus assumes control as it did when the left hypoglossus was cut. Here too, though, the resulting song is less accomplished than that found in normal birds.

## IN SUMMARY

Comparative research with non-human species may help to answer two fundamental questions about brain lateralization: (1) why are there asymmetries in the first place? and (2) why are such asymme-

---

†Notice that control of the syrinx is same-sided, or ipsilateral, in contrast with the crossed, or contralateral, control we have come to expect.

tries generally consistent in their direction — that is, why is speech usually represented in the left and not the right hemisphere?

The evidence we have reviewed points to the existence of anatomical, pharmacologic, and/or behavioral asymmetries in a wide range of animals. Much work remains to be done, however, to firmly establish the existence of these asymmetries and to determine what their relationship might be to the asymmetries found in human beings. Norman Geschwind, one of the researchers primarily responsible for current interest in the biological foundations of laterality, has speculated on some of the more far reaching implications of animal asymmetry research.

Geschwind argued that the widespread belief that humans have certain completely distinctive characteristics, such as language and high levels of artistic and musical abilities, would be discredited as more is learned about asymmetries in animals.[18] He was particularly interested in the recent scientific debate as to whether chimps could be taught "true" language. Chimpanzees had been specially trained to communicate via sign language, but much controversy remains over whether this represents language in the same sense as language used by humans.

Geschwind proposed a hypothetical experiment that would help resolve the issue. If the chimpanzee language abilities were impaired by a left-sided lesion in the region of the brain comparable to the human language centers, whereas a bilateral lesion in other locations did not disrupt performance, the results would be consistent with the idea that the chimpanzee's "language" and human language were similar in mechanism. If the chimpanzee's ability were impaired as a result of the bilateral lesions in areas not homologous to human language centers, however, and were not impaired with the left-sided lesion, he argued that this would be evidence against the linguistic nature of the chimpanzee's performance.*

The fact that asymmetries are found in animals that do not seem to possess linguistic abilities does not weaken the argument, Geschwind claimed. He postulated that perhaps there is a forerunner of language that does not involve communication among individuals, but rather is useful to the individual animal. "It is clearly conceivable," Geschwind stated, "that such an internal method of coding

---

*We agree with Geschwind that a "positive" outcome to this hypothetical study would be powerful indirect evidence for the linguistic nature of the chimpanzee's performance. However, we believe the failure to demonstrate hemispheric asymmetry in chimpanzees of the same sort found in humans would not necessarily rule out the possibility that chimpanzee language was linguistic in the same manner as human language.

might have appeared very early in evolution and could have been used by individual non-human animals. The ability to communicate, although of great interest, might be a later 'technical' development that enabled transmission of the code from one individual to another, but the essential step in the development of the internal code might have occurred much earlier."[19]

Although these ideas are speculative, they are representative of the problems that neuroscientists wishing to understand lateralization are starting to confront. By extending the search for asymmetries beyond human beings, researchers have begun the process of discovering the answers.

# The Role of Asymmetry in Developmental Disabilities and Psychiatric Illness

Research in the area of hemispheric differences has had an impact on many fields involved in the investigation of human function and dysfunction. In Chapters 1 and 6 we discussed the clinical symptoms of injury to the right and left hemispheres. In this chapter, we consider other disabilities and abnormalities in human behavior that have been related to the division of function between the hemispheres. Although not the consequence of any obvious physical damage, these disabilities may in fact arise from subtle problems in either the left or the right side of the brain.

Is stuttering the result of competition for control of speech by the two hemispheres in a less than normally lateralized individual? Does incomplete lateralization predispose a child to reading problems, despite otherwise normal intelligence? Why does psychiatric depression seem to respond better to right-hemisphere rather than left-hemisphere shock treatment? These are a few of the questions investigators have pursued in an attempt to determine the role of the left brain and right brain in pathological processes.

There are at least two ways in which pathological processes can be related to hemispheric asymmetry of function. The pathology can be directly related to dysfunction in one of the hemispheres — that is, to dysfunction of one or more of the hemisphere's specialized abilities. Alternatively, the pathology can be associated with *patterns* of hemispheric asymmetry that differ from normal. Both kinds of dysfunction have been claimed to play a role in pathology.

## READING DISABILITY: A FAILURE OF DOMINANCE?

One of the first investigators to propose a link between lateralization and reading disability was Samuel T. Orton. Orton was a physician who had worked during the early decades of this century with children suffering from reading and writing problems. In the course of his work, he noticed that these children sometimes wrote in mirror form, reversing the orientation of individual letters as well as their sequence within a word. For example, the word *cat* might be written "ɹʌɔ," such as it would appear if one viewed "cat" in a mirror. Similarly, these children often reversed letter sequences in reading, so that *saw* was read as "was."

Orton observed that children who made mirror-image reversals in reading and writing also tended to have unstable preferences for one hand. He interpreted this finding as a sign of incomplete cerebral dominance. This association of reading disability and incomplete cerebral dominance led him to propose that the two are related:

> Since the normal pattern in the adult is a concentration of control of the functions under discussion in the hemisphere opposite to the master hand, and since our clinical observations show so wide a variation both in time and degree in the development of a selective preference for either side in many children, it is suggested that these disorders may derive from a comparable variation affecting the essential language areas of the brain and thus rest on a basis largely physiological in nature.[1]

Because the two sides of the brain are symmetrical about the mid-line, information about the visual world, he suggested, is represented in mirror-image form on each side: "The exact symmetrical relation-ship of the two hemispheres would lead us to believe that the group of cells irradiated by any visual stimulus in the right hemisphere are the exact mirror counterpart of those in the left." Figure 10.1 shows the result.

Orton argued that information represented in the dominant hemi-sphere was oriented correctly, whereas information in the nondom-inant hemisphere was in mirror-image form. In the absence of suffi-ciently developed cerebral dominance, the two representations, one normally oriented and one reversed, would cause confusion in read-ing and writing. Orton used the term *strephosymbolia* to describe the resulting condition.

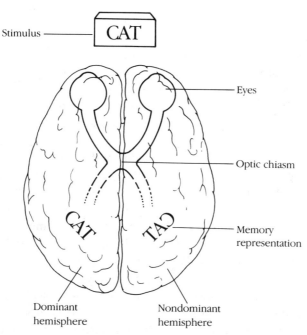

**Figure 10.1** Schematic representation of Orton's theory. Orton assumed that a visual stimulus is represented in opposite orientations in the two hemispheres. [From Corballis, "The Left–Right Problem in Psychology," *Canadian Psychologist* 15 (1974)]

Orton's term for this type of reading and writing difficulty is no longer used, and his ideas of how representations are laid down in mirror-image fashion in each hemisphere have been shown to be incorrect. Nevertheless, the basic notion that reading disability may be linked to hemispheric asymmetry is still under active investigation. With the development of behavioral tools to study hemispheric asymmetry, it has become possible to test more directly the idea that reading disability is linked to atypical brain asymmetry. It turns out that Orton may have been right, but for the wrong reasons.

### Behavioral Studies with Normal and Impaired Readers

Dichotic listening tasks have been popular in studies investigating the relationship between lateralization and reading. One of the first studies to use this approach compared the dichotic listening performance of 14 normal fourth-graders with that of 14 boys who had been classified as dyslexic.[2] *Dyslexia* is the term applied in cases where reading disability is present but is not associated with other problems, such as sensory impairment, retardation, or emotional difficulties.

The dichotic digits tasks showed a significant right-ear advantage for the normal children and a weak, nonsignificant left-ear advantage for the dyslexics. Consistent with this finding are other studies showing a higher incidence or magnitude of right-ear advantage among good readers than among poor readers.[3]

Lateralized tachistoscopic presentation has also been used to investigate hemispheric asymmetry in dyslexic children. Using letters and words as stimuli, several studies have pointed to a greater right-visual-field superiority in normal readers than in dyslexic readers.[4]

In contrast to the findings suggesting that dyslexia may be related to the direction and degree of hemispheric asymmetry are a number of studies reporting no differences between normals and dyslexics on behavioral tests. Both dichotic listening and tachistoscopic studies have reported comparable asymmetries for both groups using verbal stimuli.[5] One study even reported a right-visual-field effect larger for dyslexic subjects than for normal ones.[6] The authors proposed that too much lateralization can adversely affect reading ability. This, of course, is the opposite of Orton's view, which stated that too little lateralization poses a problem for reading.

What can we make of this diversity of findings? A review of the literature leads to the conclusion that much of the conflict between studies is traceable to the way in which the investigators defined their subject populations. Dyslexia is not a unitary disorder; it may take different forms, each probably having different causes. The dyslexic children most likely to show reduced asymmetry in behavioral tests appear to be those with deficits that extend beyond reading difficulties to include auditory–linguistic deficits, that is, problems with the sounds of language and with language more generally.

Up to this point we have concentrated on the hemispheric organization of linguistic functions. Do differences exist between normal and dyslexic children in hemispheric specialization for spatial functions? Witelson's large-scale study using dichaptic stimulation, discussed in Chapter 7, suggests that there are.[7]

When given two novel forms to feel simultaneously, one in each hand, normal children were better able to make a visual match to the form held in the left hand. Dyslexic children, however, showed no differences. The same study failed to find any differences between the groups on a verbal dichotic listening task. Witelson concluded that developmental dyslexia may be associated with bilateral representation of spatial functions and left-hemispheric representation of language functions. She argued that the existence of spatial functions in both hemispheres may disrupt left-hemisphere language functions during the reading process.

Still other work suggests that when the recognition of faces is studied with lateralized tachistoscopic presentation, the performance of dyslexic children is similar to that of normal readers.[8] Thus, dyslexics may show bilateral representation of certain aspects of presumed right-hemisphere function (visual–tactile matching of forms), but other aspects (face recognition) are lateralized to the same degree as in normal subjects. These findings emphasize the importance of the specific task in the outcome of lateralization studies. Certain tasks may lead to one set of conclusions; others can lead to very different conclusions.

## Anatomical Asymmetries in Dyslexics

Some anatomical evidence pointing to a relationship between brain asymmetry and dyslexia have been reported recently.[9] Computerized brain scans were obtained for 24 patients classified as developmentally dyslexic and ranging in age from 14 to 47. Six were left-handed.

Measurements of the width of the brain in the region where the parietal and occipital lobes meet were made on each side and then compared. Results showed that 42 percent of the patients had brains with parieto-occipital regions wider on the right side than on the left, and 33 percent had brains wider on the left; 25 percent showed virtually no asymmetry.

When data from dyslexic patients was subdivided by handedness, 50 percent of the left-handers and 39 percent of the right-handers showed a reversal of the asymmetries found in normal subjects. Only 9 percent of the normal left-handers examined showed wider parieto-occipital regions on the right. It is also interesting to note that the patients with reversals of brain asymmetry had lower scores on tests of verbal intelligence than did the patients with normal patterns of asymmetry, although there were no differences between the two groups in performance or nonverbal IQ.

The authors emphasize that a reversal of brain asymmetry alone is not sufficient to produce dyslexia. The incidence of dyslexia in the population is from 1 to 3 percent; brain-asymmetry reversal is considerably more frequent. They suggest that reversal interacts with other factors to produce dyslexia. From their data, though, they estimate that individuals with reversals in brain asymmetry are at five times greater risk for dyslexia than are other individuals.

### Evaluating the Evidence

The data just presented are highly suggestive of a relationship between brain lateralization and reading disability, although differences among subjects and tasks clearly play an important role in the outcome of such studies. Even if this relationship were to be reliably established, however, we could not be sure that the extent or type of brain lateralization *determined* reading abilities.

Orton assumed that weak cerebral dominance caused reading disability. One could easily argue, however, from the data reviewed above, that some third factor is responsible for the relationship we observed and that there is no direct causal link between lateralization and reading skill. It is even possible to argue that reading ability itself may affect lateralization. Good readers may spend more time reading than poor readers, and this could conceivably affect brain lateralization.

Each of these alternatives must be considered speculative at best, and much additional work will be necessary before these possibilities will be disentangled. For now, it is important to keep two points in mind when considering the relationship between lateralization and reading ability. First, most subjects who show little evidence of asymmetry (or even reversed asymmetry) on dichotic listening tests and other measures of lateralization do not show evidence of reading problems. Second, many subjects with such problems have normal lateralization as measured by these tests. Thus, reduced lateralization is neither a necessary nor a sufficient condition for reading problems. Reading difficulties are a complex class of problems to which many different factors may contribute. Similarly, brain lateralization is but one aspect of a complex of brain functions that provide the neurological substrate for reading.

## STUTTERING: THE CASE FOR COMPETITION FOR CONTROL OF SPEECH

Most people have probably heard the claim that it is unwise for parents to force a child showing a natural preference for the left hand to use the right hand. It has been argued that such attempts have potentially serious consequences for the child's overall adjustment, including increasing the chances that the child will stutter.

Samuel Orton played an important role in establishing this idea. Orton believed that in some cases stuttering is the result of competition between the hemispheres for the control of speech. In individuals with well established cerebral dominance, the left hemisphere assumed control, whereas those with poorly established dominance were at risk for stuttering. Forcing a child to switch hands against his or her natural preference could disrupt the establishment of dominance and result in a stuttering problem. In his own practice with stutterers, Orton observed that children allowed to use their naturally preferred hand after having been forced to use the right hand would stop stuttering.

What evidence links hemispheric organization to stuttering? One piece of evidence sometimes mentioned is the purported higher incidence of left-handedness and ambilaterality among stutterers than in the general population. Because left-handers and ambidextrous people tend to be less lateralized for language functions than right-handers, the increased incidence of left-handedness and ambilaterality among stutterers is certainly consistent with Orton's ideas. Recent studies, however, have challenged the figures showing a higher incidence of left-handedness among stutterers.[10]

The general consensus now appears to be that the frequency of left-handedness is not significantly higher among stutterers than among nonstutterers. In any case, the status of the relationship between hemispheric organization and stuttering should not rest solely on handedness data. Before a convincing case can be made that stuttering is a disorder of cerebral organization, direct evidence is needed bearing on the hemispheric asymmetry of stutterers themselves.

Some evidence addressing this question has come from behavioral studies of brain asymmetry. Again, dichotic listening has been a popular technique. One of the first studies showed that 55 percent of adult stutterers had a left-ear advantage in a dichotic task, whereas only 25 percent of normal subjects showed a left-ear advantage.[11] Later studies, however, have been unable to replicate these findings with either adults or children. No differences were found between normal subjects and stutterers in the size of the ear-asymmetry effect.[12]

Another interesting approach has involved stutterers tested with sodium amobarbital. One study looked at four stutterers who underwent sodium amobarbital testing for an unrelated neurological problem.[13] All four of the patients, three left-handers and one right-hander, showed evidence of bilateral control of speech. Sodium amobarbital was injected on each side on successive days. Speech impairment followed injection on either side.

This is in contrast to the typical sodium amobarbital finding, in which transient aphasia follows injection on one side (usually the left) but not on the other. Moreover, in each case, stuttering was reported to have stopped after the surgical removal, for medical reasons, of one of the presumed speech centers. This finding is perhaps the strongest evidence linking stuttering to the bilateral distribution of speech.

An attempt to replicate the sodium amobarbital work, however, failed to obtain similar results.[14] The subjects in this study were four right-handers, only one of whom showed any evidence of bilateral representation of speech. The fact that even one of the right-handers showed bilateral speech is important, however, for it is extremely rare in normal right-handers. The sodium amobarbital data can thus be viewed as a partial, but certainly not total, confirmation of the idea that stutterers have speech bilaterally represented in the brain.

One might argue, based on the Wada test, that tests sensitive to the lateralization of speech production, rather than speech perception, are best suited to the search for possible differences between stutterers and normal control subjects. In another effort to study lateralization of speech production, Harvey Sussman and Peter Mac-Neilage have developed a task called *pursuit auditory tracking*. In this task, a subject hears two tones simultaneously — a target tone in one ear and a cursor tone in the other ear. The subject's task is to track the frequency of the randomly varying target tone with the cursor tone, which the subject can vary through movements of the jaw.

Sussman and MacNeilage found that normal subjects tracked more accurately when the cursor was presented to the right ear and the target was presented to the left ear than in the reverse arrangement.[15] In contrast, when a group of 28 stutterers was tested, no laterality effects were found.[16] The investigators interpreted these findings as being consistent with the hypothesis that stutterers have bilateral control of speech production.

The case for the role of brain asymmetry in stuttering is not as strong as that for its role in reading disability. First, far fewer studies have looked for such a relationship in stutterers. Second, stuttering is now viewed as a disorder with many possible causes, only one of which may be related to brain organization. Differences in subject populations could be a major factor in failures to replicate results, and until we are able to identify specific subgroups, the replication problem will persist.

What of the claim that forcing a child to switch hands increases the likelihood that the child will stutter? At this point, no conclusive evidence exists linking brain lateralization and stuttering, let alone if switching hand usage at an early age has important consequences for the distribution of language functions between the hemispheres. One older study reported that the incidence of stuttering in college students with an early, forced hand switch was no higher than that found in control populations.[17] However, observations such as Orton's persist.

There may well be a link between stuttering and forced switching that is independent of brain lateralization. A general increase in stress may be caused by insisting the child use a hand she or he is not comfortable with. This stress, in turn, may be the factor that is causally related to the stuttering. Relevant to this point is the observation that the incidence of stuttering is not reported to be particularly high in the People's Republic of China, a society that has exerted considerable pressure toward the use of the right hand. This would argue against the neurological basis for the link between hand switching and stuttering and would suggest that any association is the result of processes of a different sort.

## AUTISM

Autism is one of the most puzzling of all behavioral abnormalities in children. The classic symptoms of autism include inability to use speech to communicate in a normal way, stereotyped and obsessive movements, and social aloofness. The first signs of autism are usually noticed when the child is an infant. Such children are frequently unresponsive to parental handling and do not seem to react to their environment. Until relatively recently, autism was seen primarily as a disorder having psychodynamic origins. Faulty patterns of interaction established by the parent were believed to be the basis of the disorder, and attention was focused on the characteristics of the parents of autistic children.

Current approaches to autism focus on its origins in brain dysfunction. Although the nature of that dysfunction is far from clear, several investigators have suggested that the disorder may differentially involve the left hemisphere. One source of evidence that these investigators point to comes from the behavior of autistic children. A salient characteristic of autism is the failure of these children to acquire language normally. Intelligence per se does not seem to be a factor, because even severely retarded (but not autistic) children learn to speak without special training. This has suggested to some that some special, left-hemisphere problem may be present in autistic children.

In contrast to their having depressed language skills, autistic children sometimes show considerable artistic or musical ability or extraordinary memory abilities in selected areas. It is not uncommon to find autistic children who are able to tell the days on which a particular date falls over several centuries. The ability to perform elaborate mental arithmetic problems has also been reported. A case history of an autistic girl with extraordinary drawing ability has recently been documented.[18] At the age of 3½, Nadia was producing lifelike drawings with considerable detail (see Figure 10.2). Like the skills that characterize other autistic children, Nadia's performance was quick and almost without conscious effort. It has been suggested that the nature of these special abilities is a reflection of the contributions of the right hemisphere. Nadia's drawing skills

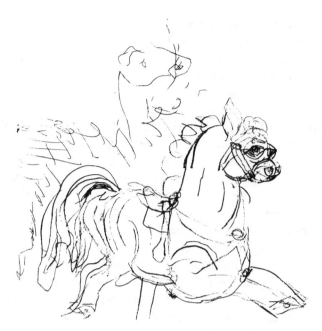

**Figure 10.2** Horses were among Nadia's favorite subjects. She drew this merry-go-round horse before she was 4 years old. [From Selfe, *Nadia — A Case of Extraordinary Drawing Ability in an Autistic Child*, (London: Academic Press, 1977)]

diminished as therapy continued; however, it is impossible to tell whether the change was a consequence of the therapy or would have resulted naturally as she matured.

A limited amount of other evidence is consistent with the hypothesis that abnormal patterns of hemispheric asymmetry are involved in autism. A recent review of the literature that combined the findings of a number of studies on handedness in autistic children reported that 52 percent were left-handed or did not have an established hand preference.[19] These figures point, albeit indirectly, to differences in hemispheric asymmetry between normal and autistic children. They do not, of course, provide any information about the reasons for the differences; early brain damage and genetic factors are both possibilities.

A recent EEG study compared EEG activity of autistic subjects with age- and handedness-matched normal controls during the performance of several verbal and spatial tasks.[20] Data were analyzed in terms of the ratio of alpha activity recorded from the right hemisphere to alpha activity in the left hemisphere (R/L ratio). As alpha activity is reduced when a hemisphere is engaged in a task, higher ratios indicate relatively greater left-hemisphere activation, whereas lower ratios indicate relatively greater right-hemisphere involvement. Results showed that the autistic and control groups did not differ significantly in the pattern of hemispheric activation during the spatial tasks, but the autistic subjects showed greater right-hemisphere activity in the linguistic tasks. In order to look at patterns of lateralization for individual subjects, the difference between the mean ratio for the verbal tasks and the mean ratio for the spatial tasks was used. Negative scores, thus, represented "reversals" in asymmetry, and positive scores, the "normal" pattern of lateralization. A reversal was seen in 7 of the 10 autistic children, compared with 3 out of 10 control subjects.

Dichotic listening has also been used to explore hemispheric asymmetry in autistic children. In one study, 19 autistic children ranging in age from 8 to 14 were presented with dichotic word pairs. Although the autistic children as a group did not show a left-ear advantage, they did show less right-ear superiority than a control group. Five had a right-ear advantage, 7 a left-ear advantage, and 7 showed no advantage.[21]

What can be concluded about the role of atypical hemispheric asymmetry of function in autism? A recent review of this topic called for considerable caution in reaching conclusions.[22] In reviewing each of the sources of evidence and data raised here, the investigators point out that alternative explanations may account for each of the findings. For example, they challenge the notion that language deficits and, hence by inference, left-hemisphere dysfunction, is primary in autism.

Delay in language development, rather than deficits as such, characterize much of autistic speech, the researchers argue, making the case for left-hemisphere dysfunction weaker. Moreover, they maintain that this type of analysis ignores the deficits of autistic children in the areas of prosody, the social use of language, and the ability to read emotional expression in language. To the extent these functions are lateralized in normal adults, it is the right hemisphere, and not the left, that is involved.

In drawing conclusions from their review, the authors argue that the hypothesis of left-hemisphere dysfunction can be useful if it is pursued on an individual-by-individual basis, rather than looking at entire groups. Although the hypothesis may be useful in some cases, they believe that the neurological deficits in autism may be more variable and more pervasive than what is assumed by the left-hemisphere dysfunction hypothesis.

We agree with this call for caution. Although the data are suggestive of some relationship between autism and left-hemisphere dysfunction, considerably more research will be needed before the relative role of dysfunctions in each hemisphere can be determined. It is possible that this research will lead to better classifications or discriminations of the various behavioral abnormalities we now group together under the label "autistic."

## HEMISPHERIC ASYMMETRY AND PSYCHIATRIC ILLNESS

Within the last decade, investigators have begun to explore the possibility that certain psychiatric disorders, particularly schizophrenia and depression, may involve the hemispheres asymmetrically. The first evidence suggesting such a link came from the clinical study of patients with brain lesions. It was noted that schizophrenia-like symptoms were more likely to occur after lesions on the left side, and symptoms of affective disorders (depression) were more likely to arise after lesions on the right side. Other clinical evidence also pointed to an asymmetric role of the hemispheres in mental illness.

Although the evidence from clinical work was not particularly strong, it meshed well with general notions about the functions of the left and right hemispheres. The thought disorders and verbal hallucinations that are frequently symptoms of schizophrenia fit with the view of the left hemisphere as the analytic, language half of the brain. The mood disorders characteristic of affective illness are consistent with the conceptualization of the right hemisphere as the one controlling nonverbal functions.

### Observations From the Clinic

One of the first attempts to link psychopathology with a model of hemispheric specialization was made by psychiatrist Pierre Flor-Henry about 20 years ago.[23] Flor-Henry compared 50 cases of temporal lobe epilepsy that also showed psychotic symptoms with 50 cases without psychotic symptoms. When both groups were subdivided on the basis of left-hemisphere, right-hemisphere, or bilateral location of the epileptic focus, he found significant differences between the groups. The psychotic group had a greater incidence of left-hemisphere focus than the nonpsychotic group. A further break-down of the psychotic group into four subgroups based on the nature of their illness suggested that a left-hemisphere focus was more common in schizophrenia and a right-hemisphere focus was more common in affective psychoses.

This work has been criticized on the grounds that the results are weak statistically; other studies, however, have produced results pointing in the same general direction. One large study looked at the effect of head injury sustained during World War II.[24] The Minnesota Multiphasic Personality Inventory (MMPI) was administered to all participants, who were classified into one of two groups on the basis of whether they showed any language deficits as a result of their injury. The investigators found an increased frequency of high scores on the schizophrenic scale of the MMPI in the group with language disturbances. By dividing subjects on the basis of language impairment rather than by side of injury, this study more directly addressed the question of the link between impaired language centers and schizophrenia.

Additional clinical evidence pointing to right-hemisphere involvement in affective illness comes from findings on unilateral electroconvulsive shock (ECS), in which current is delivered through electrodes placed on the scalp. Electroconvulsive shock is occasionally used in the treatment of depression and is quite effective in many cases. Although the conventional treatment generally has been bilateral, numerous reports have suggested that post-treatment confusion and memory loss frequently accompanying ECS can be reduced by using electrodes placed on only one side of the head. Furthermore, when unilateral shock is used, it is more effective when applied to the right hemisphere.

These claims have important implications for lateralization of function in affective illness. If the effectiveness of ECS as a treatment for depression varies as a function of the side of the brain to which it is administered, the result is strong evidence for the lateralized nature of the disorder.

Of three carefully conducted studies comparing the therapeutic effect of left, right, or bilateral ECS, two found the left-hemisphere-only condition to be less effective in relieving depression than the right-hemisphere-only treatment. One study found no difference.[25] The studies assessed the effectiveness of ECS at least one month after the last treatment by means of a blind evaluation of each patient.

Results in this area are not totally consistent, but the general picture that emerges is one in which depression responds more effectively to right-hemisphere ECS than to left-hemisphere ECS. Thus, we have another piece of evidence pointing to the lateralized nature of certain forms of mental illness.

## Behavioral and Electrophysiological Studies

A variety of behavioral and electrophysiological techniques have been used to explore the role of brain organization in mental illness. Some support for the lateralized dysfunction model of mental illness has come from studies of the orienting response measured by skin conductance. When a subject is alert and presented with a novel stimulus, the resistance of the skin on the arm to mild electric current decreases. This is one of several peripheral physiological changes that take place when a person is alerted to something new or different. With repeated presentation, this response diminishes and is said to have *habituated*.

John Gruzelier and his colleagues studied the skin conductance of both schizophrenic and depressed patients in response to repeated auditory stimuli.[26] Among the schizophrenics, most showed little, if any, conductance response in the left hand. In contrast, the response amplitudes of depressed patients were smaller for the right hand than for the left. Gruzelier notes that these orienting responses are believed to be controlled by the ipsilateral hemisphere, so that a left-hemisphere disorder and a right-hemisphere disorder are implicated by his findings in schizophrenia and depression, respectively.

Some evidence consistent with a relationship between brain organization and psychiatric illness has come from work on lateral eye movements. In Chapter 3, we reviewed evidence suggesting that the direction of lateral eye movements (LEMs) after the presentation of a question reflects differential hemispheric activation. Several studies have reported a greater frequency of left LEMs following spatial questions.

In a study of 29 schizophrenic and 31 control subjects, all right-handed, a series of verbal–nonemotional, spatial–nonemotional, verbal–emotional, and spatial–emotional questions were presented, and LEMs were recorded. Results showed that schizophrenics produced more right LEMs than controls to all but the spatial–emotional questions.[27] If one interprets LEMs as a measure of cerebral activation, these findings suggest that schizophrenic patients utilize the left hemisphere to a greater extent than the right, both for questions for which left-hemisphere processing is presumed more appropriate and for questions for which it is not.

A somewhat different approach to the relationship between brain organization and mental illness has been taken by Graham Beaumont and Stuart Dimond.[28] Evidence from postmortem examinations shows a significant increase in the size of the corpus callosum in chronic schizophrenics. Beaumont and Dimond speculated that the increase reflects compensation for defective interhemispheric communication. To test this hypothesis, they used tachistoscopically presented material lateralized to one hemisphere at a time, and they asked subjects to identify the stimuli, which were letters, digits, and abstract shapes. In this condition, the schizophrenic subjects performed as well as nonschizophrenic patients and nonpsychiatric medical patients.

When two stimuli were presented simultaneously, however, and the task was modified to require judgments of "same" or "different," differences between the schizophrenic and control patients appeared. The largest differences were found when each of the two stimuli in a pair was presented to separate hemispheres. Smaller differences between schizophrenic and normal subjects were observed when the two stimuli on each trial were presented to the same hemisphere. Figure 10.3 shows the test procedures. Beaumont and Dimond argue that the difficulty encountered by schizophrenic patients in the task involving both hemispheres is the result of a defect in communication between the two sides, which is greater than what can be accounted for on the basis of deficits within each hemisphere.

Electroencephalographic measures have been used by Flor-Henry in a study with 28 schizophrenic, 18 manic–depressive, and 19 control subjects performing verbal and visuo-spatial tasks.[29] Schizophrenic subjects had significantly more EEG power in the left-temporal region than normal subjects; power in the right-temporal region was comparable with that in normal subjects. Manic–depressives, however, had more power on both sides of the head in parts of the EEG than did normal subjects, with the right side showing greater power than the left.

## Some Theoretical Considerations

In our brief review of evidence suggesting a relationship between brain lateralization and psychiatric disorder, we have looked at a number of different ways in which the question has been studied experimentally and clinically. Investigators have proposed three dif-

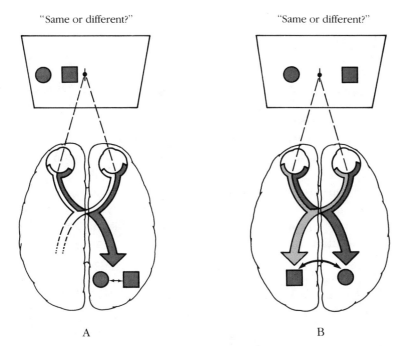

"Same or different?" "Same or different?"

A B

**Figure 10.3** Intrahemispheric versus interhemispheric "same"—"different" judgments. A. When both stimuli are presented in one half of the visual field, they project directly to one hemisphere. B. When the stimuli to be compared are presented to each side of the fixation point, they are initially processed by separate hemispheres. Comparing them involves some amount of information transfer across the corpus callosum.

ferent models of the nature of that relationship. Each of the studies we have reviewed can be interpreted in terms of one or more of these models.

1. The *lateralized-deficit model* holds that deficits in one hemisphere are associated with particular forms of mental illness. These deficits are believed to be quite subtle, requiring highly sensitive measures of lateralization to detect them.

2. The *cognitive-style model* views certain forms of mental illness as characterized by atypical modes of information processing that result from nonoptimal utilization of hemispherically linked functions. There are no hemispheric deficits per se; rather, the illness is the result of inappropriate patterns of hemispheric involvement.

3. The *interaction model* ties psychopathology to a problem between the hemispheres, rather than to a deficit in either hemisphere alone

or the pattern of their involvement. Here, the difficulty is seen to lie in the faulty exchange of information between the halves of the brain.

It is clearly premature to argue strongly for one model over the other. In fact, although all the evidence reviewed points to some involvement of brain lateralization in psychopathology, each piece alone is not particularly compelling. Like reading disability and stuttering, mental disorders probably have a number of different causes, many of which produce the same overall symptomatology. Perhaps brain asymmetry is involved in some forms of schizophrenia and affective illness but not in all. We need better ways to subdivide patients into appropriate groups. It is even possible that the measures of lateralization themselves may be useful in this task.

## THE ROLE OF THE LEFT BRAIN AND THE RIGHT BRAIN IN PATHOLOGY

The pathologies considered in this chapter are diverse, ranging from stuttering to schizophrenia. In each case a lateralized abnormality of some sort is believed to exist but has not been unequivocally demonstrated. Before attempts are made to apply research findings to the treatment of persons with the sort of problems just considered, we must be sure that the findings are firmly established.

We repeatedly noted the importance of recognizing that many dysfunctions probably have more than one cause. To assume that similar symptoms always result from the same cause is to grossly oversimplify the intricacies of human brain–behavior relationships. Lateralized dysfunction may be involved in some, but not all, forms of a disorder. It is also important to remember that lateralized dysfunction may not be sufficient by itself to result in a particular problem; other factors may have to operate at the same time before a deficit will occur. We have noted that a full range of patterns of lateralization are observed in normal persons, suggesting that particular patterns of lateralization per se are not sufficient causes for certain deficits.

# 11

# Hemisphericity, Education, and Altered States

The rapidly growing body of knowledge dealing with the nature of hemispheric asymmetry has led quite naturally to speculation about the consequences of asymmetry for everyday behavior. Does the specialization seen in the hemispheres of normal individuals correspond to distinct modes of thought? Do some people rely more on the left side of the brain, others more on the right? Are there cultural differences in hemisphericity? Do the educational systems of western civilization emphasize so-called left-brain thinking and perhaps neglect the potential of the right brain?

These are some of the popular issues raised by the discoveries discussed in earlier chapters. In this chapter, we consider several such issues.

## TWO BRAINS, TWO COGNITIVE STYLES?

We have seen evidence that, after the surgical division of the two hemispheres, learning and memory can continue separately in the left brain and the right brain. Each half of the brain of a split-brain patient is able to sense, perceive, and perhaps even conceptualize independently of the other. Furthermore, in virtually every approach to the study of hemispheric processes, including approaches using normal individuals, findings support the existence of hemispheric differences. In earlier chapters, we discussed the difficulty in characterizing the differences. Some talk of a verbal–nonverbal distinction. Others argue that the halves of the brain differ in terms of how they deal with information in general.

Since the first split-brain operations, a progression of labels have been used to describe the processes of the left brain and right brain. The most widely cited characteristics may be divided into five main groups, which form a kind of hierarchy. Each designation usually includes and goes beyond the characteristics above it:

| Left Hemisphere | Right Hemisphere |
|:---:|:---:|
| Verbal | Nonverbal, visuo-spatial |
| Sequential, temporal, digital | Simultaneous, spatial, analogical |
| Logical, analytical | Gestalt, synthetic |
| Rational | Intuitive |
| Western thought | Eastern thought |

The descriptions near the top of the list seem to be based on experimental evidence; the other designations appear more speculative. The verbal–nonverbal distinction, for example, was the earliest to emerge from split-brain studies and behavioral research with normal subjects. The sequential–simultaneous distinction reflects a current, though not universally accepted, theoretical model holding that the left hemisphere tends to deal with rapid changes in time and to analyze stimuli in terms of details and features, whereas the right hemisphere deals with simultaneous relationships and with the more global properties of patterns. In this model, the left hemisphere is something like a digital computer, the right like an analog computer.

Many investigators speculating on these issues have attempted to go beyond these distinctions. A popularly accepted view of the differences between the hemispheres is that the left brain operates in a logical, analytical manner and the right brain works in a Gestalt, synthetic fashion.

Once one starts using such labels to describe the operation of the hemispheres, several questions come to mind. Are they just convenient descriptions of how the hemispheres deal with information? Or do they imply that the hemispheres differ in their styles of thinking? Is it possible to view the specialized functions of the left brain and the right brain as distinct modes of thought?

Historically, philosophers and students of the mind have shown a tendency to divide intellectual faculties into two types. For example, consider the following quotation from a yogic philosopher who wrote, in 1910:

> The intellect is an organ composed of several groups of functions, divisible into two important classes, the functions and faculties of the right hand, the functions and faculties of the left. The faculties of the right hand are comprehensive, creative, and synthetic; the faculties of the left hand critical and analytic. . . . The left limits itself to ascertained truth, the right grasps that which is still elusive or unascertained. Both are essential to the completeness of the human reason. These important functions of the machine have all to be raised to their highest and finest working-power, if the education of the child is not to be imperfect and one sided.[1]

Many Western thinkers have also talked of mental organization as if it were divided into two parts. Rational versus intuitive, explicit versus implicit, analytical versus synthetic are some examples of these dichotomies. More are listed in Table 11.1. Although these terms are quite varied, they do seem to have something in common. Perhaps, as some have suggested, they correspond to the separate processes of the two cerebral hemispheres.

Why so many two-part divisions? Do they label truly distinct and separate qualities, or do they just describe the extremes of a set of continuous behaviors? In other words, are we dealing with all-or-none differences, or are there gradations in between? Some have insisted on the former view because, they claim, it conforms best to a neuroanatomical reality—the existence of a left brain and a right brain capable of operating independently. Another view is that the formulation of dichotomies or opposites is just a convenient way of viewing complex situations.

The idea that different modes of knowing are reflected in hemispheric functions has become associated in recent years with psychologist Robert Ornstein. In addition to his electroencephalographic (EEG) studies of hemispheric asymmetry, Ornstein has been

Table 11.1

*Dichotomies*

| | |
|---|---|
| Convergent | Divergent |
| Intellectual | Intuitive |
| Deductive | Imaginative |
| Rational | Metaphorical |
| Vertical | Horizontal |
| Discrete | Continuous |
| Abstract | Concrete |
| Realistic | Impulsive |
| Directed | Free |
| Differential | Existential |
| Sequential | Multiple |
| Historical | Timeless |
| Analytical | Holistic |
| Explicit | Tacit |
| Objective | Subjective |
| Successive | Simultaneous |

interested in the nature of consciousness and its relation to hemispheric function.

In 1970, Ornstein published a book entitled *The Psychology of Consciousness*. In it, he set forth the message that Western men and women have been using only half of their brains and, hence, only half of their mental capacity.[2] He noted that the emphasis on language and logical thinking in Western societies has ensured that the left hemisphere is well exercised. He went on to argue that the functions of the right hemisphere are a neglected part of human abilities and intellect in the West and that such functions are more developed in the cultures, mysticism, and religions of the East. In short, Ornstein identified the left hemisphere with the thought of the technological, rational West and the right hemisphere with the thought of the intuitive, mystical East.

Many outlandish claims and misinterpretations have followed in the wake of Ornstein's book. For example, some have equated the left hemisphere with the evils of modern society. Ornstein, however, has stressed that the cerebral hemispheres are specialized for different types of *thought*. He also insists that schools spend most of their time training students in what seem to be left-hemisphere skills.

Ornstein has become an advocate of the existence of alternate ways of knowing and alternate forms of consciousness. He feels that our intellectual training unduly emphasizes the analytical,

> . . . with the result that we have learned to look at unconnected fragments instead of at an entire solution. . . . As a result of this preoccupation with isolated facts, it is not surprising that we face so many simultaneous problems whose solutions depend upon our ability to grasp the relationship of parts to wholes. . . . Split- and whole-brain studies have led to a new conception of human knowledge, consciousness, and intelligence. All knowledge cannot be expressed in words, yet our education is based almost exclusively on its written or spoken forms. . . . But the artist, dancer, and mystic have learned to develop the nonverbal portion of intelligence.[3]

As we have seen, ideas about the nature of hemispheric differences are diverse. They have evolved from verbal–nonverbal distinctions to ever more abstract notions of the relationship between mental function and the hemispheres. In this process, ideas concerning hemispheric differences have moved further and further away from basic research findings. Some have found this progression disconcerting because the distinction between fact and speculation is often blurred. The term *dichotomania* has been coined to refer to the avalanche of popular literature fostered by the most speculative notions. One investigator has noted:

> It is becoming a familiar sight. Staring directly at the reader— frequently from a magazine cover— is an artist's rendition of the two halves of the brain. Surprinted athwart the left cerebral hemisphere (probably in stark blacks and grays) are such words as "logical," "analytical," and "Western rationality." More luridly etched across the right hemisphere (in rich orange or royal purple) are "intuitive," "artistic," or "Eastern consciousness." Regrettably, the picture says more about a current popular science vogue than it does about the brain.[4]

## HEMISPHERICITY

The idea that the two hemispheres are specialized for different modes of thought has led to the concept of hemisphericity—the idea that a given individual relies more on one mode or hemisphere than on the other. This differential utilization is presumed to be reflected in the individual's "cognitive style" — the person's preferences and approach to problem solving. A tendency to use verbal or analytical approaches to problems is seen as evidence of left-sided hemisphericity, whereas those who favor holistic or spatial ways of dealing with information are seen as right-hemisphere people.

Hemisphericity has been claimed by different sources to extend not only to perception but to all kinds of intellectual and personality dimensions. Several years ago, a cartoon appeared in a well-known magazine showing a very fancy country club with a little sign outside reading, "Left Hemisphere People Only." The idea that differences among people may be related to differences in the degree to which they use their two hemispheres is a very appealing one that has captured the fancy of the popular media. Culture and occupation are two areas that have been studied experimentally.

## The Role of Culture

Some attempts by anthropologists to characterize the cognitive processes of different cultures and subcultures seem similar to many notions about the left brain and right brain. One school of thought suggests that there are qualitatively distinct intersocietal, interclass, and interindividual ways of thinking. Most anthropologists, however, insist that "average" human minds function in the same way, regardless of cultural differences. Some have suggested that there is an inconsistency in simultaneously asserting that the human mind functions the same way everywhere and that fundamental ways of thinking differ radically with cultural background.[5]

One way out of the dilemma is to say that every human brain is capable of more than one kind of logical process, and that cultural differences exist with respect to the processes used to deal with various situations. The idea that two different structures within the brain are capable of qualitatively distinct logical processes appealed to investigators interested in resolving the "culture–cognition" paradox.

Can differences in cognitive style between cultures be accounted for on the basis of differences in left- versus right-hemisphere usage? One study compared the performance of 1,220 persons of varied backgrounds, including Hopi Indians, urban blacks, and rural and urban whites, on two tests considered reasonably selective in the hemispheric performance they tap. One test, the Street Gestalt Completion Test, is believed to involve primarily processing in the right hemisphere (see Figure 11.1). The other test, the Similarities Subtest of the Wechsler Adult Intelligence Scale, is thought to involve processing primarily in the left hemisphere. A sample question in the latter test is, "How are a screwdriver and a hammer alike?"

The investigators estimated the relative "right- versus left-hemisphere mode of thought" in each subject group by constructing a ratio of the average Street Gestalt/Similarities scores for each group. High ratios (larger numerator) were interpreted as signifying more right-hemisphere thought; lower ratios (larger denominator) were believed to signify greater left-hemisphere thinking. The results showed rural Hopi Indians to have the highest ratio, followed by urban black women, urban black men, rural whites, and urban whites. The investigators concluded that Hopis and blacks rely relatively more on their right hemispheres in thinking than do the other groups.[6]

A critique published soon after this research appeared argued convincingly that the reported cultural differences were a restatement of cultural differences on verbal IQ tests, rather than evidence for greater right-hemisphere thinking among often deprived groups. The authors stated that no appreciable differences exist between the groups on the Street Gestalt ("right-hemisphere") Test and that the groups differ only on the verbal Similarities Subtest. If one is to interpret the findings in hemispheric terms, they conclude, the only thing that can be said is that "the right hemisphere appears to develop similar levels of ability in radically different cultural groups

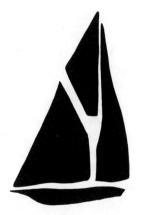
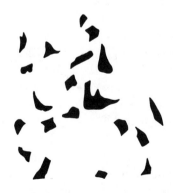

**Figure 11.1** Examples from the Street Gestalt Completion Test. What do these figures depict?

whereas development of the left hemisphere is depressed by lack of educational opportunity."[7]

Another problem with this and many studies that claim to show patterns in the use of the two sides of the brain is the questionable nature of the measures employed. Although tests such as the Similarities Test certainly seem verbal rather than spatial, it is by no means certain that they are just testing the abilities of the left hemisphere. The situation is even more questionable with many of the standardized nonverbal tests. Many so-called tests of spatial ability have been shown to involve a large and sometimes essential verbal component. At the present time, there are no confirmed right-hemisphere-only or left-hemisphere-only tests.

Of course, these criticisms do not rule out the possibility that in certain situations there are cultural differences in hemispheric involvement. In Chapter 3, we considered the importance of the subject's strategy in determining the outcome of laterality studies. If specific groups consistently use different strategies in a wide variety of tasks, we would expect to find some evidence of those differences in laterality studies. Studies looking specifically for these effects, however, require the use of tests that are sensitive to small differences in hemispheric utilization.

A small number of studies have suggested that this is an area worthy of further exploration. One study supportive of cultural differences used dichotic listening to compare native Navajo and Anglo college students matched for age, sex, and handedness.[8] The stimuli were the syllables "pa," "ta," "ka," "ba," "da," and "ga." The right-ear advantage was found for the Anglo subjects, whereas a left-ear advantage was found for the Navajo subjects. The investigators tentatively suggest that the difference may be attributable to the fact that Navajo is a very literal and concrete language, characteristics that may favor processing in the right hemisphere. Although the stimuli employed were English syllables, Navajo–English bilinguals may also use the right hemisphere for processing English.

A different task also believed to be sensitive to hemispheric asymmetry for language has been used by Walter McKeever to address the same issue.[9] Subjects viewed laterally presented drawings of outlines of familiar objects and were asked to name the objects in English. Reaction time was recorded. Navajo college students showed the same right-visual-field advantage (presumably reflecting left-hemisphere specialization for language) as groups of Anglo subjects did in earlier studies. When the 20 Navajo subjects were further broken down into groups based on their utilization of English and Navajo, comparable results were obtained for the 13 who described themselves as competent speakers of both English and Navajo, as well as for the 7 who described themselves as primarily English–speaking. Thus, these results provide no support for the idea that right-handed Navajo subjects show right-hemisphere specialization for the processing of English, although McKeever notes that this task involves vocal output, whereas the dichotic listening task is believed to be sensitive primarily to auditory receptive language. Perhaps these functions may be lateralized in different hemispheres in the Navajo. A more likely explanation, he suggests, is that culturally determined ear-report-order differences are responsible for the left-ear advantage found in Navajo subjects. Although he has no basis for assuming that such differences should exist, McKeever proposes that it is as plausible an explanation as one that calls for right-hemisphere specialization for language in Navajo subjects.

Using EEG as a measure, another study has reported evidence for greater right-hemisphere activity in Hopi children listening to a story in Hopi, compared with that when the story is presented in English.[10] Relatively less alpha activity was recorded over the right hemisphere when the children listened to Hopi than when they listened to English. Hopi, like Navajo, is a more concrete language than English, which is rather abstract. The investigators note that a primary feature of Hopi is its involvement with the perceptual field, linking speech immediately with its context. English, in contrast, orients its users to separation from the perceptual field. These differences, they believe, are responsible for the differential hemispheric involvement observed for the two languages.

Like many issues dealing with hemispheric asymmetry, the evidence for cultural hemisphericity is scanty but intriguing. Much more work is needed to determine if cultural differences in hemispheric utilization are real and, if so, to what they are attributable.

## Occupational Differences in Hemisphericity?

Do artists make greater use of the right hemisphere than lawyers? The evidence for this and related questions is controversial. Robert Ornstein and David Galin recorded and compared EEG activity over the right and left hemispheres of lawyers and clay modelers (ceramists) while they performed several tasks. The tasks included assembling blocks into specified patterns and tracing a complex pattern viewed through a mirror, both supposedly involving the right hemisphere more than the left. The subjects were also asked to write a description of a passage of prose from memory and to copy a similar passage—tasks thought to involve primarily the left hemisphere.

The investigators expected the lawyers to show more left-hemisphere activity than the ceramists in all these situations. They found that the lawyers showed a greater change in left-hemisphere activity as the task changed. The relationship between differential EEG activity, occupational group, and task, however, was complex and difficult to interpret with any simple generalization.[11]

Some studies were performed to determine if there is differential utilization of the hemispheres in college students pursuing different majors at Simon Fraser University by Paul Bakan.[12] Bakan monitored lateral eye movements (LEMs). Among the undergraduates he tested, those who had the most left LEMs were most likely to be majoring in literature or the humanities. Science or engineering majors tended to be right-lookers. If we assume that left LEMs reflect greater right-hemisphere involvement and vice versa, these findings point to differences in occupational hemisphericity—that is, differences in the degree to which individuals in different occupations utilize each cerebral hemisphere.

Cerebral blood flow has also been studied in an attempt to find evidence for occupational hemisphericity. James Dabbs, using a technique that measured very small differences in the temperatures on the two sides, has reported that the amount of blood flow to each side of the brain differs between English majors and architecture majors.[13] He found a higher level of blood flow in the left hemisphere for English majors and a higher level in the right hemisphere for architecture majors. These findings presumably reflect the overall resting level of hemispheric activity in the two groups. Because of its potential significance, extension and replication of this study to more conventional regional cerebral blood flow techniques are needed.

It is important to keep in mind that effects suggesting differential hemispheric involvement as a function of occupation are generally weak and have failed to be replicated in some studies. Differences in the sensitivity of the tests used, as well as variability in the subject populations tested, no doubt contribute to these problems. Further work is needed before a strong statement for or against the notion of occupational hemisphericity can be justified.

It is also important to remember that findings suggesting the possibility of differential hemispheric utilization as a function of occupation do not necessarily support the idea that hemispheric organization per se is different for different groups. In a study employing the visual half-field procedure with lawyers and sculptors, a right-visual-field superiority was found for both groups when letter stimuli were used, and a left-field-superiority was found for both when the task involved discrimination of faces.[14] Thus, both groups showed the same distribution of functions between the hemispheres. Studies supporting the notion of hemisphericity are consistent with the view that the pattern of activation of the hemispheres may vary among groups as a function of occupation, but that the underlying asymmetric brain organization is comparable.

## Can Hemisphericity Be Measured with Questionnaires?

A number of people have developed paper-and-pencil tests that claim to assess hemisphericity. They assert that by completing one of these tests and having it scored (sometimes for a substantial fee) an individual can determine his or her preferred hemisphere. In turn, they promise, this will be useful information when selecting a career, a spouse, or in any other choice where hemispheric compatibility seems desirable.

One hemisphericity questionnaire that has undergone the scrutiny of persons other than its developers is "Your Style of Learning and Thinking."[15] A careful look at the questionnaire shows that the scores correlate highly with tests designed to measure creativity. This is not surprising in view of the logic underlying such tests. As the "nonverbal" hemisphere, the right hemisphere is seen as responsible for intuition which, in turn, is seen as a core characteristic underlying creativity. According to this line of reasoning, a test measuring creativity would reflect the degree of right-hemisphere involvement and hence, hemisphericity.

A major problem with this approach, however, is that there is little in the way of scientific evidence linking creativity to the right hemisphere, let alone evidence tying degrees of creativity to the degree of right-hemisphere utilization. Before the idea of hemisphericity can be fairly evaluated, we will need good measures of differential hemispheric activity. There are a number of possible candidates for such a measure—ear asymmetries in dichotic listening, evoked potential measures, regional cerebral blood flow—but each currently has problems that limit its usefulness as a measure of hemispheric activity in a particular individual. Should technical and interpretational difficulties be resolved, however, such measures, and perhaps others, may prove useful in testing the notion that each of us relies more on one hemisphere than the other. Without a way to measure hemisphericity, however, its existence remains an interesting but untested hypothesis.

## ALTERED STATES

In the preceding section, we explored the possibility of differential hemispheric involvement in different groups of subjects. The premise underlying this approach is that certain characteristics of individuals are predictive of the degree to which the two hemispheres will be brought into play in a particular task. In this section, we consider a related idea: that differences in a given individual's mental state will be associated with differences in hemispheric activity. Thus, although the first approach deals with differences between subjects, the second considers differences within a subject at different times. The hypnotic trance and dreaming are two altered states that have received the most attention from the standpoint of hemispheric differences.

### Dreaming and the Hemispheres

The association between hemispheric activation and dreaming found its origin in occasional reports that patients with brain damage in the posterior region of the right hemisphere no longer had dreams.[16] The right-hemisphere effect fit nicely with the idea that dreams are frequently nonlogical and involve visual images and emotional ideas. Because data depended on the patients' reports, however, the results could be explained in terms of the inability of the patients to remember the dreams that they actually had, rather than in terms of lack of dreams per se. A direct test of the notion that it is the right hemisphere only that is involved in dreaming came from an investigation with split-brain patients discussed in Chapter 2. As the patients slept, their EEGs were monitored for occurrence of the activity that indicated a dream was in progress. Whenever such activity was identified, the patients were awakened and asked to report the dreams. The patients were able to do so, indicating that the left hemisphere had access to the content of the dreams.[17]

The nature of dreams in split-brain patients has been studied by Klaus Hoppe, a psychoanalyst. Hoppe analyzed the dreams of 12 split-brain patients and reported that "patients after commissurotomy reveal a paucity of dreams, fantasies, and symbols. Their dreams lack the characteristics of dream work; their fantasies are unimaginative, utilitarian, and tied to reality; their symbolization is concretistic, discursive, and rigid."[18]

This description suggests that the left hemisphere lacks access to imagery and fantasy, functions presumably localized in the disconnected right hemisphere. It should be remembered, however, that these patients had epilepsy of long standing, and it would be important to determine how much of these results could be attributed to hemispheric disconnection and how much to other factors. The research necessary to answer these questions has not yet been done.

## Hypnosis and Hypnotizability

The possibility of differential hemispheric involvement during hypnotic trance first received attention in studies of hypnotic susceptibility. Subjects differ widely in how easily they can be hypnotized, and investigators have tried to determine what factors are involved. The abilities to concentrate and to be absorbed by a novel are two of the factors that positively correlate with hypnotizability. The similarity between these abilities and what is thought to be characteristic of the right hemisphere led naturally to the hypothesis that hypnotic susceptibility correlates with right-hemisphere activation.

Some evidence consistent with this idea has come from a study of lateral eye movements.[19] In these studies, greater hypnotizability was found in subjects showing a preference for leftward eye movements. Eye movements, as discussed in Chapter 3, have been studied as an indicator of hemispheric activity; however, it remains to be determined if they are truly reflective of hemispheric asymmetry. Thus, it would be premature to conclude that the association between hypnotizability and right-hemisphere activation had been conclusively demonstrated.

Another study looking at the neuropsychological correlates of hypnotizability measured EEG during the performance of a variety of tasks, including spatial orientation, tonal memory, verbal categorization, and mental arithmetic. It was expected that the first two tasks would suppress alpha activity more in the right hemisphere, whereas the second two tasks would suppress alpha activity more in the left hemisphere. The results showed that subjects classified as highly hypnotizable showed a greater shift of cortical activation between the cerebral hemispheres appropriate to the tasks than low-hypnotizable subjects, although most subjects in both groups showed a shift in the appropriate direction. In contrast to the eye-movement data pointing to greater right-hemisphere involvement in highly hypnotizable subjects, these data suggest greater task specific hemispheric involvement in such subjects.[20]

Bakan has studied the relationship between handedness and hypnotizability.[21] Using a 10-point scale of hypnotic susceptibility, he divided performance into three categories: 0–3, low hypnotizability; 4–7, medium hypnotizability; and 8–10, high hypnotizability. Bakan observed that half of all right-handed subjects tested fell in the middle category, while for left-handed subjects there was an over-representation in the low- and high-hypnotizability groups. Because of the relationship between handedness and hemispheric asymmetry, these findings are intriguing, although their meaning remains unclear.

Another approach to hypnosis and hemispheric activity has involved looking at hemispheric involvement during hypnosis. In one study, subjects listened to dichotically presented speech before, during, and after a hypnotic trance. The right-ear advantage obtained before and after the trance was significantly reduced during the trance, owing to improvement in the left-ear scores.[22] These results suggest that hypnosis may involve differential activation of the hemispheres. Considerably more research needs to be done, however, before any firm link can be drawn between hypnosis — or any other altered state — and hemispheric asymmetry.


## EDUCATION AND THE HEMISPHERES

Does an elementary school program restricted to reading, writing, and arithmetic educate mainly one hemisphere and leave half of an individual's potential unschooled? Is the entire educational system biased against developing right-hemisphere talents?

Joseph Bogen, one of the pioneers of the commissurotomy procedure, has been an especially avid proponent of developing what he calls "appositional thinking" in school.[23] The word *propositional* was adopted by neurologist John Hughlings Jackson in the nineteenth century to describe the left hemisphere's dominance for speaking, writing, calculation, and related tasks. In contrast, Bogen coined *appositional* to refer to the information processing of the right hemisphere in well-lateralized right-handers.

In Bogen's view, society has overemphasized propositionality at the expense of appositionality. IQ tests, for example, are aimed at propositional left-hemisphere abilities. Their use is justified by the claim that they predict success in a society that most often measures success monetarily and in terms of productivity. Bogen argues that such measures are very narrow and do not take into account artistic creativity and other right-hemisphere skills that are not easily quantifiable.

The idea that half — more precisely, the right half — of our mental capability is neglected has been appearing with increasing frequency in educational journals, self-help manuals, and a variety of other publications. Articles usually include a background summary of some of the data on laterality along with the author's personal interpretation of what the data mean. Some end with advice about "boosting right-hemisphere thinking" or "training the right hemisphere."

The major business of the left hemisphere, these articles often claim, is the logical representation of reality and communication with the external world. Thinking, reading, writing, counting, and worrying about time are also usually attributed to the left hemisphere. The business of the right hemisphere, in contrast, is said to be understanding patterns and complex relationships that cannot be precisely defined and may not be logical. The qualities of the right hemisphere, an author will state, are essential for creative insight but tend to be inadequately developed.

One writer's statement is representative of a common interpretation of why the right side of the brain is neglected:

> Because we operate in such a sequential-seeming world and because the logical thought of the left hemisphere is so honored in our culture, we gradually damp out, devalue, and disregard the input of our right hemispheres. It's not that we stop using it altogether; it just becomes less and less available to us because of established patterns.[24]

Later in the same article, this author proposes "Ten Ways to Develop Your Right Brain." Here are four examples:

> When presenting information, have a musical background that occasionally drowns out the presentation.
>
> Give a 30 second explanation of something, and ask people to guess what you're getting at.
>
> One day a week, make it a rule that no one in the office or plant can use the word no. (The right hemisphere has no equivalent of no.)

If something is not acceptable, the person must deal with it by saying, "yes, if . . ."

Before a meeting when new speculative thinking is needed, have a ritual idea "dance" and light some punk so you can each read an idea in the smoke.[25]

Our educational systems may be deficient and may limit a broad spectrum of human capabilities. We question, however, the division of styles of thinking along hemispheric lines. It may very well be that in certain stages the formation of new ideas involves intuitive processes independent of analytic reasoning or verbal argument. Preliminary schemes ordering new data or reordering pre-existing knowledge could possibly arise from even aimless wanderings of the mind during which a connection is seen between a present and a past event or a remote analogy is established. But are these right-hemisphere functions? We do not think it is as simple as that, and there is certainly no conclusive evidence to that effect. Our educational system may miss training or developing half of the brain, but it probably does so by missing out on the talents of both hemispheres.

## From Theory to Practice

The ideas concerning education and the hemispheres considered up to this point have been very general. In this section, we consider two approaches that are much more specific in their recommendations.

Betty Edwards, a California art teacher, has presented her method of teaching people to draw in a book entitled *Drawing on the Right Side of the Brain*.[26] Her basic premise is straightforward: under ordinary conditions, it is the right hemisphere of the brain that has the ability to draw. When left alone, the right hemisphere will produce very respectable drawings, even in untrained adults. The catch is that for most of us, the right brain is not given the opportunity to display its talents. The verbal, analytical, left hemisphere (lacking in artistic ability) becomes involved and interferes. The natural tendency to label and analyze a picture or a scene before drawing it, in Edwards' view, is the source of this interference.

Edwards' method of instruction is designed to reduce the amount of left-hemisphere involvement in the drawing process. One of her first exercises involves having students copy a drawing of a person—with the picture held upside down. The reasoning is simple. Held upside down, the picture is no longer easily recognizable. In fact, it is difficult to label any part of it. Thus, Edwards proposes, the copying task is one in which the right hemisphere may proceed without interference from the left. According to Edwards, most adults will be pleasantly surprised when they finish their drawings and rotate them 180 degrees. It will be, she claims, a very acceptable copy of the original drawing.

Edwards' method has several stages, and we cannot do it justice here. Briefly, however, it involves creating conditions in the drawing situation that minimize the likelihood of left-hemisphere involvement. As part of this process, she suggests verbally reassuring the left hemisphere that it is not being abandoned and that a new technique is being tried out just temporarily.

Does Edwards' method work? We know of no research that addresses this question, but her book is filled with before-and-after drawings produced by her adult students. The differences are striking. If they are truly representative, Edwards has devised a method that works, and we do not wish to quarrel with success. We do note, however, that at this point there is no way of knowing if her methods work for the reasons she indicates. We know from split-brain research that the left hemisphere is inferior to the right in its ability to draw; no firm basis exists for believing, however, that in the intact brain the left hemisphere interferes with the expression of right-hemisphere artistic ability. Although it is not clear whether this is a serious part of her method, we are doubtful about the value of "talking" to the left hemisphere to keep it from feeling abandoned. Such a notion suggests that the two hemispheres each contain something like a "little person" who can be talked to and reasoned with — an idea that we hope is as implausible to the reader as it is to us.

The fact is, however, that Edwards' method appears to work. It will remain for future research to demonstrate why. For now, the value of the method is independent of its hypothesized mechanism. It is not increased because of the neuropsychological rationale offered to explain it, nor does the rationale receive any support because of the method's success.

The idea that atypical patterns of hemispheric asymmetry may be present in certain disorders such as reading disability and stuttering (see Chapter 10) led naturally to the development of educational programs described to be therapeutic. Beginning with an emphasis on the need for a child to develop a dominant hemisphere, Glen Doman, a physical therapist, and Carl Delacato, an educational psychologist, have developed and promoted an educational program specifically designed for retarded and handicapped children. They argue that "man has achieved cortical dominance wherein one side of the cortex controls the skills in which man outdistances lower forms of animals."[27] Further, they propose that cortical dominance is subject to maturational development and that disruption of this development results in language and communication problems.

The program of treatment they propose is known as "patterning" and is based on the assumption that normal cortical dominance develops through a series of stages. The program is individualized for each child depending on what point in "level of neurological organization" the child has reached without skipping any developmental stages. Children who are not yet walking are required to spend most of their day on the floor, with crawling emphasized. A team of therapists, parents, and volunteers take turns manipulating the head and limbs of a child who is unable to make the necessary movements alone. Other techniques used in particular children include restricting the use of one arm, occluding one eye, and prohibiting singing and listening to music. The rationale is to develop total cortical dominance extending not only to language but to a dominant eye, hand, and foot.

Although the Doman and Delacato method is still in use, it has been severely criticized on many grounds.[28] First, many of the assumptions they make are known to be false. For example, hemispheric asymmetry, as seen in Chapter 8, most likely is present at birth and does not develop over time. Moreover, occluding the left eye and restricting musical activities are unlikely to result in development of a dominant left hemisphere. The left eye projects to both hemispheres, as seen in Chapter 2, and there is no reason to believe that specialization of the right hemisphere for music would interfere at all with the specialization of the left hemisphere for language.

Doman and Delacato's methods have been criticized on other grounds as well. Critics point out that the methods have been promoted in such a way that parents cannot refuse treatment without calling into question their adequacy as parents, and unsubstantiated claims of success have been made, extending even to claims of making normal children superior.[29]

It may well be the case that the "patterning" treatment does have some residual benefits. It is totally unclear at this point, however, whether those benefits are specific to the treatment. After all, any "close supervision, repeated testing, structured environment, and a favorable atmosphere also may produce substantial benefits in IQ and social functioning."[30]

## SCIENCE, CULTURE, AND THE CORPUS CALLOSUM

After accepting the distinction that the left hemisphere is analytic and the right is intuitive, astronomer–biologist Carl Sagan has gone on to speculate about how the two modes have interacted to generate the accomplishments of our civilization. In his book *The Dragons of Eden*, Sagan describes the right hemisphere as a pattern recognizer that finds patterns, sometimes real and sometimes imagined, in the behavior of people as well as in natural events. The right hemisphere has a suspicious emotional tone, for it sees conspiracies where they do not exist as well as where they do. It needs the left hemisphere to analyze critically the patterns it generates in order to test their reality:

> There is no way to tell whether the patterns extracted by the right hemisphere are real or imagined without subjecting them to left hemisphere scrutiny. On the other hand, mere critical thinking, without creative and intuitive insights, without the search for new patterns, is sterile and doomed. To solve complex problems in changing circumstances requires the activity of both cerebral hemispheres: the path to the future lies through the corpus callosum.[31]

Sagan goes on to suggest that intuitive thinking does well in situations where we have had previous personal or evolutionary experience. "But in new areas — such as the nature of celestial objects close up — intuitive reasoning must be diffident in its claims and willing to accommodate to the insights that rational thinking wrests from Nature."[32] Sagan describes science as paranoid thinking applied to nature, a search for natural conspiracies, for connections in data:

> Our objective is to abstract patterns from Nature (right hemisphere thinking), but many proposed patterns do not in fact correspond to the data. Thus all proposed patterns must be subjected to the sieve of critical analysis (left hemisphere thinking). The search for patterns without critical analysis, and rigid skepticism without a search for patterns, are the antipodes of incomplete science. The effective pursuit of knowledge requires both functions.[33]

He concludes that the most significant creative activities of a culture — legal and ethical systems, art and music, science and technology—are the result of collaborative work by the left and right hemispheres. We completely agree. Sagan also suggests, "We might say that human culture is the function of the corpus callosum."[34] This may be true, not so much because the corpus callosum interconnects "analytic" with "intuitive" thinking, but because every structure in the brain plays a role in human behavior, and human culture is a function of human behavior.

# 12

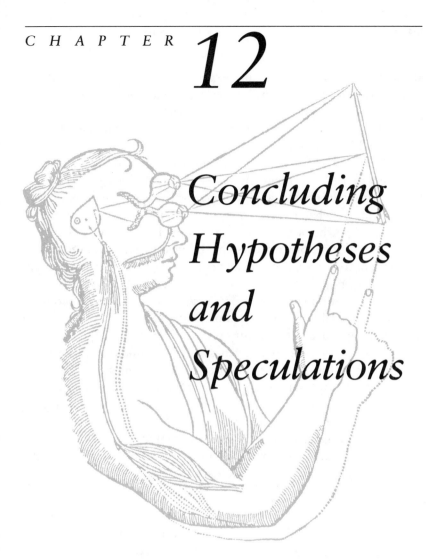

# Concluding Hypotheses and Speculations

A great deal more has been said about the left brain and right brain than we have reported in the preceding chapters. Speculation concerning the implications of hemispheric asymmetry has followed closely behind discoveries with split-brain patients and other investigations into the functioning of the halves of the brain. This is not surprising, for great indeed is the temptation to account for observations about our own minds and the varieties of human experience in light of discoveries about the brain.

Much speculation has touched on the nature of consciousness. What does laterality research have to offer the age-old question about the relationship between mind and body (or between mind and brain)? Does it provide any experimental evidence for Freud's concept of the "unconscious"? Does each hemisphere in a split-brain patient possess a consciousness of its own?

In addition, researchers have posed and attempted to answer on a provisional basis a great many theoretical questions concerning the "how" and "why" of hemispheric specialization. Why is language localized in the left brain? What is the evolutionary reason for lateralization? Just how much of one hemisphere is different from the other? To what extent are the many observed asymmetries a consequence of hemispheric differences in language capacity rather than a sign of some other processing differences? Does the verbal left hemisphere truly dominate behavior? Is it instrumental in creating a feeling of mental unity?

The issues are diverse, and discourse about even one topic may operate at several levels. For example, consciousness is an especially confusing topic because the word means different things to different investigators. One calls consciousness a style of thinking or a way of viewing the world. Another may use the term to mean "self-awareness." Yet another may mean all the information of which one is aware at a given moment. Despite these and other problems, in this chapter we survey some of the complex and controversial ideas that have emerged as investigators have attempted to theorize about hemispheric differences as well as to extend the implications of left brain and right brain beyond the data.


## THE "WHY" AND "HOW" OF HEMISPHERIC SPECIALIZATION

Although much has been said about what each hemisphere can and cannot do, there is still little understanding of the reasons for hemispheric specialization in the first place. There is also little knowledge about the physiological mechanisms that may underlie these fundamental differences. Dealing with these "why" and "how" issues should help answer the "what" of specialization, a question that has preoccupied us throughout much of this book. It is not clear which question is more important or should be answered first. Insight into any one helps reformulate ideas about the other two. An ultimate understanding of hemispheric specialization undoubtedly will arise from the interaction of successively better answers to all three questions.

In earlier chapters, we mentioned different investigators' speculations concerning the evolution and the mechanisms of hemispheric asymmetry. We now try to bring these speculations together as well as to consider some more recent hypotheses about the nature of hemispheric specialization and callosal function.

## An Evolutionary Perspective

Why is the hemisphere that controls speech also the one that usually controls a person's dominant hand? Is it a coincidence, or is there a profound relationship that should tell us something about what is involved in both speech and manipulative skills?

Doreen Kimura and her colleagues have obtained evidence that the left hemisphere may be essential for certain types of hand movement.[1] Patients with damage to the left hemisphere but without paralysis of the right side may have difficulty copying a sequence of hand movements and complex finger positions with either the left or the right hand. Kimura suggests that this finding bears a relationship to reports in the clinical literature of deaf-mutes who sustained left-hemisphere damage in addition to their earlier speech and hearing disabilities. These individuals had used hand movements for communication, but after damage to the left hemisphere displayed disturbances of these movements similar to the disruption of speech suffered by normal speakers who sustain such damage.

Kimura has also studied the gestural hand movements of a group of normal subjects, including individuals with right-hemisphere speech dominance as determined by dichotic listening tests. If speech is controlled by the left hemisphere, as it is in most people, the right hand makes more of the free hand movements, whereas if speech is controlled by the right hemisphere, the left hand makes more of those movements.

Kimura and others have proposed that left-hemisphere specialization for speech is a consequence not so much of an asymmetric evolution of symbolic functions as of the evolution of certain motor skills "that happen to lend themselves readily to communication."[2] In other words, the left hemisphere evolved language, not because it gradually became more symbolic or analytic per se, but because it became well adapted for some categories of motor activity.

It is possible that the evolutionary advantages offered by the development of a hand skilled at manipulation also happened to be a most useful foundation on which to build a communication system, one that at first was gestural and utilized the right hand but later came to utilize the vocal musculature. As a result, the left hemisphere came to possess a virtual monopoly on control of the motor systems involved in linguistic expression, whether by speech or writing.

Although the differences are considerably less striking than in the case of expression, the left hemisphere also appears to be somewhat superior to the right in its comprehension ability. Researchers at the Haskins Laboratories have shown that the left hemisphere is better at decoding the extremely rapid transitions in frequency that are part of certain speech sounds. Using the dichotic listening technique, they found that right-handed subjects show a right-ear advantage for consonant–vowel syllables such as "ba," "da," and "ga." These differ only in terms of the rapid frequency changes taking place in the first 50 milliseconds or so of the syllable, so the left hemisphere appears to have an advantage in processing this quickly changing information.[3]

Some evidence directly implicating the left hemisphere in the processing of this rapidly changing frequency information comes from a study in which the duration of this information was increased using computer-synthesized speech. In one set of syllables, the frequency changes occurred within the first 40 milliseconds of the stimulus, and in the second set, the information was extended synthetically to 80 milliseconds. Overall identification was not affected by this process, and a significant right-ear advantage for both types of syllables was found when they were presented dichotically. The magnitude of the right-ear advantage, however, was significantly reduced when the rapidly changing frequency information was extended from 40 to 80 milliseconds. Subjects produced fewer correct right-ear responses and more correct left-ear responses with the 80-millisecond set than they did with the 40-millisecond set.[4]

But is the left-hemisphere advantage simply one of being able to track rapid frequency changes in speech? There is reason to believe that more is involved. Investigators at Haskins have discovered that the rapid frequency changes that signal *b* in the syllable "ba" are different from those that signal *b* in "be" or "bo." Similarly, the acoustic configuration of other consonants also changes as a function of the vowel in the syllable.[5] Figure 12.1 shows the nature of these changes for *d*.

What do all the different *b*s or *d*s have in common that allow our perceptual systems to hear them as identical sounds? Haskins researchers have noted that they are similar in terms of the way they are *produced*. The similarity in production, they argue, is responsible for the similarity in perception.

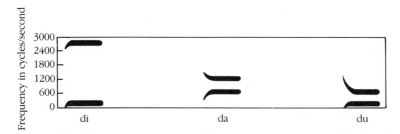

**Figure 12.1** Idealized spectrogram of sound frequencies produced in voicing "di," "da," and "du." Each sound consists of air vibration concentrated mainly within two frequency ranges, called the first and second formants. Recognizing these sounds involves perceiving the rapid change at the beginning of the formant. Even this early part of the formant changes as the vowel sound changes, despite the fact that all sounds start with *d.*

This idea, the motor theory of speech perception, holds that to perceive speech sounds, the human brain actually figures out what it would have had to do to produce them. Speech researchers have worked hard to explain what allows speech pronounced in so many different ways to be understood so readily. One quality that seems invariant across any particular sound is the way the throat, mouth, lips, and tongue are controlled in its production. The Haskins researchers have proposed that in perceiving speech, a listener is in some manner figuring out how he or she would produce the same sounds. Although this theory is not universally accepted, it is of interest to our discussion, for it suggests that finely controlled motor sequences may be an inseparable part of our language communication system, in terms of both production and perception.

What about the right hemisphere? Has it changed during the period in which the left hemisphere acquired its motor and communication skills? Abilities unique to the right hemisphere remain elusive and difficult to define, although spatial ability is strongly implicated. Just as the left hemisphere evolved language, a symbolic system surpassing any single sensory modality, perhaps areas in the right hemisphere evolved ways of representing abstractly the two- and three-dimensional relationships of the external world grasped through vision, touch, and movement. In addition to the spatial tasks considered in earlier chapters, the ability to visualize a complex route or to find a path through a maze seems to depend on the right hemisphere. Although it is usually characterized as more spatial than the left, it is probably more accurately described as more manipulo-spatial—that is, possessing the ability to manipulate spatial patterns and relationships.

We have just considered how verbal skills may have grown out of the fine movement skills of the left hemisphere. Perhaps the spatial skills of the right hemisphere are due to another kind of motor skill: the ability to manipulate spatial relationships. Our ability to generate mental maps, rotate images, and conceptualize mechanical contraptions could very well be an abstract, internalized, right-brain counterpart to the motor skills of the left brain.

Are these right-hemisphere skills a result of evolutionary specialization that developed in a complementary fashion to those occurring in the left brain? Or are they more ancient abilities that were at one time bilaterally represented but were essentially displaced in the left by the emergence of language? As mentioned in Chapter 2, different investigators hold different views on this issue. Jerre Levy, for example, has argued that the cognitive processes used for language and for spatial-perceptual functions are incompatible and, therefore, had to develop in separate areas. By analyzing the tasks and questions most difficult for each hemisphere of split-brain patients, she inferred that the left and right modes of processing would mutually interfere if they existed within the same hemisphere.

These kinds of data yield insights into why lateralization took place, but they do not necessarily invalidate the idea that it was mainly the left hemisphere that changed. The issue is not readily decided. Its resolution will depend on much more complete knowledge of what is both common and different about the two hemispheres, as well as the neural mechanisms behind the similarities and differences. Even when we achieve this knowledge, however, it is likely that several equally plausible evolutionary schemes for hemispheric specialization will remain.

## THE NATURE OF HEMISPHERIC SPECIALIZATION AND CALLOSAL FUNCTION: SOME RECENT IDEAS

### The Routine and the Novel

Learning and new task performance clearly involve dealing with situations in terms of codes and organizational schemes already present in the brain, that is, dealing with "what is out there" in terms of an already established repertoire of ways of describing and organizing events. This "repertoire" of ways in which an individual brain organizes and understands consists of a whole continuum ranging from biologically fixed visual pattern identification cells to natural language, musical notation, and culturally determined rules of games. Neuropsychologists Elkhonen Goldberg and Louis Costa call these built-in organizational schemes "descriptive systems" and propose that hemispheric differences in function are rooted in the extent to which an individual's "descriptive systems" are or are not applicable to ongoing events. They hypothesize that the left hemisphere is highly efficient at processing that takes advantage of well routinized codes, such as the motoric aspects of language production, and that the right hemisphere is crucial for situations for which no readily apparent code ("descriptive system") is available, that is, more novel situations. Their model also predicts a shift in the hemisphere involved in a particular task, depending on the extent to which the task becomes efficiently performed and routine.[6]

Their model is based partly on observation of the nature of tasks where discrepancies from "expected" hemisphere involvement seem to appear, and partly on some neuroanatomical considerations. As discussed in earlier chapters, not all language-related functions are in the realm of the left hemisphere, nor are all visuo-spatial functions the realm of the right hemisphere. They note that it is more the repetitive aspects of language—syntax (grammar) and phonology (sound structure)—that most clearly depend on left-hemisphere function. The right hemisphere appears to have some role in semantics (meaning) and a great deal to do with the contextual aspects of language.

Beyond mentioning these and several other generally accepted limits on simply labeling the left hemisphere the "verbal" hemisphere, Goldberg points out some interesting observations concerning the domain of the right hemisphere, such as what appear to be inconsistencies in the lateralization of figure and picture perception. Goldberg[7] mentions reports that the recognition of line drawings of meaningful objects seems to suffer predominantly after posterior left-hemisphere lesions, whereas the recognition of full photograph-like pictures may suffer after either left- or right-hemisphere lesions. Furthermore, the impairment of line-drawing recognition is greater than that of full picture recognition in left-hemisphere patients. This difference in the involvement of the two hemispheres in processing these two types of materials cannot be explained in terms of language codability—both are pictures of meaningful objects. It can be explained, however, from a perceptual point of view. Line drawings are the visual models of a whole set or class of real objects, whereas pictures are unique representations (or representations of unique objects).

"Classes of materials may differ in the degree of their relevance to existing descriptive systems, thus forming gradients of relative left–right hemispheric involvement in their processing," according to Goldberg. The data just described lead to an example of such a gradient for visual perception, ranging from line drawings of meaningful objects to detailed pictures of meaningful objects, to nonsense shapes, to human faces, with line-drawing interpretation being most left-hemisphere dependent and face recognition most right-hemisphere dependent (see Figure 12.2).

Cultural and individual differences may influence the available repertoire of pre-existing codes or descriptive systems. Speakers of Thai, a tonal language, show a right-ear dichotic listening advantage (indicating left-hemisphere processing) for tonal differences in vowels, whereas English speaking subjects do not.[8] As noted in Chapter 6, there have been reports of a right-ear preference for recognition of musical patterns by trained musicians, but a left-ear preference in nonmusicians.[9] Goldberg and Costa view this finding as consistent with the hypothesis that there is a right-to-left shift of hemispheric superiority as a function of increased competence with respect to a particular type of activity.

Goldberg and Costa discuss evidence for differences in neuroanatomical organization of the two hemispheres that may account for two fundamental distinctions in processing. They bring together data suggesting that areas devoted to sensory- and motor-specific function are greater in the left hemisphere[10] whereas the right hemi-

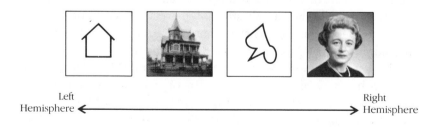

Left                                                                                      Right
Hemisphere ←—————————————————————————————→ Hemisphere

**Figure 12.2** An example of visual stimuli that fall into a continuum in terms of left- versus right-hemisphere processing, as suggested by Goldberg et al.

sphere is characterized by greater areas of "associative" (higher level, integrative) cortex[11] (see Appendix for a brief discussion of sensory – motor versus associative cortical areas). Combining the data from a study that suggested there is more tissue in the right hemisphere[12] with a study suggesting an asymmetry in the ratio of grey to white matter in each hemisphere,[13] Goldberg and Costa propose that there is relatively more white matter in the right hemisphere, indicating greater connections between regions in that hemisphere. Thus, "it appears that there is relatively greater emphasis on *inter*regional integration inherent in the neuronal organization of the right hemisphere, and on *intra*regional integration in the left hemisphere." In Chapter 1 we mentioned a related conclusion by Josephine Semmes, who proposed that mental processes are distributed over larger regions of brain tissue in the right half of the brain than in the left half.[14]

Goldberg and Costa conclude that as a result of these anatomical differences the right hemisphere has a greater capacity for dealing with informational complexity and for processing many modes of representation within a single task, whereas the left hemisphere is superior at tasks requiring detailed fixation on a single, often repetitive, mode of representation or execution. According to them, additional, indirect support for this viewpoint comes from data concerning the different ability of each of the two hemispheres to perform the functions of both. Evidence indicates that the right hemisphere is better able to take on language functions after left-hemisphere damage in infants, than the left hemisphere is able to take on visuo-spatial skills after right hemisphere damage.[15] Thus, the right hemisphere seems more flexible and able to handle greater informational complexity.

In summary, Goldberg and Costa argue against assigning fixed hemispheric specificities for particular materials or tasks and emphasize that "there is a gradient of relative hemispheric involvement in a wide range of cognitive processes, reflecting the degree of their *routinization*." Because of this they also emphasize individual differences in relative hemispheric contributions to performing different tasks. They place no value judgement on the relative "importance" of either hemisphere and argue that the left is "dominant" only insofar as it may have to do with elaborate or highly skilled functions in a cultural sense. In addition they suggest that:

Various views of the nature of hemispheral asymmetry need not be seen as mutually exclusive, but rather as examples of the *entire set of consequences* which stem from fundamental biological differences in hemispheral organization and function.[16]

## A Model of Callosal Function

In our discussions of models of hemispheric asymmetry of function up to this point, only minimal attention has been paid to the functions of the corpus callosum. In Chapter 2 we talked of the corpus callosum as a means of updating each hemisphere regarding information received by the other or perhaps suppressing one hemisphere while the other "takes over" some activity. At first glance this seems reasonable and consistent with the idea of the corpus callosum as an "interhemispheric integrator."

Actually, statements such as "the callosum integrates hemispheric activity by providing information from one hemisphere to the other" are vague and explain little if anything in terms of specific mechanisms. The notion of the interhemispheric fibers serving to either largely duplicate information between hemispheres or to generally suppress a hemisphere's activity lead to some paradoxical questions. As Jerre Levy has observed, if in fact the corpus callosum provides carbon copy-like information (e.g., something seen in the left visual field by the right hemisphere is sent over to the left hemisphere), why have the corpus callosum, "if all you need to do is move your eyes around."[17] After all, most split-brain patients seem to do quite well after they recover from the operation. On the other hand, if the corpus callosum only inhibits, allowing each hemisphere to function independently, why is it so complex, so intricate in its connections of so many regions of the brain? We need to develop a model that explains the need for its detailed connections, as the "carbon copy" model does, but which also explains how these connections provide unique or truly useful information.

We will now consider some hypotheses that look a little more carefully at these issues and propose more specific mechanisms for callosal function (as well as hemispheric asymmetries) at both a theoretical and anatomical/physiological level.

*Excitation or Inhibition? Regional or Global?* Psychologist Norman Cook considers four possible neurophysiological roles for the corpus callosum, two involving reducing neural activity (inhibition) and two involving increasing neural activity (excitation) in the hemisphere opposite to where activity starts.[18] Either inhibition or excitation can operate at the global (diffuse) level, slowing down or activating the entire hemisphere, or at the regional level, doing so only in specific regions in a "point in one hemisphere" to a "point in the other hemisphere" manner (callosal fibers do connect corresponding regions of the two hemispheres in a point-to-point or "topographic" manner). Thus, the four possibilities are: diffuse excitation, topographic excitation, diffuse inhibition, and topographic inhibition. Cook contends that neither excitation model is sufficient — diffuse excitation would amount to using the callosum for purposes of arousing or alerting the other hemisphere, and topographic excitation would provide carbon-copy information between hemispheres. In either case, the corpus callosum would tend to accentuate or duplicate what was already happening in the other hemisphere; Cook believes it must do more than that.

Cook similarly rejects the diffuse inhibition possibility, arguing that it is absurd to imagine so large a nerve fiber tract simply serving to shut down one hemisphere while the other is active. Besides, he argues, there is no electrophysiological or metabolic (e.g., blood flow) evidence that there is any suppression of overall activity in one hemisphere as the other becomes more active. This leaves Cook with the topographic inhibitory model, which he discusses in terms of how it can account for sharing of information between hemispheres in a manner that can serve to accentuate functional asymmetries. Contrary to first expectations, he argues, inhibition does *not* mean an absence of information. Cook shows how topographic inhibition can result in activation of complementary aspects of almost any function in the two hemispheres.

To understand his model we must first accept two assumptions, both of which have considerable support from experimental data. The first is that arousal and attentional mechanisms located deep in the brain tend to activate regions of both hemispheres symmetrically. The brain's main arousal system, the *reticular activating formation*, does in fact consist of subcortical groups of cell bodies and pathways that are not separated by cutting the callosum. As mentioned in Chapter 4, cerebral blood flow data have also shown that when there are increases in metabolism, they tend to occur in regions of both hemispheres, even during speech production. The other assumption is that related aspects of some item in memory are represented in the brain anatomically near each other, or at least that access to these related aspects is provided by neighboring neurons.

Cook contends that topographic inhibition across the corpus callosum suppresses in one hemisphere the exact same neuronal pattern of activity that originated in the other, but at the same time allows activity to develop in surrounding neurons representing complementary, e.g., contextual, aspects of the original information. Figure 12.3 illustrates how this might occur.

In most language-related activity, for example, it would be excitation in the left that inhibits equivalent neurons in the right and promotes surrounding context-associated processing. As an example, excitation of the cortical neurons that represent "cat" in the left hemisphere would inhibit "cat" in the right hemisphere while allowing excitation of peripheral cat-related neural assemblies ("kitten, lion, dog," etc.) in that hemisphere. If the ongoing language is, "The cat pounced on the mouse," then not only would individual words produce related contextual items in the right but also the meaning of the left hemisphere's sentence, as a whole, would generate right-hemispheric contextual meaning.

Where "the cat pounced on the mouse" denotes a specific act of predation, the pattern in the right hemisphere would be inhibition of that specific act of predation (cat and mouse), but excitation of

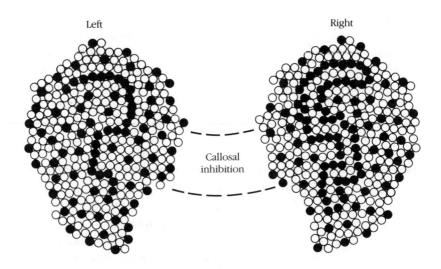

Figure 12.3 An example of topographic inhibition, mediated by the corpus callosum, creating a suppression of activity in the same grouping of cells of the right hemisphere that are active in the left. This is accompanied by increased activity in the immediately surrounding neurons in the right hemisphere that are thought to encode related or contextual information. Dark circles represent neurons or columns of neurons that are firing. [From Cook, "Callosal Inhibition: The key to the Brain Code," Fig. 1, p. 102, in *Behavioral Science*, 1984]

classes of similar predator–prey relationships — connoting the dominance of the strong over the weak, the surprise and desperation of the attack, etc.[19]

These complementary aspects of whatever item is being processed are the result of a "mirror-image negative relationship" between equivalent areas of the two hemispheres, created or at least accentuated by continuous topographic inhibition across the cerebral commissures. In the case of language, this implies that whatever the left hemisphere asserts explicitly, the right hemisphere connotes in a more generalized pattern with the explicit message omitted. Thus, by producing two distinctly different patterns of neural excitation within bilaterally identical regions (each of which was aroused by the general attentional system), "callosal homotopic inhibition allows the 'two brains' momentarily to hold different perspectives on the same information."

Language-related examples are just one type of example of how this system works, according to Cook. The idea of complementary functions of equivalent areas extends to other functions including perception where, for example, perception of a visual figure versus its contextual background also operates in a similar manner. Cook's assumption that equivalent (homotopic) areas of the two hemispheres end up active for complementary aspects is supported by what is known about subtle language and cognitive deficits after right hemisphere injury — such as the deficits in context, metaphor, and humor discussed in Chapter 6.

### Do the Hemispheres Make Use of Different Neural Circuits?

A recent paper by psychologist S.H. Woodward has proposed a relationship between two different patterns of neuronal connectivity and the specialized functions of the two cerebral hemispheres. Bringing together some theoretical concepts of memory storage and some basic neurophysiological data, Woodward proposes that left-hemisphere processing relies primarily on tight connections between vertical columns of neurons, whereas right hemisphere processing depends on weaker and longer horizontal connections.[20] Figure 12.4 illustrates the prominent horizontal and vertical dimensions evident in the major layers of cortical neurons and their interconnections (see Chapter 4 for a brief discussion of the cortical layers). Both vertical and horizontal circuitry have been well studied by neuro-

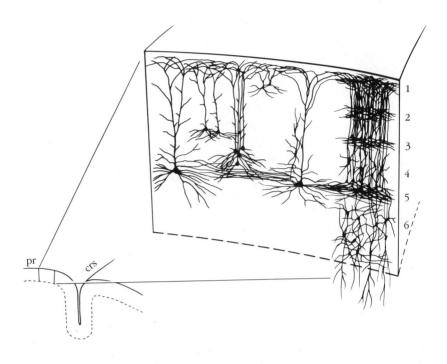

**Figure 12.4** A cross-section through a cortical gyrus illustrating the prominent horizontal and vertical dimensions of assemblies of cortical neurons and their interconnections. The six layers of different types of neurons are the same as those discussed in Chapter 4. The interconnections are formed by both axons and dendrites, mostly from pyramidal cells. [Adapted from Scheibel, Davies, Lindsay, and Scheibel, "Basilar dendritic bundles of giant pyramidal cells," Fig. 1, p. 309, in *Experimental Neurology, 42,* 307–319, 1974]

physiologists and there is no conclusive evidence that the connections actually differ in some way in the two hemispheres. What could differ, however, is which kind of circuitry is more utilized in each hemisphere.

Woodward reviews several modern theories concerning ways to store information and notes the striking parallel between alternative models of memory storage and the kinds of processing horizontal and vertical neuronal connections can offer. Several theorists have examined ways of coding information while concentrating on the extent to which each way is accurate and efficient. As expected, there is an "accuracy/efficiency trade off" in any design—the most accurate storage systems are usually the most cumbersome and inflexible. Two theoretically different ways of storage that seem relatable to anatomical processes are "conjunctive encoding" and "coarse encoding."[21]

"Conjunctive encoding" uses a separate definite unit of memory or memory trace (for example a connection between cells) to stand for every aspect and every important relationship (conjunction) between items. Such an encoding scheme is highly specific but quickly runs out of units. In "coarse encoding" each elementary unit of memory is broadly tuned so that properties or features specified by a unit overlap in varying degrees with those specified by others. Any part or feature of, say, a visually presented item, is then represented by activity in a group of units within whose overlapping representational boundaries it falls. Although efficient and quite flexible in terms of situations it can approximately code, coarse encoding has limitations. A coarse encoding system breaks down when it has to encode large numbers of highly similar, co-occurrent events.

This is the situation with the encoding necessary for language articulation, where, as discussed earlier, complex and highly similar speech sounds co-occur continuously. This limitation may apply even more strongly to the codes necessary for fine motor movements of the dominant hand. The motor memory codes for either require highly similar, often simultaneous movements whose representation in memory cannot be achieved via coarse, overlapping patterns. Much of the material considered to be the realm of the left hemisphere requires a memory system capable of highly specific, very compactly organized representations. This appears to be more in line with the potential of conjunctive encoding and the characteristics of columnar "vertical" organization.

Figure 12.5 schematically illustrates the two types of neuronal connecting circuits as if they were completely segregated to the left and the right hemisphere. The right-hemisphere anatomy is presumed to be dominated by overlapping horizontal connections, thought to involve greater distances, and to be weaker or less precise than the tight vertical columns of neurons in the left. Diagrams illustrating the concepts of "coarse encoding" type memory have looked very similar to the overlapping connections drawn on the right side of Figure 12.5; thus, this kind of memory storage may be associated with patterns coded by horizontal neuronal connections. The efficiency of "coarse encoding" increases as features of a stimulus are more dispersed and variable. "These characteristics appear to

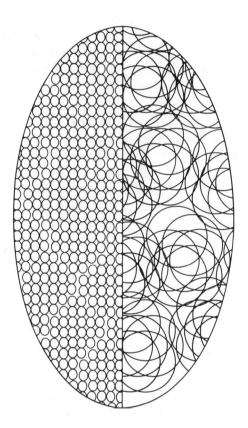

**Figure 12.5** This diagram represents an idealization of differences in the way neural circuitry is utilized by right- and left-hemisphere functioning. In the left, it is mostly highly coupled, nonoverlapping connections between vertically arranged cell neighbors that are important. Precision coding of small differences, like those needed for fine motor movements, would depend on this type of columnar organization. In the right, horizontal axonal connections dominate, and cell groups over large distances overlap in their connections, which are "weaker" than the vertical connections that the left tends to depend on. The encoding potential of this kind of anatomy seems to be more applicable to encoding more diffuse, less repetitive information, as in most visuo-spatial stimuli. [Adapted from Woodward, 1988.]

correspond closely to classical notions of the right hemisphere as excelling in the integration of spatially and temporally disparate features and the representation of stimulus 'wholes and continuities.'"[22]

What establishes the left hemisphere's use of "vertical" neuronal connections and the right hemisphere's use of "horizontal" connections? Because the vertical and horizontal anatomy does not appear to be lateralized, Woodward has to account for lateralization of their activities, that is, a hemispheric difference in physiological use rather than in anatomy itself. Neurophysiologists have shown that activities within a hemisphere tend to suppress or inhibit horizontal connections (through "lateral inhibition" and "positive feedback") and that vertical circuitry tends to dominate local cortical patterns. (In fact, in Norman Cook's model of callosal function previously discussed, the surrounding "contextual" neurons are suppressed in the left hemisphere by inhibition created by initial processing of the stimulus material.)

If vertical cortical circuitry dominates the response to a stimulus, how does horizontal circuitry prevail in some situations? Woodward proposes that this happens through inhibitory signals carried over to the right hemisphere by the corpus callosum (the reader may note some similarity with Cook's model). He suggests that in the absence of hemispheric specialization, it is the vertical mode that prevails or is more primary, that is, it is the left hemisphere's kind of specialization that is the "unmarked case" and that transcallosal input to the right hemisphere permits increasing utilization of horizontal, "coarse coding" type of storage and processing.

Woodward claims clinical evidence from cases of callosal agenesis and hemispherectomies performed in infants (see Chapter 8) supports that left-hemisphere (language) functions can develop in either hemisphere but that right-hemisphere (visuo-spatial) skills only seem to develop well when there are two intact hemispheres.[23] Thus, the left hemisphere imposes specialization on the right and this, Woodward proposes, is done via callosal inhibition of vertical circuitry and the subsequent utilization of horizontal processes. Woodward suggests that a class of cells called "double-bouquet" cells, to which the callosum projects, could conceivably mediate the relative dominance of vertical and horizontal circuitry in favor of the latter.[24]

*Some Comments* It is interesting to consider how similar, yet different, some aspects of these models are. For example, consider how the same evidence — differential recovery from early left- versus early right-hemisphere damage — is interpreted differently by Goldberg and Costa and by Woodward.

Goldberg and Costa interpret this evidence as a "differential ability of each of the two hemispheres to perform the function of both." Thus, because the right hemisphere develops good language skills after left-hemisphere damage in infants, but the left hemisphere does not seem to be able to develop good nonverbal skills after right-hemisphere damage, Goldberg and Costa suggest that the right hemisphere is *better able* to subserve the functions of both hemispheres. This, they claim, is indirect support that the right hemisphere has increased capacity for dealing with complexity, whereas the left hemisphere is superior at tasks requiring "fixation."

Woodward sees the same difference in recovery data as evidence that left-hemisphere organization is primary, that is, always has to be present before "right-hemisphere type" functions develop. Thus, Goldberg and Costa's view attributes more initially fixed or "hard wired" differences to the hemispheres, whereas Woodward views these differences as arising from a progression that first establishes one kind of processing which, in turn, alters how processing is done on the other side. The fact that it is almost always the left side that starts this in Woodward's model still requires some biologically-based "hard wired" bias in development.

It is also interesting to note the similarities in the function of the corpus callosum postulated by Cook and by Woodward. In both cases the information transferred is mostly inhibitory in nature. In Cook's model the callosal signals suppress "identical patterns" of activity and foster activity in adjacent neurons thought to represent related or contextual information. In Woodward's model, callosal signals suppress vertical neuronal circuitry allowing the other kind of connections, horizontal, to be used to a greater degree. In both models callosal inhibition serves to suppress in the other hemisphere the exact same pattern of activity started on one side of the brain and foster some other kind of activity. In Cook's model, this other activity is highly related to the initial stimuli, so the hemispheres end up dealing with different aspects of the same information. In Woodward's model the callosal signals bias the way in which the right hemisphere deals with information in general.

## TWO BRAINS, TWO MINDS?

More than four centuries ago, the great French philosopher René Descartes concluded that the pineal gland, at the base of the brain, is the seat of consciousness. He based his conclusion on his belief in the unity of consciousness and on the fact the pineal gland was the only brain part he could find that was not double in structure.

Assigning consciousness to part of the body seems an inconsistent twist in Descartes' thinking if one examines his writings on the relationship between body and mind. Although Descartes enjoyed mechanically analyzing some of the functions of living things and had great interest in human anatomy (see Figure 12.6), he felt there was something about human beings that could not be explained in these terms. He saw the human body as similar to the bodies of animals, but he questioned whether the human mind could be part

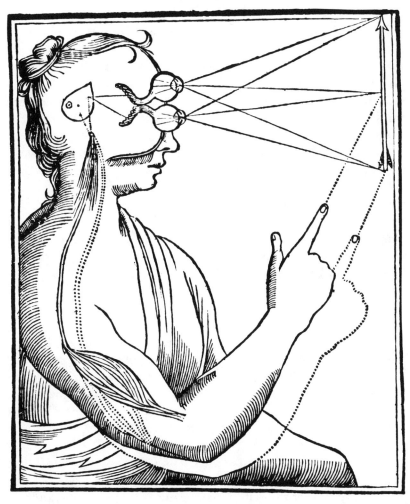

**Figure 12.6** Descartes' diagram illustrating the interaction of mechanistic and mental processes in the pineal body. Light reflected from an object (an arrow) is imaged on the retinas of the eyes and conducted by the optic nerves to the brain. There, it is apprehended by the soul at the pear-shaped pineal body, which also initiates responsive movements. [Reprinted by permission of Sandford Publications, Oxford, England.]

of the same physical world. An analysis of one's own thought, he felt, cannot prove the existence of anything outside personal experience. Descartes concluded that an absolute distinction must be made between the mental and the physical.

The assertion that the mind is independent of the body came to be known as *Cartesian dualism*. Some modern skeptics have referred to it as the "ghost in the machine" idea. The philosophical issues revolving around the relationship between body and mind in general are referred to as the *mind–body problem*.

Within the past two and a half decades, work with split-brain patients has raised questions about the implications of split-brain surgery for the mind–body problem. If the surgeon's knife accomplishes a separation of consciousness, then splitting the brain *is* splitting the mind. One is then forced, the argument goes, to accept the fact that mind is brain, or at least that mind arises from the workings of the brain.

Although one can argue with the premise that split consciousness implies mind is brain, most of the controversy in this areas focuses on whether such patients can actually be shown to possess two realms of consciousness, at least some of the time. In Chapter 2 this question was discussed on a theoretical level by Gustav Fechner and William McDougall. Fechner argued that the split-brain operation would result in a doubling of consciousness. McDougall argued that consciousness would remain unaffected by such a procedure.

Roger Sperry has argued that the results of split-brain research point to a doubling of consciousness in these patients:

> Everything we have seen so far indicates that the surgery has left these people with two separate minds, that is, two separate spheres of consciousness. What is experienced in the right hemisphere seems to lie entirely outside the realm of experience of the left hemisphere. This mental dimension has been demonstrated in regard to perception, cognition, volition, learning, and memory.[25]

For Sperry, the impression of mental unity in split-brain patients is an illusion, a consequence of the sharing by the two sides of the brain of the same position in space, the same sensory organs, and the same experiences in everyday situations outside the lab.

In contrast, Sir John Eccles, also a Nobel laureate for his work in physiology, does not believe that there are two separate minds in a split-brain patient or that consciousness is in any way split by commissurotomy.[26] He claims that the right hemisphere cannot truly think. He makes a distinction between "mere consciousness," which humans share with animals, and the world of language, thought, and culture, which is uniquely human and essential to any idea of a mind.

In Eccles' opinion, everything that is truly human derives from the left hemisphere, where the speech center resides and where interactions between brain and mind occur. The split-brain patient who blushes or smiles when a pinup is flashed to her right hemisphere not only cannot report why she did so but truly does not *know* why she blushed. The right hemisphere cannot know because only the left hemisphere can have thoughts or knowledge.

Although such controversies are highly confounded by subjective definitions of *consciousness*, some attempts have been made to be more precise in using this term. One approach is to form an operational definition, which is a definition in terms of the procedures that may be used to measure a concept. Along these lines, Donald McKay, who theorizes about artificial intelligence, has noted that the split brain cannot be viewed as a split mind until it can be shown that each separated half has its own independent system for assigning values to events, setting goals, and establishing response priorities.

An experiment to address this point was conducted by Joseph LeDoux and Michael Gazzaniga with their unique commissurotomy patient, P.S. The study took advantage of the considerably greater than usual linguistic capabilities in P.S.'s right hemisphere, which is discussed in Chapter 2. P.S.'s right hemisphere was able to express itself by arranging Scrabble letters with the left hand in response to questions. LeDoux and Gazzaniga's intention was to ask subjective questions of each hemisphere separately and to compare the results.

On each trial, P.S. was asked a question orally. The key word or words were replaced by the word "blank." The missing word or words were then visually presented in either the left visual field (to the right hemisphere) or in the right visual field (to the left hemisphere). The questions included "who *(are you)*?" "Would you spell the name of your favorite *(hobby)*?" "What is *(tomorrow)*?" The italicized items were the key words actually flashed in the respective visual field. When they were presented to the right hemisphere, P.S. was asked to spell out his answers using the Scrabble letters.

P.S. was also asked to rate how he felt about a particular word by pointing to a number from 1 ("like very much") to 5 ("dislike very much"). Some of the words were chosen because of their personal significance to the patient. They included "Paul" (his name) and

"Liz" (his girl friend's name). A sample question is, "How much do you like _____?" A word would then appear in either the left or the right visual field.

The results showed both that P.S.'s right hemisphere could answer the questions asked and that its answers and evaluations sometimes differed from those of the left hemisphere. For example, ratings by the right hemisphere were consistently closer to the "dislike" end of the scale in the word-rating test than were ratings by the left hemisphere. When asked the job he would pick, the right hemisphere spelled out "automobile race," in contrast to P.S.'s normal left-hemisphere verbal assertion that he wanted to be a draftsman.

LeDoux and Gazzaniga further noted that the answers to a few questions varied in several different testing sessions. Sometimes the answers given by the left and the right were similar; sometimes they were discordant. P.S. appeared to be in a better mood on the days when the opinions and values of the left brain and the right brain overlapped.

Regarding the issue of double consciousness, the investigators stated:

> Each hemisphere in P.S. has a sense of self and each possesses its own system for subjectively evaluating current events, planning for further events, setting response priorities, and generating personal responses. Consequently, it becomes useful now to consider the practical and theoretical implications of the fact that double consciousness mechanisms can exist.[27]

Although P.S. is a special case because of the extent of verbal capabilities in both his hemispheres, the theoretical implications of demonstrating an apparent double-consciousness in the same person extend beyond this one case. In addition to illustrating the older claim that splitting the brain can split the mind, LeDoux and Gazzaniga feel that their observations suggest "the nature and origin of those mental qualities unique to man." These, they feel, are dependent on an active language system:

> When this system is absent, as in the right hemisphere of most split brain patients, . . . the organism functions mainly at the perceptual motor level. Though certain cognitive skills can be demonstrated in such instances, the richness and characteristic flexibility of human behavior seems to be lacking in the absence of linguistic sophistication. . . . Add a rich linguistic system to an isolated mass of non-

verbal tissue as in the right hemisphere of P.S., and a human being with the capacity to value, aspire, and reflect on life experience emerges.[28]

The idea that consciousness is dependent on language or linguistic processes is not entirely new. Several philosophers and linguists have subscribed to so-called verbal access theories of consciousness. These theories have in common the concept that the brain events experienced as conscious are the events processed by the language system of the brain.

## CONSCIOUSNESS AND THE HEMISPHERES

### The Origins of Consciousness: Verbal Access Theories

Until as recently as 3,000 years ago, members of the group *Homo sapiens* were virtually automatons, lacking both a concept of self-fulfillment and a sense of the brevity of life. They heard voices inside their heads and called them gods. These gods told them what to do and how to act. Their minds were divided into two parts: an executive part called "god" and a follower part called "man." When writing and more complex human activity started weakening the authority of the auditory hallucinations, this "bicameral mind" slowly broke down. The voices of the gods fell silent, and what we call consciousness was born.

This is the radical theory of Princeton psychologist Julian Jaynes. Jaynes proposes that the speech of the gods occurred in the right hemisphere and was heard by the auditory and speech centers of the left hemisphere by means of the cerebral commissures. Perhaps, he suggests, the pattern-recognition and spatial processing mechanisms of the right hemisphere were communicating with the left hemisphere through primitive language.

Jaynes supports many of his contentions by reference to ancient literature and to history. He feels that the *Iliad*, for example, describes a people who are not conscious. They do not decide to fight, and they do not plan strategy or do anything else without the intervention of a god or some hallucination.

These auditory and visual hallucinations, occurring whenever a novel situation arose, show us the structure of the bicameral mind. Achilles, like all bicameral people, had a split mind. One part, the executive god part, stored up all admonitory experience and fitted things into a pattern and told the follower or person part what to do through an auditory hallucination.[29]

To Jaynes, consciousness depends on linguistic processes and the creation of an internal, metaphorical "I." Consciousness is a smaller part of our mental life than previously assumed. A great deal of our mental activity is not conscious but automatic: we do not think about it. This is one reason why it should not be so difficult to imagine ancient humans going through life without the "self-consciousness" we have developed. They may not have been able to view themselves at a distance or to imagine themselves doing something in the future.

> Consciousness is learned on the basis of language and taught to others. It is a cultural invention rather than a biological necessity. . . . We know now that the brain is more plastic, more capable of being organized by the environment than we previously supposed. . . . We can assume that the neurology of consciousness is plastic enough to allow the change from the bicameral mind to consciousness to be made largely on the basis of learning and culture.[30]

Although there is considerable controversy concerning Jaynes' theory, the idea of connecting the voices of gods in ancient times to a stage in the cultural development of language is fascinating. In addition to his view, there are other ways in which the development of language may have been responsible for some of the earlier beliefs of human beings. Instead of equating the voices of the gods with the right hemisphere's attempt to speak to the left, ancient men and women can be viewed as having misinterpreted internalized speech developing in the left hemisphere. It is possible that in the early phases of the evolution of language, humans were caught off guard by the fact that they could speak to themselves.

Jaynes' theory is a bold example of theories dealing with the topic of consciousness in terms of linguistic mechanisms. Because verbal skills are the most clearly lateralized functions of the brain, such verbal access theories of consciousness lead to questions about the relationship between hemispheric function and consciousness.

## The Right Hemisphere and the Unconscious

Arthur Koestler, a well-known writer, argued that the "creative act" usually occurs through other than conscious analytic intention. In his book *The Act of Creation*, Koestler mentions the idea of incubation periods: putting a problem aside for a time in the hope of coming up with an insight later. He also suggests that the unconscious does a great deal of matchmaking or forming of analogies.

Several famous scientists have told how they found a solution to a problem during a dream. Otto Loewi, who won the 1936 Nobel Prize in Physiology or Medicine for showing that nerve impulses are transmitted by means of chemical agents, described how the critical experiment came to him in a near-sleep state. He had come up with the idea of chemical transmission 17 years earlier but had put it "aside" for lack of a way to test it. Fifteen years later he performed experiments (unrelated to his old idea) for which he had designed a technique to detect fluids secreted by a frog's heart. One night, two years later:

> I awoke, turned on the light, jotted down a few notes on a tiny slip of thin paper. Then I fell asleep again. It occurred to me at six o'clock in the morning that during the night I had written down something most important, but I was unable to decipher the scrawl. The next night, at three o'clock, the idea returned. It was the design of an experiment to determine whether or not the hypothesis of chemical transmission that I had uttered seventeen years ago was correct. I got up immediately, went to the laboratory, and performed a simple experiment on a frog heart according to the nocturnal design.[31]

Loewi isolated two frog hearts, the first with its nerves intact, the second without. He stimulated the vagus nerve of the first heart. The vagus nerve has an inhibitory effect on the heart, so its beat slowed down. He immediately removed some of the salt solution in which the heart was bathed and applied it to the second heart. It slowed down. By going a few steps further, Loewi unequivocally proved that nerves influence the heart (and most other tissue) by releasing specific chemical substances from their terminals.

A careful review of the chain of events leading to Loewi's experiment dispels any notion that it was an accidental or purely intuitive discovery. The background for it had been set by years of rigorous work. However, the act of connecting two critical ideas apparently came while he was in an unconscious or semiconscious state.

Koestler attributes a role to the unconscious in discovery, calling it the "type of thinking prevalent in childhood and in primitive societies, which has been superseded in the normal adult by techniques of thought which are more rational and realistic."[32] As for the incubation period (such as the 17-year period in Loewi's case), Koestler calls it "thinking aside" or a rebellion against constraints that is "a temporary liberation from the tyranny of overprecise verbal concepts, of the axioms and prejudices ingrained in the very texture of specialized ways of thought."[33]

The temptation to reinterpret such ideas in terms of the laterality data is obviously great. Several investigators have suggested that dreaming is part of the realm of the right hemisphere. Some believe that the right hemisphere does all the dreaming; others feel that the dream state allows the right hemisphere to express itself more freely than usual because the left hemisphere does not dominate or interfere. Sigmund Freud, the father of psychoanalysis, believed that the qualities of the unconscious mind are revealed through the logic of dreams.

Do the discoveries with split-brain patients have any consequences for Freud's theories? David Galin thinks they do. He believes they provide a neurological validation for Freud's notion of an unconscious mind. Galin points out that the right hemisphere's mode of thought is similar to Freud's description of the "unconscious," and he notes a parallel between the functioning of the isolated right hemisphere and mental processes that are repressed, unconscious, and unable to control behavior directly: "Certain aspects of right hemisphere functioning are congruent with the mode of cognition psychoanalysts have termed primary process, the form of thought that Freud originally assigned to the system Ucs (unconscious)."[34] These include the extensive use of images, lesser involvement in the perception of time and sequence, and a limited language of the sort that appears in dreams and slips of the tongue.

Galin believes that the two hemispheres usually operate in an integrated fashion, but at certain times they may be blocked from communicating with each other. As a result, a situation similar to what is found in split-brain patients may occur in a normal individual. Galin describes several ways in which the two hemispheres of an ordinary person could function as if they had been surgically disconnected. In one interesting example, he talks of the inhibition of information transfer because of conflict: "Imagine the effect on a child when his mother presents one message verbally, but quite another with her facial expression and body language; 'I am doing it because I love you, dear' say the words, but 'I hate you and will destroy you,' says the face."[11]

Galin believes that although each hemisphere is exposed to the same sensory input, it effectively receives a different input because each emphasizes only one of the messages. The left will attend to the verbal cues, and the right will attend to the nonverbal cues. He continues with the following conjecture:

> In this situation, the two hemispheres might decide on opposite courses of action; the left to approach and the right to flee. . . . The left hemisphere seems to win control of the output channels most of the time, but if the left is not able to "turn off" the right completely, it may settle for disconnecting the transfer of the conflicting information from the other side. . . . Each hemisphere treats the weak contralateral input in the same way in which people in general treat the odd discrepant observation that does not fit with the mass of their beliefs; we first ignore it, and then if it is insistent, we actively avoid it.[36]

Galin believes that during such moments of disconnection, the left hemisphere alone governs consciousness. Mental events in the right hemisphere, however, continue a life of their own and act as a "Freudian" unconscious, as an "independent reservoir of inaccessible cognition," which may create uneasy emotional states in a person.

It is interesting to note that LeDoux and Gazzaniga make some anecdotal observations about their patient P.S. that seem psychodynamic in nature. They refer to the experiments where they addressed subjective questions to P.S.'s left and right hemispheres separately:

> The day that case P.S.'s left and right hemispheres equally valued himself, his friends, and other matters, he was a calm, tractable, and appealing adolescent. On the days that the right and left sides disagreed on these evaluations, case P.S. became difficult to manage behaviorally. Clearly, it is as if each mental system can read the emotional differences harbored by the other at any given time. When they are discordant, a feeling of anxiety, which is ultimately read out by hyperactivity and general overall aggression, is engendered. The crisp surgical instance of this dynamism raises the question of whether or not such processes are active in the normal brain, where different mental systems, using different neural codes, coexist within and between the cerebral hemispheres.[37]

## The Role of Verbal Mechanisms in Mental Unity, or the Chicken and Snow Shovel Experiment

Gazzaniga and LeDoux conducted another series of experiments on P.S., which they claim provides a clue to a major mechanism of personal thought—the process by which we construct a reality based on actual behavior.

P.S. was tested with pairs of visual stimuli presented simultaneously to each side of a fixation point located on a projection screen. The picture falling into each visual field was thus processed by the hemisphere normally receiving input from that side of the fixation point. P.S. was asked to use his hands to point to pictures that were related to what he had seen flashed on the screen from among several placed in front of him. Figure 12.7 shows the procedure.

He did this quite well. His right hand pointed to a picture related to one that had been flashed in his right visual field (to the left hemisphere), and his left hand pointed to a picture related to one that had been flashed in his left visual field (to the right hemisphere). Of particular interest was the way in which P.S. verbally interpreted these double responses:

> When a snow scene was presented to the right hemisphere and a chicken claw was presented to the left, P.S. quickly and dutifully responded correctly by choosing a picture of a chicken from a series of four cards with his right hand and a picture of a shovel from a series of four cards with his left hand. The subject was then asked, "What did you see?" "I saw a claw and I picked the chicken, and you have to clean out the chicken shed with a shovel."
>
> In trial after trial, we saw this kind of response. The left hemisphere could easily and accurately identify why it had picked the answer, and then subsequently, and without batting an eye, it would incorporate the right hemisphere's response into the framework. While we knew exactly why the right hemisphere had made its choice, the left hemisphere could merely guess. Yet, the left did not offer its suggestion in a guessing vein but rather a statement of fact as to why that card had been picked.[38]

Gazzaniga and LeDoux see in these results the suggestion that the major task of the "verbal self" is to construct a reality based on actual behavior. They feel that verbal mechanisms are not always

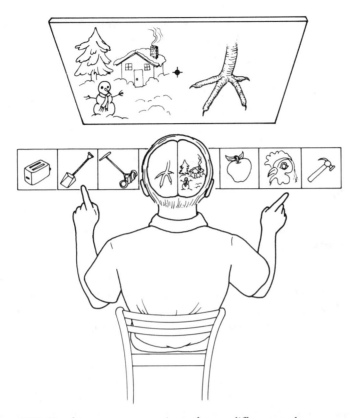

**Figure 12.7** Simultaneous presentation of two different tasks, one to each hemisphere of patient P.S. The patient's left hemisphere saw the chicken claw, and the right hemisphere saw a snow scene. Each hemisphere responded by choosing, with the contralateral hand it controlled, a picture related to what it had seen. The patient was then asked to "explain" his choices. [From Gazzaniga and LeDoux, *The Integrated Mind*, Fig. 42, p. 149 (New York: Plenum Press, 1978)]

privy to the origin of our actions and can attribute cause to actions not actually accessible to them: "It is as if the verbal self looks out and sees what the person is doing, and from that knowledge it interprets a reality." They raise the question of whether we indeed know whence our many separate behaviors arise.

They also offer the hypothesis that a developing organism contains a constellation of mental systems — emotional, motivational, and perceptual — each with its own values and response probabilities:

Then, as maturation continues, the behaviors that these separate systems emit are monitored by the one system we come to use more and more, namely, the verbal, natural language system. Gradually, a concept of self-control develops so that the verbal self comes to know the impulses for action that arise from the other selves, and it either tries to inhibit these impulses or free them, as the case may be.[39]

They conclude that the left hemisphere, in most of us, contains that which makes us feel like single, purposeful beings — that is, our language system.

### From Split Brain to Normal Brain: A Case for Mental Duality in Both

When the word *teacup* is projected tachistoscopically on a screen, with *tea* presented to the left and *cup* to the right of a fixation point, a split-brain patient cannot read the whole word. Instead, the patient will say the word was *cup*, because the verbal left hemisphere saw what was to the right of fixation (the right visual field). The patient's left hand, under control of the mute right hemisphere, will point to the word *tea* in an array of words that includes *cup* and *teacup*. Some theorists feel this situation is a convincing argument for the duality of mind in the split-brain patient; otherwise, one gets into difficulty answering simple questions about the experiment:

Q: Did the patient see the word *teacup*?

A: Of course he did.

Q: Then why did he say he saw *cup*?

A: His left hand pointed to *tea*, so if you put the two responses together . . .

Q: But the left hand passed over *teacup* in favor of *tea*, just as he said he saw, not *teacup*, but *cup*.

A: Well, it's all the same patient, isn't it?

Q: Yet you or I would say *teacup* and point to *teacup* with the left hand. Surely there is some difference between our responses and his. And that difference seems to be that his left hemisphere sees only *cup*, the right only *tea*.

A: If you insist . . .[40]

Roland Puccetti argues that the patient's responses indicate a true perceptual experience in each hemisphere. "So here it appears that what is going on in each hemisphere is not just an initial registration of the visual material but a reading out—verbally in one case, manually in the other—of what was actually seen."[41]

But Puccetti goes beyond the issue of whether there are two minds in a split-brain patient to propose that, in fact, double consciousness is the *normal* situation in humans without the operation. In the intact human brain, under the same experimental conditions, the word *teacup* is seen at the same time in both hemispheres, one half of the word coming directly to each hemisphere and the other half coming indirectly via the corpus callosum (see description of the visual system in Chapter 2). Why then, Puccetti asks, does not the subject not see *teacup teacup* instead of just *teacup*, if consciousness spans both hemispheres?

Some would answer that the duplication is only in the initial sensory registration of the stimulus that is not at a conscious level— the double sensory representations are fused in the processing that leads to our "seeing" the stimulus. Puccetti contends, however, that each hemisphere normally does "see" the whole visual field; that is, each hemisphere is conscious of *teacup* just as each hemisphere is conscious of half that word when the corpus callosum is split. Thus, cutting the corpus callosum does not in itself produce a divided mind but, rather, only deprives two existing minds of half their normal visual input (the ipsilateral half-field), subsequent to which the separate consciousnesses become evident. In the intact brain, neither half-brain has introspective access to the conscious contents of the other. The callosal connections do not provide this; rather, they provide transfer of more basic sensory information.

Puccetti explains his view of two separate centers of visual awareness by drawing an analogy with two side-by-side observers of a football game. Each observer sits in a booth that provides a direct window view of half the field and a television view, similar in size and adjoining the window, of the other half. The window-view half for each observer is the television view for the other. If the television cables are cut, each observer loses sight of the half of the football field that the other sees directly through the window.

Yet nothing in the visual experience of either of the viewers, before or after the cables are cut, provides any introspective evidence that there are really two of them, side by side. Indeed as Gazzaniga [1970] has pointed out, following split-brain surgery, the speaking viewer to the left initially does not even notice that half the field is gone.[42]

But why this duplication of conscious experience? Puccetti claims, as others have, that duplication has to occur at the sensory level, that each half-brain must supply information about what it is seeing to the other half. "How much more efficient it is if nature wires in a relay system so that each half brain sees the same visual target in the same place in extrabodily space at almost the same time."[43] But at the same time, he contends, conscious unity must be confined to each hemisphere; otherwise, there would be a doubling of the sensory field at a conscious level, and this would be counterproductive when dealing with any visual target. Thus, there is no overall mind spanning the two half-brains.

Why is it that we are not aware of two separate conscious entities within our heads? Why do the two half-brains seem to work so well together? Puccetti feels that the cross-cuing phenomenon provides part of the answer. Experiments with split-brain patients have shown that the disconnected left (verbal) hemisphere will actually claim possession of material presented to only the right hemisphere. A transcript from a session with commissurotomy patient L.B., whose mute right hemisphere had just been shown a picture of his mother, helps illustrate this:

Examiner: "Do you know who it is?"

L.B.: "Uh-huh," in an affirmative tone.

Examiner: "Can you name it? Who is it?" When subject hadn't answered after several seconds examiner added "Don't know who?"

L.B.: "I know who, but I can't verbalize it."

Examiner: "Can you give the name?"

L.B.: "I know I can spell it but you won't let me spell."[44]

L.B.'s left hand could spell out "Mom" under control of the mute right hemisphere, but the examiner did not allow this. The right hand could not do this, even though it is the talking left hemisphere that claims it can be done. What is significant is that "the verbal half brain insists it has this knowledge, under the surface somewhere, and implies that there is no other conscious center that has it."[45]

Puccetti also argues that the right hemisphere's continuing to faithfully cue the speaking hemisphere, as in a game of charades, under such experimental conditions attests to its lifetime role in a secondary position to the left hemisphere in most matters of communication with the outside world. Little is changed for the mute right hemisphere after commissurotomy. Occasionally it can undertake an independent action with the left arm or leg but on the whole has no way of expressing itself except through providing information to the left hemisphere.

Puccetti's hypothesis of duality of consciousness in the normal brain, as one may expect, has a large number of critics. Nevertheless it is an interesting approach to questions brought to mind by split-brain research.

### What Kind of "Selves" Are Hemispheres?

Philosopher–psychologist Daniel N. Robinson of Georgetown University argues that issues pertaining to the unity of consciousness are largely unaffected by split-brain data.[46] He reminds us that the issue is older and deeper than contemporary commentators generally acknowledge, and that examination of historical versions of the dispute reveal insights and confusions similar to those now filling the pages of contemporary journals. Much of the confusion has to do with questions of definition — words that have quite different meanings are used interchangeably, leading not only to confusion but to subtle deceptions.

Robinson acknowledges the scientific merit of new findings and theories regarding the lateralization of psychological processes. However, he sees only one consistent finding in research with split-brain patients that can be claimed to have relevance to issues of "split selves" or "double consciousness." This, he says, is the personal state of "epistemic contradiction," the contradictory knowledge–claims sometimes encountered in the testing of commissurotomized patients. The same patient, often at nearly the same time, will assert and deny a specific claim or fact of memory: "The left hand, as the expression goes, may not know what the right one is doing, or as today's commentator would say, the left brain doesn't know what the right one is saying, because the right one cannot speak." These contradictions "are used in defense of the notion of the disunity or multiplicity of self or," Robinson goes on, "the duality of self, apparently because there happen to be two hemispheres."

The plain fact, Robinson argues, is that any number of experimental operations produce just this state in perfectly normal observers. For example, observers under certain cueing conditions will "recall" a number or letter which, after it was initially presented briefly in an array, they could not recognize at all.[47] In certain psychophysical experiments observers will respond just as quickly to a flash they claim they do not "see" as to the same flash when it is presented alone.[48] Robinson mentions other examples such as "hysterical" patients who adopt entirely distinct identities, sleep walkers who complete elaborate actions and do not recall anything about it afterwards, and hypnotic subjects who deny what they know.

> For those who would use such findings as proof of a multiplicity of selves, there is an embarrassment of riches to which commissurotomies add very little, but for those committed to the duality thesis, the findings are actually too good for the thesis to be true. States of epistemic contradiction are, as it happens, not limited to two per person. Recall Eve's *three* faces, and Binet[49] turned up cases involving many more. Needless to say, however, none of these cases included any evidence of more than two hemispheres.[50]

The real problem, Robinson contends, has to do with meanings and interchangeable use of such words as "self," "self-identity," "personal identity," and "person." A *person* is a human being, often of unknown identity, possessing certain attributes not present to the same degree in the rest of the animal kingdom—a collection of attributes shared by *many* entities of a certain kind. One can answer "it is a person" to a *what* question.

To know *who* that person is we must go beyond the attributes that established personhood and establish the *personal identity*. If we inquire as to name, occupation, address and details of a person's life we may assert that we know the actual identity of the person—the *personal identity*. This is different from *self-identity*, however, because, for example, that specific person may be amnesic and therefore ignorant of the very identity we established. Nevertheless, the amnesic is not doubtful of existing and "surely must be granted a *self*, and will claim as much whether we grant it or not."

Robinson contends that some of the effects observed in split-brain patients and the other examples of contradictory knowledge claims *may* be taken as evidence of multiple *personal identities* and even multiple *self-identities*, but in no case are they evidence of multiple *selves*.* Robinson concludes:

> The separate personal identities and the different self-identities ascribed to and adopted by a person may be shocking to that person when subsequently discovered. But the basic fact of existence as a conscious entity cannot be shocking, for this is never news. As of now logic, language, and data leave the "moi" (me) intact and preserve the unity of self as an issue of continuing interest, and even of mystery.[51]

## LEFT AND RIGHT IN BIOLOGY AND PHYSICS

French biologist Louis Pasteur discovered in the nineteenth century that molecules of tartaric acid could assume either of two mirror-image forms and that a certain plant mold could act on one, but not on the other, form of the acid. This meant that the plant mold, in effect, could tell left from right! Pasteur assumed that this implied that a fundamental asymmetry exists in the molecular structure of the plant mold itself and wrote, "This important criterion (of molecular asymmetry) constitutes perhaps the only sharply defined difference which can be drawn at the present time between the chemistry of dead or living matter." He went on to speculate that "life is dominated by asymmetrical actions. I can even imagine that all living species are primordially, in their structure, in their external forms, functions of cosmic asymmetry."[52]

Are the origins of asymmetry in humans and in certain other life forms to be found in more fundamental aspects of nature — in the fundamental forces operating in biology and physics? The forces of nature have long been assumed to preserve *parity*, a concept derived from physics that means, in its most general sense, that phenomena remain unchanged if reflected through a plane or viewed in a mirror; that is, natural interactions in the world look just as normal viewed in a mirror as they do viewed directly. It is only the presence of human artifacts (such as writing) or the knowledge of the exact arrangements of an original scene that can give away whether a

---

*And, we add, it may be most reasonable to view them simply as laboratory manifestations of the many unconscious processes going on within a person's head that psychology and physiology have been attempting to document over the last hundred years.

picture is mirror-reversed or not. The laws governing a mirrored scene, including how objects interact, appear to be exactly the same as those governing the original. Pasteur's idea of a cosmic asymmetry, however, though perhaps not justified by the limited data on which it was based, was nevertheless prophetic of some recent developments in biology and physics.

## Molecular Biology

The discovery of deoxyribonucleic acid (DNA) as the genetic material in cells and the discovery of DNA's helical structure was heralded as a major contribution to biology and genetics. The double strands of each DNA molecule encode genetic information in terms of the sequencing of component amino acids. The two long strands are wound around each other in a clockwise spiral; thus, the DNA molecule cannot be superimposed on its mirror reflection. Some investigators have speculated that this and other asymmetries at the molecular level underlie the gross asymmetry in some organisms, including the leftward displacement of the heart and, perhaps, handedness and cerebral lateralization in humans. They argue that these gross asymmetries must lie in the molecular mechanisms that control the development of the organism's structure.[53] Although each cell contains identical DNA molecules containing all of the information necessary to form the complete organism, the cells differentiate to form different kinds of tissue (muscle, bone, blood, neurons, etc.). It is thought that the genetic information in each cell interacts with some other source of "positional" information in the growing embryo that determines the cell type and ultimately the actual shape and structure of the organism.[54]

The mechanisms regulating the growth of structure and form are not known, and the existence of a positional code is only hypothesized. Psychologists Corballis and Beale suggest that any systematic differences in the formation of left and right would be part of this code and that genes themselves do not encode the direction of asymmetry. They argue that the positional code must consist of a structural asymmetry at the molecular level. Whether or not the asymmetries are expressed depends on interaction of the positional code with the genetic code. As noted in Chapter 5, Corballis and Beale propose that in most people, handedness and cerebral lateralization are under the influence of a left–right gradient contained in the positional code that results in right-handedness and the left-cerebral control of speech. In some minority, however, this positional code gradient "is denied expression, and the directions of handedness and cerebral lateralization are assigned randomly and independently."[55]

### Parity in Nuclear Physics

As previously mentioned, the forces of nature have long been assumed to preserve parity; that is, normal interactions in the world do not in any way define left and right in the sense that such concepts could be derived from asymmetries in the way things work (or forces operate). Even the deflection of a compass needle to the left or the right by a parallel current carrying wire could not be used to define these directions, because the designations of the needle's "north" and "south" poles are essentially arbitrary. A mirror image of an experiment set up to deflect a compass needle with an electric current would look perfectly normal because the observer would assume the needle's poles were reversed.

In 1957, however, physicists discovered that some instances of the so-called weak nuclear force (or weak interaction) involving radioactive emissions from atoms did not conserve parity. The nucleus of the cobalt-60 atom was shown to emit electrons more frequently from one end than from the other. The north and south poles of a magnetic field, thus, could be defined in an absolute way by stating that if cobalt-60 nuclei are lined up in the field, then the south pole is that toward which the greater number of electrons are emitted.[56] This would also allow distinguishing between a compass needle's deflection (in the presence of a current carrying wire) in the real world and in a mirror.

The issue of whether a fundamental distinction exists between left and right in the physical laws of the universe remains a debated one. Some physicists have appealed to "deeper" principles to argue that parity is still preserved, such as the essentially arbitrary nature in which "positive" and "negative" electric charge is defined, along with the consequent labeling of the direction of current flow. Even the direction of time flow is brought in as a factor to help preserve the sense of absolute symmetry in natural interactions. Nevertheless, there is a sense now that, at least at relatively fundamental levels of analysis of physical interactions, natural asymmetries do occur.

Are these more or less fundamental physical asymmetries the basis for the asymmetries evident at the level of molecular biology? At first glance it seems unlikely, because it is not evident how asymmetries at the level of weak nuclear interactions have any influence at the biochemical level, for chemical interactions depend on the electro-magnetic force, a much stronger force than that associated with nuclear decay. It is thought that the influence of these asymmetries at the level of chemical interactions is negligible, yet some theorists have speculated that, given the time scale of biochemical evolution on earth, the influence would be substantial.[57] In addition, there is some evidence that parity is not conserved at the level of electromag-netic and, therefore, chemical interactions.[58]

In reviewing these and other data for asymmetries in nature, Corballis and Beale conclude that "they do strengthen our convic-tion that the systematic asymmetries of morphology, molecular biol-ogy, and subatomic interactions are ultimately linked, and that there is, after all, an absolute, universal distinction between left and right."[59]

## POSTSCRIPT

In the process of reviewing the literature for this book and reflecting on our own direct involvement in the area of hemispheric specializa-tion for many years, we have become increasingly aware of the "dichotomania" problem. One symptom of the problem is to exag-gerate hemispheric differences and to ignore other forms of brain organization, such as the orderly differences within a hemisphere.

At the same time, we have become even more impressed with the reality of hemispheric differences and with their potential for helping us understand the brain mechanisms underlying higher mental func-tions. It is possible that some of the most profound human mental abilities are a result of nature's forfeiting, to an extent, a very old, stable, and successful method of changing the brain: bilaterally sym-metric evolution. Why so much of nature involves mirror-symmetri-cal structure, and why the brain has for the most part evolved in a mirror-symmetrical fashion, is a theoretical issue that largely remains a subject of conjecture.

One suggestion is that a doubled structure is less subject to damage. Mechanisms in one side can easily take over functions lost in the other because they are basically doing the same thing. Once asymmetries developed, this advantage was lost. Substituting for this loss of redundancy, however, was the added survival value of lan-guage, sophisticated mental mapping capabilities, and whatever other talents the integrated action of the asymmetric components of the two hemispheres can generate.

In studying these asymmetries, researchers are going beyond what is different about the halves of the brain. They are uncovering ways in which the brain deals with different kinds of information in the environment and ways in which it generates some of our behavior. The discovery of different processes and mechanisms in the brain encourages the idea that mental abilities may be explained in these ways. Investigators have touched on issues of consciousness, emotion, and the unity of experience. Some of these may be premature attempts using insufficient data and inappropriate definitions, but they are steps, first steps, in the long endeavor to understand the brain and, perhaps, ourselves.

# *Appendix*

*Functional*
*Neuroanatomy:*
*A Brief Review*

Modern functional mapping of the human brain has been attempted through the study of the effects of brain damage, electrical stimulation, neurosurgical procedures, and neuroanatomical studies coupled with animal research. The history of thought on the relationship between neuroanatomy and behavior has revolved around two opposing views. At one time, fanciful maps of the brain were drawn allotting specific regions to "thrift," "love of family," "greed," "memory," and so on. At the other extreme was the view that the brain operates as a unit and that within the brain, there are no relationships between particular regions and specific mental functions.

Brain researchers today have moved away from these extremes. The brain is now thought to be organized in both a focal and a diffuse manner, depending on what functions are being studied. Basic sensory and motor functions are controlled by very specific regions, whereas higher mental functions involve a constellation of regions across the brain.

In this Appendix, we review some basic neuroanatomy, concentrating on the cortical regions of the cerebral hemispheres — the regions of the human brain involved in most of the debate about asymmetry of function. We have tried to present views that represent a consensus among brain researchers, although considerable controversy remains in many instances. Because of these uncertainties, it is necessary to consider the newest "maps" of the brain as a rough guide rather than as a definitive road atlas.

The central nervous system consists of the spinal cord and the brain. The brain is conventionally divided into three major regions: the hindbrain, the midbrain, and the forebrain. These areas and some of the structures within them are demarcated in Figure A.1.* The major divisions are made on an embryological basis. Each develops from a different embryonic layer and is roughly related to different evolutionary stages in the development of the vertebrate nervous system.

Hindbrain and midbrain structures have traditionally been thought to control the more automatic, unconscious aspects of behavior. These include basic functions essential to life, such as breathing, the sleep–wake cycle, and levels of arousal or degrees of responsiveness to external events. It is becoming more apparent that these deeper structures of the brain also contribute to the processing of information necessary for higher mental functions.

The forebrain is the largest and most highly developed section of the brain in humans and the higher animals. It consists of a complex of anatomically distinct groups of nerve-cell bodies called nuclei, which are surrounded by nerve fibers sheathed in myelin and covered by the cerebral cortex.† The cortex forms the familiar convoluted surface of the brain and consists of multiple layers of com-

---

*Reference is often made to the brain stem and to the cerebrum. The brain stem includes the hindbrain and midbrain structures, excluding the cerebellum. Some anatomists also include the very central nuclei of the forebrain (the thalamus), located immediately above the midbrain. The cerebrum refers to the forebrain.

†The nerve fibers sheathed in myelin are known as "white matter" because of their white appearance in fresh brain tissue. The cortex, which has a gray appearance, is known as "gray matter."

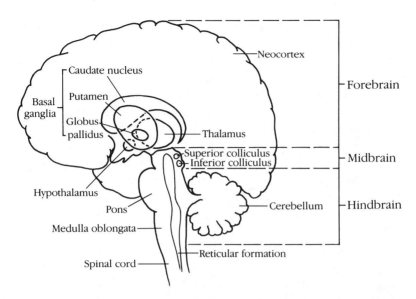

**Figure A.1** Schematic view of the brain showing the basic relationships of deep nuclear groups and brain-stem structures. [From Gazzaniga, Steen, and Volpe, *Functional Neuroscience*, Fig. 3.13, p. 61. (New York: Harper & Row Publishers, 1979).]

plexly interconnected neurons. It is the "newest" structure, in evolutionary terms, and is well developed only in mammals; it is most expansive and convoluted in humans. The neocortex, as most of the human cortex is called, contains approximately 9 billion of the 12 billion neurons of the central nervous system. It is generally considered to be responsible for the highest functions of the human brain, such as abstract thought and language.

The entire central nervous system is essentially bisymmetric. A sagittal plane (front to back) through the middle of the human body will divide the nervous system into two mirror-image sections. The left and right halves of the brain stem do not physically separate until the thalamus of the forebrain. The forebrain looks like separate mirror-image halves connected by fiber bundles. These halves are the cerebral hemispheres.

## Functional Areas of the Cortex

Almost the entire surface of each cerebral hemisphere consists of neocortex. Each hemisphere can be divided into four lobes, using the major folds of the cortex, called gyri (ridges) and sulci (valleys), as landmarks. Figure A.2 shows the divisions along the surface of one hemisphere. The central sulcus separates the frontal lobe from the parietal lobe. It also serves as the landmark for separating the anterior, or front, half of each hemisphere from the posterior areas.

The other major fissure, called the lateral sulcus (sylvian fissure), separates the temporal lobe from the frontal and parietal lobes. The most posterior portion of the cortex is called the occipital lobe.

Each lobe is known to serve a different sensory or motor function. The occipital lobe is a visual center. Parts of the temporal lobe are involved with hearing. The anterior part of the parietal lobe is concerned with somatosensory function. The posterior part of the frontal lobe mediates motor function. Figure A.3 shows the areas involved.

The areas of the cortex receiving input from the sense organs or controlling the movements of particular body parts are called primary zones or primary projection areas. The primary motor areas of the frontal lobe control specific parts of the body (see Figure A.4). The primary sensory areas in the parietal, temporal, and occipital lobes are said to possess high modal specificity: each is active only when there is stimulation in its particular modality. In addition, within each primary sensory area, smaller areas respond only to highly specific properties or parts of its "sensory window."

All primary areas are topologically arranged so that there is a systematic, orderly representation in the cortex of different parts of the body, different auditory qualities, and specific parts of the visual

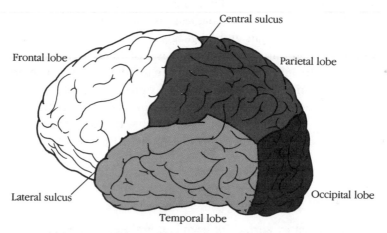

**Figure A.2** Division of the cerebral hemisphere into lobes.

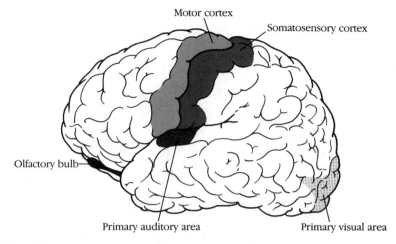

**Figure A.3** Primary sensory and motor areas of the brain. The remaining areas are often termed "uncommitted" or "association" cortex.

field. Lesions in these areas lead to highly specific deficits, such as blindness in one part of the visual field, selective hearing loss, loss of sensation in one part of the body, or partial paralysis. The extent of the damage will determine the amount of the "sensory window" that is lost.

Figure A.5 shows the primary projection areas in the brains of four animals and in the human brain. In lower animals, most of the brain is devoted to sensory and motor functions; there is little else. In higher animals, and especially human beings, a great deal of the cortex does not seem to be committed to the specific senses. These areas are known as "uncommitted" cortex or "association" areas.

## The Association Areas of the Parietal, Occipital, and Temporal Lobes

Some investigators make a distinction between secondary and tertiary association cortex. Secondary zones are the areas adjacent to the primary projection areas and are still considered to have some modal specificity; that is, they are higher-level processing centers for the specific sensory information coming into the primary area. Modality-specific information becomes integrated into meaningful wholes in secondary zones. Single sensory stimuli are combined and

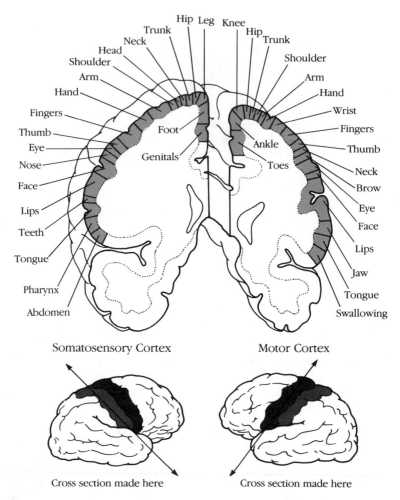

Figure A.4 The motor and somatosensory areas of the cortex are projections of areas of the body. Some areas, such as those representing the face, tongue, and fingers, are disproportionately large because the amount of cortical surface devoted to a given part of the body reflects the requirements of that body part. The lips take up more space in the motor cortex than they do in the somatosensory cortex, as the lips do more muscle-controlled moving than they do sensing. [From Lassen, Ingvar, and Skinhoj, "Brain Function and Blood Flow," Scientific American, Inc., 1978. All rights reserved.]

elaborated into progressively more complicated patterns. Damage to secondary zones gives rise to perceptual disorders restricted to a specific modality. In visual agnosia, for example, a patient can see but does not recognize or comprehend what is being looked at. There are also auditory and tactile agnosias.

Tertiary zones* lie at the borders of the parietal, temporal, and occipital secondary zones. In these association areas, or "zones of overlapping," modal specificity disappears. Neural activity does not seem to depend on stimulation of any single sensory modality. Various sensory fields overlap, and combinations of sensations become perceptions of a progressively higher order. Tactile and kinesthetic impulses are built up into perceptions of form and size and are associated with visual information from the same objects. It is thought that objects come to be represented ultimately by a constellation of memories compounded from several sensory channels. Damage to areas such as the parietal–occipital junction and parietal–temporal junction result in disorders transcending any single modality.

It is at this level that hemispheric asymmetries appear. Damage to the right hemisphere within these zones may produce disorders of manipulo-spatial abilities or the neglect syndrome, in which a patient ignores the left half of space. Damage within these zones in the left hemisphere may interfere with language comprehension or the ability to name objects. Thus, the association areas of the posterior of the brain seem to be concerned with high-level perceptual processes and more abstract "manipulation" of these processes. The left and right hemispheres seem to differ in what processes they handle best.

## The Association Areas of the Frontal Lobes

The rear of the frontal lobe is the primary motor area. The secondary motor area, analogous to the secondary sensory zones of the posterior of the brain, lies immediately in front of the motor strip and is called the premotor area. This area is involved in higher-level motor organization. Damage to this region leads to disturbances in the organization of movements. (Damage to the motor strip itself leads to paralysis.) In the left hemisphere, damage to specific parts of the premotor area (Broca's area) leads to disorganization of speech—the expressive dysfunction known as Broca's aphasia.

The functions of the remaining areas of the frontal lobes seem more elusive. The areas in the anterior part of the frontal lobes (called prefrontal) are no longer directly tied in to motor control and are believed to serve higher integrative functions. This prefrontal

---

*The definition of *tertiary zones* is from A. R. Luria, *Higher Cortical Functions in Man* (New York: Basic Books, 1966).

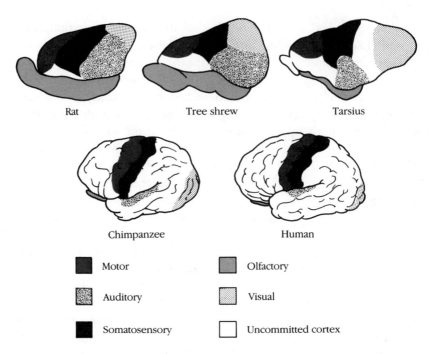

Rat                    Tree shrew                  Tarsius

Chimpanzee                    Human

■ Motor                    ■ Olfactory

▨ Auditory                    ▨ Visual

■ Somatosensory                    □ Uncommitted cortex

**Figure A.5** The brains of five mammals, showing differences in the proportions of "uncommitted" cortex to areas devoted primarily to sensory and motor functions. [From Penfield, *Brain and Conscious Experience*, ed. J. C. Eccles (New York: Springer-Verlag, Inc., 1966), Pontifica Academia Scientiarum.]

area is often referred to as frontal granular cortex because of the characteristic "granular" neurons of which it is mostly composed. As shown in Figure A.6, these areas are particularly enlarged in the human brain. They account for humans' distinctively high forehead when the shape of their skulls is compared with the skulls of other primates.

Damage to these prefrontal areas can result in both intellectual and personality changes. Although patients still seem capable of performing many different tasks, deficits in executing sequences of operations or solving complex problems becomes evident. A patient may have trouble shifting "set" and become stuck on a task. There is an inability to inhibit the first tendency aroused by a problem. Having done one step properly, the patient may continue to use the same strategy in totally inappropriate contexts. This is often referred to as perseveration. These syndromes suggest that the frontal lobes are involved in the planning and organization of actions.

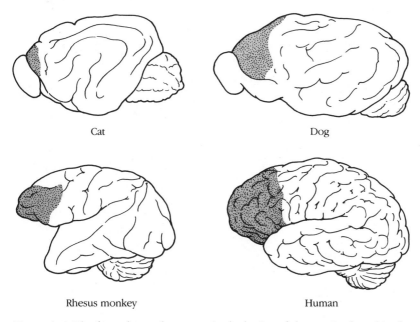

Cat                              Dog

Rhesus monkey                    Human

**Figure A.6** The frontal granular cortex in the brains of three animals and in the human brain (not drawn to scale). [From Walsh, *Neuropsychology—A Clinical Approach* Fig. 4.1, p. 110. (Edinburgh: Churchill Livingstone Ltd., 1977).]

The inflexibility seen in certain frontal syndromes has often been called a deficit in abstract thinking, but this label is controversial. Some investigators claim a "dissociation between thought and action." The patient can verbalize what he or she should be doing yet is unable to carry it through.

The personality and emotional changes associated with damage to the frontal lobes are even more elusive than the intellectual deficits. Earlier in this century, the frontal regions were the object of many experimental surgical procedures that attempted to control several forms of mental illness. Despite a great deal of literature on the subject, the question of how the frontal lobes function and the actual effects of the operations remain controversial.

In general, it appears that the frontal association areas not only play a major role in planning and controlling action, but may also control or inhibit emotional tendencies. Luria has suggested that the frontal areas serve as a tertiary integrative zone for the motor system as well as for the limbic system, an older region deeper in the forebrain believed to play a major role in emotion.

# Notes

## Chapter 1  A Historical Overview of Clinical Evidence for Brain Asymmetries

[1] R. W. Sperry, "Brain Bisection and Consciousness," in *Brain and Conscious Experience*, ed. J. Eccles (New York: Springer-Verlag, 1966).

[2] R. Ornstein, *The Psychology of Consciousness*, 2nd Ed. (New York: Harcourt Brace Jovanovich, 1977).

[3] R. Ornstein, "The Split and Whole Brain," *Human Nature* 1 (1978): 76–83.

[4] P. Bakan, "The Eyes Have It," *Psychology Today* 4 (1971): 64–69.

[5] J. E. Bogen, "The Other Side of the Brain. VII: Some Educational Aspects of Hemispheric Specialization," *UCLA Educator* 17 (1975): 24–32.

[6]W. Gibson, "Pioneers in Localization of Brain Function," *Journal of the American Medical Association* 180 (1962): 944–951.

[7]P. Broca (1863), cited in R. J. Joynt, "Paul Pierre Broca: His Contribution to the Knowledge of Aphasia," *Cortex* 1 (1964): 206–213.

[8]P. Broca (1864), cited in M. Critchley, *Aphasiology and Other Aspects of Language* (London: Edward Arnold, 1970).

[9]P. Broca (1865), cited in S. Dimond, *The Double Brain* (London: Churchill-Livingstone, 1972).

[10]J. H. Jackson, *Selected Writings of John Hughlings Jackson*, ed. J. Taylor (New York: Basic Books, 1958).

[11]Ibid.

[12]Ibid.

[13]Ibid.

[14]T. Weisenberg and K. E. McBride, *Aphasia: A Clinical and Psychological Study* (New York: Commonwealth Fund, 1935).

[15]H. Hecaen and M. Albert, *Human Neuropsychology* (New York: Wiley, 1978).

[16]O. Dalin (1745), cited in A. L. Benton and R. J. Joynt, "Early Descriptions of Aphasia," *Archives of Neurology* 3 (1960): 205–222.

[17]A. Gates and J. Bradshaw, "The Role of the Cerebral Hemispheres in Music," *Brain and Language* 4 (1977): 403–431.

[18]J. Semmes, "Hemispheric Specialization, a Possible Clue to Mechanism," *Neuropsychologia* 6 (1968): 11–26.

[19]B. Bramwell, "On Crossed Aphasia," *Lancet* 8 (1899): 1473–1479.

[20]W. Penfield and L. Roberts, *Speech and Brain Mechanisms* (Princeton, N.J.: Princeton University Press, 1959).

[21]J. A. Wada and T. Rasmussen, "Intracarotid Injection of Sodium Amytal for the Lateralization of Cerebral Speech Dominance: Experimental and Clinical Observations," *Journal of Neurosurgery* 17 (1960): 266–282.

[22]T. Rasmussen and B. Milner, "The Role of Early Left-Brain Injury in Determining Lateralization of Cerebral Speech Functions," in *Evolution and Lateralization of the Brain*, ed. S. Dimond and D. Blizzard (New York: New York Academy of Sciences, 1977).

## Chapter 2 The Human Split Brain: Surgical Separation of the Hemispheres

[1]T. C. Erikson, "Spread of Epileptic Discharge," *Archives of Neurology and Psychiatry* 43 (1940): 429–452.

[2]W. Van Wagenen and R. Herren, "Surgical Division of Commissural Pathways in the Corpus Callosum," *Archives of Neurology and Psychiatry* 44 (1940): 740–759.

[3]G. Fechner (1860), cited in O. Zangwill, "Consciousness and the Cerebral Hemispheres," in *Hemispheric Function in the Human Brain*, ed. S. Dimond and G. Beaumont (New York: Halsted Press, 1974).

[4]J. Akelaitis, "Studies on the Corpus Callosum. II: The Higher Visual Functions in Each Homonymous Field Following Complete Section of the Corpus Callosum," *Archives of Neurology and Psychiatry* 45 (1941): 789–796.

A. J. Akelaitis, "The Study of Gnosis, Praxis and Language Following Section of the Corpus Callosum and Anterior Commissure," *Journal of Neurosurgery* 1 (1944): 94–102.

[5]R. E. Myers, "Function of Corpus Callosum in Interocular Transfer," *Brain* 79 (1956): 358–363.

R. E. Myers and R. W. Sperry, "Interhemispheric Communication Through the Corpus Callosum. Mnemonic Carry-Over Between the Hemispheres," *Archives of Neurology and Psychiatry* 80 (1958): 298–303.

[6]R. W. Sperry, "Hemisphere Deconnection and Unity in Conscious Awareness," *American Psychologist* 23 (1968): 723–733.

[7]M. S. Gazzaniga, *The Bisected Brain* (New York: Appleton-Century-Crofts, 1970).

[8]S. M. Ferguson, M. Rayport, and W. S. Corrie, "Neuropsychiatric Observations on Behavioral Consequences of Corpus Callosum Section for Seizure Control," in *Epilepsy and the Corpus Callosum*, ed. A. G. Reeves (New York: Plenum Press, 1985).

[9]M. White, Personal Communication.

[10]F. Bremer, "An Aspect of the Physiology of Corpus Callosum," *Journal of Electroencephalography and Clinical Neurophysiology* 22 (1967): 391.

[11]C. B. Trevarthen, "Manipulative Strategies of Baboons, and the Origins of Cerebral Asymmetry," in *Hemispheric Asymmetry of Function*, ed. M. Kinsbourne (London: Tavistock, 1974).

[12]R. W. Doty, "Electrical Stimulation of the Brain in Behavioral Cortex", *Annual Review of Psychology* 20 (1969): 289–320.

[13]J. Levy, C. Trevarthen, and R. W. Sperry, "Perception of Bilateral Chimeric Figures Following Hemispheric Disconnection," *Brain* 95 (1972): 61–78.

[14]L. Franco and R. W. Sperry, "Hemisphere Lateralization for Cognitive Processing of Geometry," *Neuropsychologia* 15 (1977): 107–114.

[15]P. Greenwood, D. H. Wilson, and M. S. Gazzaniga, "Dream Report Following Commissurotomy," *Cortex* 13 (1977): 311–316.

[16]E. Zaidel and R. W. Sperry, "Memory Impairment Following Commissurotomy in Man," *Brain* 97 (1974): 263–272.

[17]Ferguson, Rayport, and Corrie, "Neuropsychiatric Observations on Behavioral Consequences of Corpus Callosum Section for Seizure Control."

[18]J. E. LeDoux, G. Risse, S. P. Springer, D. H. Wilson, and M. S. Gazzaniga, "Cognition and Commissurotomy," *Brain* 100 (1977): 87–104.

[19]M. S. Gazzaniga and S. A. Hillyard, "Language and Speech Capacity of the Right Hemisphere," *Neuropsychologia* 9 (1971): 273–280.

[20]E. Zaidel, "A Technique for Presenting Lateralized Visual Input with Prolonged Exposure," *Vision Research* 15 (1975): 283–289.

[21]E. Zaidel, "Auditory Language Comprehension in the Right Hemisphere Following Cerebral Commissurotomy and Hemispherectomy: A Comparison with Child Language and Aphasia," in *Language Acquisition and Language Breakdown*, ed. A. Caramazza and E. Zurif (Baltimore: Johns Hopkins University Press, 1978).

[22]M. S. Gazzaniga and J. E. LeDoux, *The Integrated Mind* (New York: Plenum Press, 1978).

[23]M. S. Gazzaniga, B. Volpe, C. Smylie, D. H. Wilson, and J. E. LeDoux, "Plasticity in Speech Organization Following Commissurotomy," *Brain* 102 (1979): 805–816.

[24]M. S. Gazzaniga, "Right Hemisphere Language Following Brain Bisection: A 20 Year Perspective," *American Psychologist* 38 (1983): 525–537.

[25]E. Zaidel, "A Response to Gazzaniga: Language in the Right Hemisphere, Convergent Perspectives," *American Psychologist* 38 (1983): 342–346.

[26]N. Geschwind, "The Frequency of Callosal Syndromes in Neurological Practice," in *Epilepsy and the Corpus Callosum*, ed. A. G. Reeves (New York: Plenum Press, 1985).

[27]R. D. Nebes, "Direct Examination of Cognitive Function in the Right and Left Hemispheres," in *Asymmetrical Function of the Brain*, ed. M. Kinsbourne (Cambridge: Cambridge University Press, 1978).

[28]J. E. LeDoux, D. H. Wilson, and M. S. Gazzaniga, "Manipulo-Spatial Aspects of Cerebral Lateralization: Clues to the Origin of Lateralization," *Neuropsychologia* 15 (1977): 743–750.

[29]L. Franco and R. W. Sperry, "Hemisphere Lateralization for Cognitive Processing of Geometry," *Neuropsychologia* 15 (1977): 107–111.

[30]R. Puccetti, "The Alleged Manipulospatiality Explanation of Right Hemisphere Visuospatial Superiority," *Behavioral and Brain Sciences* 4 (1981): 75–76.

[31]H. Erlichman and J. Barrett, "Right Hemisphere Specialization for Mental Imagery: A Review of the Evidence," *Brain and Cognition* 2 (1983): 55–76.

[32]M. J. Farah, M. S. Gazzaniga, J. D. Holtzman, and S. M. Kosslyn, "A Left Hemisphere Basis for Visual Imagery?" *Neuropsychologia* 23 (1985): 115–118.

[33]M. Corballis and J. Sergent, "Imagery in a Commissurotomized Patient," *Neuropsychologia* 26 (1988): 13–26.

[34]G. L. Risse, J. E. LeDoux, S. P. Springer, D. H. Wilson, and M. S. Gazzaniga, "The Anterior Commissure in Man: Functional Variation in a Multi-Sensory System," *Neuropsychologia* 16 (1977): 23–31.

W. F. McKeever, K. F. Sullivan, S. M. Ferguson, and M. Rayport, "Hemispheric Disconnection Effects in Patients with Corpus Callosum Section," in *Epilepsy and the Corpus Callosum*, ed. A. G. Reeves (New York: Plenum Press, 1985).

[35]J. Levy-Agresti and R. W. Sperry, "Differential Perceptual Capacities in Major and Minor Hemispheres," *Proceedings of the National Academy of Science, U.S.A.* 61 (1968): 115.

[36]J. Levy, "Psychobiological Implications of Bilateral Asymmetry," in *Hemispheric Function in the Human Brain,* ed. S. Dimond and S. Beaumont (New York: Halstead Press, 1974).

[37]C. Trevarthen, and M. Kinsbourne, cited in J. Levy, "Cerebral Asymmetries as Manifested in Split Brain Man," in *Hemispheric Disconnection and Cerebral Function*, ed. M. Kinsbourne and W. L. Smith (Springfield, Ill.: Charles C. Thomas, 1974).

[38]Levy, Trevarthen, and Sperry, "Perception of Bilateral Chimeric Figures Following Hemispheric Disconnection."

[39]Levy, "Psychobiological Implications of Bilateral Asymmetry."

[40]J. Levy and C. Trevarthen, "Perceptual, Semantic Language Processes in Split-Brain Patients," *Brain* 100 (1977): 105–118.

[41]J. Levy and C. Trevarthen, "Metacontrol of Hemispheric Function in Human Split Brain Patients," *Journal of Experimental Psychology: Human Perception and Performance* 2 (1976): 299–312.

[42]Ibid.

[43]R. W. Sperry, "Lateral Specialization in the Surgically Separated Hemispheres, in *The Neurosciences Third Study Program*, ed. F. O. Schmitt and F. G. Worden (Cambridge, Mass.: MIT Press, 1974).

[44]J. D. Holtzman, J. J. Sidtis, B. T. Volpe, D. H. Wilson, and M. S. Gazzaniga, "Dissociation of Spatial Information for Stimulus Localization and the Control of Attention," *Brain* 104 (1981): 861–872.

[45]J. J. Sidtis and M. S. Gazzaniga, "Competence vs. Performance After Callosal Section: Looks Can Be Deceiving," in *Cerebral Hemisphere Asymmetry*, ed. J. Hellige (New York: Praeger, 1983).

[46]G. Ettlinger, C. Blakemore, A. D. Milner, and D. Wilson, "Agenesis of the Corpus Callosum," *Brain* 95 (1972): 327–346.

[47]R. Saul and R. Sperry, "Absence of Commissurotomy Symptoms with Agenesis of the Corpus Callosum," *Neurology* 18 (1968): 307.

[48]M. H. Jeeves, "Psychological Studies of Three Cases of Congenital Agenesis of the Corpus Callosum," in *Functions of the Corpus Callosum*, ed. A. V. S. de Reuck and R. Porter (London: J. and A. Churchill, 1965).

[49]Gazzaniga and LeDoux, *The Integrated Mind.*

## Chapter 3   Studying Asymmetries in the Normal Brain

[1]M. Mishkin and D. G. Forgays, "Word Recognition as a Function of

Retinal Locus," *Journal of Experimental Psychology* 43 (1952): 43–48.

[2]M. I. Barton, H. Goodglass, and A. Shai, "Differential Recognition of Tachistoscopically Presented English and Hebrew Words in Right and Left Visual Fields," *Perceptual and Motor Skills* 21 (1965): 431–437.

[3]G. Geffen, J. L. Bradshaw, and G. Wallace, "Interhemispheric Effects on Reaction Time to Verbal and Nonverbal Visual Stimuli," *Journal of Experimental Psychology* 87 (1971): 415–422.

G. Rizzolatti, C. Umilta, and G. Berlucchi, "Opposite Superiorities of the Right and Left Cerebral Hemispheres in Discriminative Reaction Time to Physiognomical and Alphabetic Material," *Brain* 94 (1971): 431–442.

[4]D. Kimura, "Spatial Localization in Left and Right Visual Fields," *Canadian Journal of Psychology* 23 (1969): 445–458.

[5]M. P. Bryden and C. Rainey, "Left–Right Differences in Tachistoscopic Recognition," *Journal of Experimental Psychology* 66 (1963): 568–571.

H. L. Dee and D. Fontenot, "Cerebral Dominance and Lateral Differences in Perception and Memory," *Neuropsychologia* 11 (1973): 167–173.

D. Kimura, "Dual Functional Asymmetry of the Brain in Visual Perception," *Neuropsychologia* 4 (1966): 275–285.

[6]D. Kimura, "Some Effects of Temporal Lobe Damage on Auditory Perception," *Canadian Journal of Psychology* 15 (1961): 156–165.

[7]M. R. Rosenzweig, "Representation of the Two Ears at the Auditory Cortex," *American Journal of Physiology* 167 (1951): 147–158.

[8]D. Dirks, "Perception of Dichotic and Monaural Verbal Material and Cerebral Dominance in Speech," *Acta Otolaryngologica* 58 (1964): 73–80.

[9]B. Milner, L. Taylor, and R. W. Sperry, "Lateralized Suppression of Dichotically Presented Digits After Commissural Section in Man," *Science* 161 (1968): 184–185.

S. P. Springer and M. S. Gazzaniga, "Dichotic Listening in Partial and Complete Split Brain Patients," *Neuropsychologia* 13 (1975): 341–346.

[10]D. Kimura, "Cerebral Dominance and the Perception of Verbal Stimuli," *Canadian Journal of Psychology* 15 (1961): 166–171.

[11]G. Geffen and R. Caudrey, "Reliability and Validity of the Dichotic Monitoring Test for Language Laterality," *Neuropsychologia* 19 (1981): 413–423.

[12]M. P. Bryden, "Binaural Competition and Division of Attention as Determinants of the Laterality Effect in Dichotic Listening," *Canadian Journal of Psychology* 23 (1969): 101–113.

S. P. Springer, "Hemispheric Specialization for Speech Opposed by

Contralateral Noise," *Perception and Psychophysics* 13 (1973): 391–393.

S. S. Lowe, J. K. Cullen, C. I. Berlin, C. L. Thompson, and M. Willett, "Perception of Simultaneous Dichotic and Monotic Monosyllables," *Journal of Speech and Hearing Research* 13 (1970): 812–822.

[13] J. Catlin and H. Neville, "The Laterality Effect in Reaction Time to Speech Stimuli," *Neuropsychologia* 14 (1976): 141–144.

H. Kallman and M. Corballis, "Ear Asymmetry in Reaction Time to Musical Sounds," *Perception and Psychophysics* 17 (1975): 368–370.

J. Morais, "Monaural Ear Differences for Reaction Times to Speech with a Many to One Mapping Paradigm," *Perception and Psychophysics* 19 (1976): 144–148.

[14] M. P. Bryden, "Tachistoscopic Recognition, Handedness, and Cerebral Dominance," *Neuropsychologia* 3 (1965): 1–8.

[15] D. Kimura, "Functional Asymmetry of the Brain in Dichotic Listening," *Cortex* 3 (1967): 163–178.

[16] D. Kimura and S. Folb, "Neural Processing of Backwards Speech Sounds," *Science* 161 (1968): 395–396.

M. Studdert-Kennedy and D. Shankweiler, "Hemispheric Specialization for Speech Perception," *Journal of the Acoustical Society of America* 48 (1970): 579–594.

[17] D. Kimura, "Left–Right Differences in the Perception of Melodies," *Quarterly Journal of Experimental Psychology* 16 (1964): 355–358.

[18] F. W. K. Curry, "A Comparison of Left-Handed and Right-Handed Subjects on Verbal and Nonverbal Dichotic Listening Tasks," *Cortex* 3 (1967): 343–352.

[19] R. Klatzky and R. Atkinson, "Specialization of the Cerebral Hemispheres in Scanning for Information in Short-Term Memory," *Perception and Psychophysics* 10 (1971): 335–338.

[20] J. G. Seamon and M. S. Gazzaniga, "Coding Strategies and Cerebral Laterality Effects," *Cognitive Psychology* 5 (1973): 249–256.

[21] S. Sasanuma, M. Itoh, K. Mori, and Y. Kobayashi, "Tachistoscopic Recognition of Kana and Kanji Words," *Neuropsychologia* 15 (1977): 547–553.

[22] S. Sasanuma, "Kana and Kanji Processing in Japanese Aphasics," *Brain and Language* 2 (1975): 369–383.

[23] S. Sasanuma and O. Fujimura, "Selective Impairment of Phonetic and Non-Phonetic Transcription of Words in Japanese Aphasic Patients: Kana vs. Kanji in Visual Recognition and Writing," *Cortex* 7 (1971): 1–18.

[24] Sasanuma et al., "Tachistoscopic Recognition of Kana and Kanji Words."

[25] M. P. Bryden, "Strategy Effects in the Assessment of Hemispheric Asymmetry," in *Strategies of Information Processing*, ed. G. Underwood (London: Academic Press, 1978).

[26]D. Hines and P. Satz, "Cross-Modal Asymmetries in Perception Related to Asymmetry in Cerebral Function," *Neuropsychologia* 12 (1974): 239–247.

E. B. Zurif and M. P. Bryden, "Familial Handedness and Left–Right Difference in Auditory and Visual Perception," *Neuropsychologia* 7 (1969): 179–187.

[27]S. Blumstein, H. Goodglass, and V. Tatter, "The Reliability of Ear Advantage in Dichotic Listening," *Brain and Language* 2 (1975): 226–236.

Hines and Satz, "Cross-Modal Asymmetries in Perception Related to Asymmetry in Cerebral Function."

[28]M. Kinsbourne, "The Mechanisms of Hemisphere Asymmetry in Man," in *Hemispheric Disconnection and Cerebral Function*, ed. M. Kinsbourne and W. L. Smith (Springfield, Ill.: Charles C. Thomas, 1974).

[29]M. Kinsbourne, "The Control of Attention by Interaction Between the Cerebral Hemispheres," in *Attention and Performance IV*, ed. S. Kornblum (New York: Academic Press, 1973).

[30]J. Morais and M. Landercy, "Listening to Speech While Retaining Music: What Happens to the Right Ear Advantage?" *Brain and Language* 4 (1977): 295–308.

[31]M. Moscovitch, "Information Processing," in *Handbook of Neurobiology–Neuropsychology*, ed. M. S. Gazzaniga (New York: Plenum Press, 1979).

[32]M. E. Day, "An Eye Movement Phenomenon Relating to Attention, Thought, and Anxiety," *Perceptual and Motor Skills* 19 (1964): 443–446.

[33]P. Bakan, "Hypnotizability, Laterality of Eye Movement and Functional Brain Asymmetry," *Perceptual and Motor Skills* 28 (1969): 927–932.

[34]M. Kinsbourne, "Eye and Head Turning Indicates Cerebral Lateralization," *Science* 176 (1972): 539–541.

[35]D. Galin and R. Ornstein, "Individual Differences in Cognitive Style. I: Reflexive Eye Movements," *Neuropsychologia* 12 (1974): 367–376.

K. Kocel, D. Galin, R. Ornstein, and E. Merrin, "Lateral Eye Movement and Cognitive Mode," *Psychonomic Science* 27 (1972): 223–224.

[36]G. E. Schwartz, R. J. Davidson, and F. Maer, "Right Hemisphere Lateralization for Emotion in the Human Brain: Interactions with Cognition," *Science* 190 (1975): 286–288.

[37]R. E. Gur, R. C. Gur, and L. J. Harris, "Cerebral Activation, as Measured by Subjects' Lateral Eye Movements, is Influenced by Experimenter Location," *Neuropsychologia* 13 (1975): 35–44.

[38]H. Ehrlichman and A. Weinberger, "Lateral Eye Movements and

Hemispheric Asymmetry: A Critical Review," *Psychological Bulletin* 85 (1979): 1080–1101.

[39]M. Kinsbourne and R. E. Hicks, "Mapping Cerebral Functional Space: Competition and Collaboration in Human Performance," in *Asymmetrical Function of the Brain*, ed. M. Kinsbourne (Cambridge: Cambridge University Press, 1978).

[40]M. Kinsbourne and J. Cook, "Generalized and Lateralized Effects of Concurrent Verbalization on a Unimanual Skill," *Quarterly Journal of Experimental Psychology* 23 (1971): 341–345.

[41]R. E. Hicks, "Intrahemispheric Response Competition Between Vocal and Unimanual Performance in Normal Adult Human Male," *Journal of Comparative and Physiological Psychology* 89 (1975): 50–60.

[42]M. Kinsbourne and J. McMurray, "The Effect of Cerebral Dominance on Time Sharing Between Speaking and Tapping by Preschool Children," *Child Development* 46 (1975): 240–242.

C. Krueter, M. Kinsbourne, and C. Trevarthen, "Are Deconnected Hemispheres Independent Channels? A Preliminary Study of the Effect of Unilateral Loading on Bilateral Finger Tapping," *Neuropsychologia* 10 (1972): 453–461.

## Chapter 4  Measuring the Brain and Its Activity: Some Physiological Correlates of Asymmetry

[1]D. Galin and R. Ornstein, "Lateral Specialization of Cognitive Mode: An EEG Study," *Psychophysiology* 9 (1972): 412–418.

[2]R. Cohn, "Differential Cerebral Processing of Noise and Verbal Stimuli," *Science* 172 (1971): 599–601.

A. E. Davis and J. A. Wada, "Hemispheric Asymmetry: Frequency Analysis of Visual and Auditory Evoked Responses to Nonverbal Stimuli," *Electroencephalography and Clinical Neurophysiology* 37 (1974): 1–9.

[3]M. Buschbaum and P. Fedio, "Hemispheric Differences in Evoked Potentials to Verbal and Nonverbal Stimuli on the Left and Right Visual Fields," *Physiology and Behavior* 5 (1970): 207–210.

[4]D. L. Molfese, R. B. Freeman, Jr., and D. S. Palermo, "The Ontogeny of the Brain Lateralization for Speech and Nonspeech Stimuli," *Brain and Language* 2 (1975): 356–368.

[5]C. C. Wood, W. R. Goff, and R. S. Day, "Auditory Evoked Potentials During Speech Perception," *Science* 173 (1971): 1248–1251.

[6]D. Galin and R. R. Ellis, "Asymmetry in Evoked Potentials as an Index of Lateralized Cognitive Processes: Relation to EEG Alpha Asymmetry," *Psychophysiology* 13 (1975): 45–50.

[7]A. C. Papanicolaou, A. L. Schmidt, B. D. Moore, and H. M. Eisenberg, "Cerebral Activation Patterns in an Arithmetic and a Visuospatial

Processing Task," *International Journal of Neuroscience* 20 (1983): 283–288.

[8]A. C. Papanicolaou, H. S. Levin, H. M. Eisenberg, and B. D. Moore, "Evoked Potential Indices of Selective Hemispheric Engagement in Affective and Phonetic Tasks," *Neuropsychologia* 21 (1983): 401–405.

[9]D. S. Barth, W. Sutherling, J. Engel, Jr., and J. Beatty, "Neuromagnetic Localization of Epileptiform Spike Activity in the Human Brain," *Science* 218 (1982): 891–894.

[10]G. L. Romani, S. J. Williamson, and L. Kaufman, "Characterization of the Human Auditory Cortex by the Neuromagnetic Method," *Experimental Brain Research* 47 (1982): 381–393.

[11]A. C. Papanicolaou, G. F. Wilson, C. Busch, P. DeRego, C. Orr, I. Davis, and H. M. Eisenberg, "Hemispheric Asymmetries in Phonological Processing Assessed with Probe Evoked Magnetic Fields," *International Journal of Neuroscience* 39 (1988): 275–281.

[12]N. A. Lassen and D. H. Ingvar, "Radioisotopic Assessment of Regional Cerebral Blood Flows," in *Progress in Nuclear Medicine*, Vol. 1 (Baltimore: University Park Press, 1972).

[13]J. Risberg, J. H. Halsey, E. L. Wills, and E. M. Wilson, "Hemispheric Specialization in Normal Man Studied by Bilateral Measurements of the Regional Cerebral Blood Flow: A Study with the $^{133}$Xe Inhalation Technique," *Brain* 98 (1975): 511–524.

[14]G. Deutsch, W. T. Bourbon, A. C. Papanicolaou, and H. M. Eisenberg, "Visuospatial Tasks Compared Via Activation of Regional Cerebral Blood Flow," *Neuropsychologia* 26 (1988): 445–452.

[15]M. C. Linn and A. C. Petersen, "Emergence and Characterization of Sex Differences in Spatial Ability: A Meta-Analysis," *Child Development* 56 (1985): 1479–1498.

[16]R. C. Gur, R. E. Gur, W. D. Obrist, J. P. Hungerbuhler, D. Younkin, A. D. Rosen, B. E. Skolnick, and M. Reivich, "Sex and Handedness Differences in Cerebral Blood Flow During Rest and Cognitive Activity," *Science* 217 (1982): 659–661.

[17]N. A. Lassen, D. H. Ingvar, and E. Skinhoj, "Brain Function and Blood Flow," *Scientific American* 239 (1978): 62–71.

[18]R. C. Gur, I. K. Packer, J. P. Hungerbuhler, M. Reivich, W. D. Obrist, W. S. Amarnek, and H. A. Sackheim, "Differences in the Distribution of Gray and White Matter in Human Cerebral Hemispheres," *Science* 207 (1980): 1226–1228.

[19]J. H. Halsey, U. W. Blauenstein, E. W. Wilson, and E. H. Wills, "Regional Cerebral Blood Flow Comparison of Right and Left Hand Movement," *Neurology* 29 (1979): 21–28.

[20]I. Prohovnik, K. Hakansson, and J. Risberg, "Observations of the Functional Significance of Regional Cerebral Blood Flow in 'Resting' Normal Subjects," *Neuropsychologia* 18 (1980): 203–217.

[21]G. Deutsch, A. C. Papanicolaou, W. T. Bourbon, and H. M. Eisenberg, "Cerebral Blood Flow Evidence of Right Frontal Activation in Attention Demanding Tasks," *International Journal of Neuroscience* 36 (1987): 23–28.

[22]F. Plum, A. Gjedde, and F. E. Samson, "Neuroanatomical Functional Mapping by the Radioactive 2-dioxy-d-glucose Method," *Neurosciences Research Program Bulletin* 14 (1976): 457–518.

[23]P. T. Fox, S. E. Peterson, M. I. Posner, and M. E. Raichle, "Language-Related Brain Activation Measured with PET: Comparison of Auditory and Visual Word Presentations," *Journal of Cerebral Blood Flow and Metabolism* 7, Suppl. 1 (1987): S294.

[24]J. C. Mazziotta and M. E. Phelps, "Human Neuropsychological Imaging Studies of Local Brain Metabolism and Blood Flow: Strategies and Results," *Archives of Neurology* (Abstr.) 40 (1983): 767.

[25]N. Geschwind and W. Levitsky, "Human Brain: Left–Right Asymmetries in Temporal Speech Region," *Science* 161 (1968): 186–187.

[26]J. A. Wada, R. Clark, and A. Hamm, "Cerebral Hemispheric Asymmetry in Humans," *Archives of Neurology* 32 (1975): 239–246.
S. F. Witelson and W. Pallie, "Left Hemisphere Specialization for Language in the Newborn: Anatomical Evidence of Asymmetry," *Brain* 96 (1973): 641–646.

[27]A. M. Galaburda, J. Corsiglia, G. D. Rosen, and G. F. Sherman, "Planum Temporale Asymmetry, Reappraisal Since Geschwind and Levitsky," *Neuropsychologia* 25 (1987): 853–868.

[28]S. F. Witelson, "The Brain Connection: The Corpus Callosum is Larger in Left-Handers," *Science* 229 (1985): 665–668.

[29]A. M. Galaburda and M. Habib, "Cerebral Dominance: Biological Associations and Pathology," *Discussions in Neurosciences* IV (1987).

[30]Ibid.

[31]M. LeMay and A. Culebras, "Human Brain—Morphologic Differences in the Hemispheres Demonstrable by Carotid Anteriography," *The New England Journal of Medicine* 287 (1972): 168–170.

[32]M. LeMay and N. Geschwind, "Asymmetries of the Human Cerebral Hemispheres," in *Language Acquisition and Language Breakdown*, ed. A. Caramazza and E. Zurif (Baltimore: Johns Hopkins University Press, 1978).

[33]W. H. Oldendorf, "Principles of Imaging Structure by Nuclear Magnetic Resonance," *Archives of Neurology* 32 (1983): 239–246.

[34]A. Kertesz, M. Polk, H. Howell, and S. E. Black, "Cerebral Dominance, Sex, and Callosal Size in MRI", *Neurology* 37 (1987): 1385–1388.

[35]Witelson, "The Brain Connection: The Corpus Callosum is Larger in Left-Handers."

[36]A. M. Galaburda, F. Sanides, and N. Geschwind, "Human Brain:

Cytoarchitectonic Left–Right Asymmetries in the Temporal Speech Region," *Archives of Neurology* 35 (1978): 812–817.

[37]A. M. Galaburda and V. F. Sanides, "Cytoarchitectonic Organization of the Human Auditory Cortex," *Journal of Comparative Neurology* 190 (1980): 597–610.

[38]A. M. Galaburda, M. LeMay, T. Kemper, and N. Geschwind, "Right–Left Asymmetries in the Brain," *Science* 199 (1978): 852–856.

[39]E. A. Serafetinides, "The Significance of the Temporal Lobes and of Hemispheric Dominance in the Production of LSD-25 Symptomatology in Man," *Neuropsychologia* 3 (1965): 69–79.

[40]A. Oke, R. Keller, I. Mefford, and R. N. Adams, "Lateralization of Norepinephrine in the Human Thalamus," *Science* 200 (1978): 1411–1413.

[41]L. Amaducci, S. Sorbi, A. Albanese, and G. Gainotti, "Choline-acetyl transferase (CHAT) Activity Differs in Right and Left Human Temporal Lobes," *Neurology* 31 (1981): 799–805.

[42]S. D. Glick, D. A. Ross, and L. B. Hough, "Lateral Asymmetry of Neurotransmitters in Human Brain," *Brain Research* 234 (1982): 53–63.

[43]K. H. Pribram and D. McGuinness, "Arousal, Activation, and Effort in the Control of Attention," *Psychological Review* 82 (1975): 116–149.

[44]D. M. Tucker and P. A. Williamson, "Asymmetric Neural Control Systems in Human Self-Regulation," *Psychological Review* 91 (1984): 185–215.

[45]D. N. Robinson, *The Enlightened Machine* (New York: Columbia University Press, 1980).

**Chapter 5    The Puzzle of the Left-Hander**

[1]W. Dennis, "Early Graphic Evidence of Dextrality in Man," *Perceptual and Motor Skills* 8 (1958): 147–149.

R. A. Dart, "The Predatory Implement Technique of Australopithecus," *American Journal of Physical Anthropology* 7 (1949): 1–38.

R. S. Uhrbrock, "Laterality in Art," *Journal of Aesthetics and Art Criticism* 32 (1973): 27–35.

S. Coren and C. Porac, "Fifty Centuries of Right Handedness: The Historical Record," *Science* 198 (1977): 631–632.

[2]M. C. Corballis, "The Origins and Evolution of Human Laterality," in *Neuropsychology and Cognition*, Volume 1, ed. R. N. Malateska and L. C. Hartlage (The Hague: Martinus Nijhoff Publishers, 1982).

[3]M. Barsley, *Left Handed People* (North Hollywood: Wilshire Book Co., 1979).

[4]C. Sagan, *The Dragons of Eden* (New York: Random House, 1977).

[5]Corballis, "The Origins and Evolution of Human Laterality," p. 2.

[6]R. C. Oldfield, "The Assessment and Analysis of Handedness: The Edinburgh Inventory," *Neuropsychologia* 9 (1971): 97–114.

[7]H. D. Chamberlain, "The Inheritance of Left Handedness," *Journal of Heredity* 19 (1928): 557–559.

[8]R. L. Collins, "The Sound of One Paw Clapping: An Inquiry Into the Origins of Left Handedness," in *Contributions to Behavior-Genetic Analysis — The Mouse as Prototype,* ed. G. Lindzey and D. B. Thiessen (New York: The Meredith Corporation, 1970).

[9]R. L. Collins, "When Left Handed Mice Live in Right Handed Worlds," *Science* 187 (1975): 181–184.

[10]A. Blau, *The Master Hand* (New York: American Ortho-Psychiatric Association, 1946).

[11]M. Annett, "A Model of the Inheritance of Handedness and Cerebral Dominance," *Nature* 204 (1964): 59–60.

[12]J. Levy and T. Nagylaki, "A Model for the Genetics of Handedness," *Genetics* 72 (1972): 117–128.

[13]M. Annett, "Handedness in the Children of Two Left Handed Parents," *Quarterly Journal of Psychology* 65 (1974): 129–131.

[14]R. G. Howard and A. M. Brown, "Twinning: A Marker for Biological Insults," *Child Development* 41 (1970): 519–530.

[15]H. Gordon, "Left-Handedness and Mirror Writing Especially Among Defective Children," *Brain* 43 (1920): 313–368.

[16]T. Rasmussen and B. Milner, "The Role of Early Left-Brain Injury in Determining Lateralization of Cerebral Speech Functions," in *Evolution and Lateralization of the Brain,* ed. S. Dimond and D. Blizzard (New York: New York Academy of Sciences, 1977).

[17]P. Bakan, G. Dibb, and P. Reed, "Handedness and Birth Stress," *Neuropsychologia* 11 (1973): 363–366.

[18]P. Satz, "Pathological Left-Handedness: An Explanatory Model," *Cortex* 8 (1972): 121–135.

[19]P. Satz, D. L. Orsini, E. Saslow, and R. Henry, "The Pathological Left-Handedness Syndrome," *Brain and Cognition* 4 (1985): 27–46. P. Satz, D. L. Orsini, E. Saslow, and R. Henry, "Early Brain Injury and Pathological Left-Handedness: Clues to a Syndrome," in *The Dual Brain,* ed. E. Zaidel (New York: The Guilford Press, 1985).

[20]H. Lansdell, "Verbal and Nonverbal Factors in Right-Hemisphere Speech: Relation to Early Neurological History," *Journal of Comparative and Physiological Psychology* 69 (1969): 734–738.

[21]I. Macgillivray, P. Nylander, and G. Corney, *Human Multiple Reproduction* (London: Saunders, 1975).

[22]T. Nagylaki and J. Levy, "The Sound of One Paw Clapping Is Not Sound," *Behavior Genetics* 3 (1973): 279–292.

[23]C. E. Lauterbach, "Studies in Twin Resemblance," *Genetics* 10 (1925): 525–568.

[24]Rasmussen and Milner, "The Role of Early Left-Brain Injury in Determining Lateralization of Cerebral Speech Functions."

[25]A. R. Luria, *Traumatic Aphasia* (The Hague: Mouton, 1970).

A. Subirana, "The Prognosis in Aphasia in Relation to Cerebral Dominance and Handedness," *Brain* 81 (1958): 415–425.

[26]M. P. Bryden, "Tachistoscopic Recognition, Handedness, and Cerebral Dominance," *Neuropsychologia* 3 (1965): 1–8.

P. Satz, K. Achenbach, E. Patteshall, and E. Fennell, "Order of Report, Ear Asymmetry, and Handedness in Dichotic Listening," *Cortex* 1 (1965): 377–396.

[27]H. Hecaen and J. Sauget, "Cerebral Dominance in Left Handed Subjects," *Cortex* 7 (1971): 19–48.

[28]E. B. Zurif and M. P. Bryden, "Familial Handedness in Left–Right Differences in Auditory and Visual Perception," *Neuropsychologia* 7 (1969): 179–187.

[29]W. F. McKeever and D. Van Deventer, "Visual and Auditory Language Processing Asymmetries: Influences and Handedness, Familial Sinistrality, and Sex," *Cortex* 13 (1972): 225–241.

J. A. Higenbottom, "Relationship Between Sets of Lateral and Perceptual Preference Measures," *Cortex* 9 (1973): 402–409.

[30]M. P. Bryden, "Perceptual Asymmetry in Vision: Relation to Handedness, Eyedness, and Speech Lateralization," *Cortex* 9 (1973): 418–432.

D. Hines and P. Satz, "Cross-Modal Asymmetries in Perception Related to Asymmetry in Cerebral Function," *Neuropsychologia* 12 (1974): 239–247.

[31]J. Levy and M. Reid "Variations in Writing Posture and Cerebral Organization," *Science* 194 (1976): 337.

[32]J. L. Bradshaw and M. J. Taylor, "A Word Naming Deficit in Nonfamilial Sinistrals? Laterality Effects of Vocal Responses to Tachistoscopically Presented Letter Strings," *Neuropsychologia* 17 (1979): 21–32.

W. F. McKeever, "Handwriting Posture in Left Handers: Sex, Familial Sinistrality, and Language Laterality Correlates," *Neuropsychologia* 17 (1979): 429–444.

W. F. McKeever and A. Van Deventer, "Inverted Handwriting Position, Language Laterality, and the Levy–Nagylaki Model of Handedness and Cerebral Organization," *Neuropsychologia* 18 (1980): 99–102.

[33]J. Herron, D. Galin, J. Johnstone, and R. Ornstein, "Cerebral Specialization, Writing Posture, and Motor Control of Writing in Left Handers," *Science* 205 (1979): 1285–1289.

McKeever and Van Deventer, "Inverted Handwriting Position, Language Laterality, and the Levy–Nagylaki Model of Handedness and Cerebral Organization."

L. C. Smith and M. Moscovitch, "Writing Posture, Hemispheric Control of Movement, and Cerebral Dominance in Individuals with Inverted and Non-Inverted Hand Postures During Writing," *Neuropsychologia* 17 (1979): 637–644.

[34] Herron et al., "Cerebral Specialization, Writing Posture, and Motor Control of Writing in Left Handers."

[35] M. Allen and M. Wellman, "Hand Position During Writing, Cerebral Laterality, and Reading: Age and Sex Differences," *Neuropsychologia* 18 (1980): 33–40.

[36] J. H. Halsey, V. W. Blauenstein, E. M. Wilson, and E. L. Wills, "Brain Activation in the Presence of Brain Damage," *Brain and Language* 9 (1980): 47–60.

[37] B. Milner, cited in Herron et al., "Cerebral Specialization, Writing Posture, and Motor Control of Writing in Left Handers."

[38] C. Hardyck and L. Petrinovich, "Left Handedness," *Psychological Bulletin* 84 (1977): 385–404.

[39] J. Levy, "Possible Basis for the Evolution of Lateral Specialization of the Human Brain," *Nature* 224 (1969): 614–615.

[40] E. Miller, "Handedness and the Pattern of Human Ability," *British Journal of Psychology* 62 (1971): 111–112.

F. Newcombe and G. Ratcliff, "Handedness, Speech Lateralization, and Ability," *Neuropsychologia* 11 (1973): 339–407.

[41] C. Mebert and G. Michel, "Handedness in Artists," in *Neuropsychology of Left Handedness*, ed. J. Herron (New York: Academic Press, 1980).

[42] S. Coren and C. P. Kaplan, "Patterns of Ocular Dominance," *American Journal of Optometry* 50 (1973): 283–292.

[43] S. Coren and C. Porac, "Effects of Simulated Refractive Asymmetries on Eye Dominance," *Bulletin of the Psychonomic Society* 9 (1977): 269–271.

[44] S. Coren and C. Porac, *Lateral Preferences and Human Behavior* (New York: Springer-Verlag, 1981).

[45] Ibid.

[46] Ibid.

[47] N. Geschwind and P. Behan, "Left Handedness: Association with Immune Disease, Migraine, and Developmental Learning Disorders," *Proceedings of the National Academy of Sciences* 79 (1982): 5097–5100.

[48] N. Geschwind and P. Behan, "Laterality, Hormones, and Immunity," in *Cerebral Dominance: The Biological Foundations*, ed. N. Geschwind and A. M. Galaburda (Cambridge, Mass.: Harvard University Press, 1984).

[49] N. Geschwind and N. Galaburda, *Cerebral Lateralization: Biological Mechanisms, Associations and Pathology*, (Cambridge, Mass.: MIT Press, 1987).

[50]C. P. Benbow and J. C. Stanley, "Sex Differences in Mathematical Ability: Fact or Artifact?", *Science* 210 (1983): 1262–1264.

[51]M. Corballis and M. J. Morgan, "On the Biological Basis of Human Laterality: I. Evidence for a Maturational Left–Right Gradient," *Behavioral and Brain Sciences* 2 (1978): 261–336.

[52]Ibid.

[53]N. Geschwind and N. Galaburda, *Cerebral Lateralization: Biological Mechanisms, Associations and Pathology.*

[54]M. Corballis and M. J. Morgan, "On the Biological Basis of Human Laterality: I. Evidence for a Maturational Left–Right Gradient."

**Chapter 6  Further Evidence from the Clinic: Neuropsychological Disorders**

[1]H. Hecaen and M. L. Albert, *Human Neuropsychology* (New York: John Wiley, 1978).

A. R. Luria, *Higher Cortical Functions* (New York: Basic Books, 1966).

[2]K. W. Walsh, *Neuropsychology—A Clinical Approach* (Edinburgh, London and New York: Churchill Livingston, 1978).

K. M. Heilman and E. Valenstein, *Clinical Neuropsychology* (New York: Oxford University Press, 1979).

[3]E. B. Zurif, "Language Mechanisms: A Neuropsychological Perspective," *American Scientist* 68 (1980): 305–311.

[4]A. Kreindler, C. Calavrezo, and L. Mihailescu, "Linguistic analysis of one case of jargon aphasia," *Revue Roumaine de Neurologie* 8 (1971): 209–228.

[5]J. W. Brown, *Aphasia, Apraxia and Agnosia* (Springfield, Ill.: Charles C. Thomas, 1972).

[6]A. K. Coughlan, and E. K. Warrington, "Word-Comprehension and Word-Retrieval in Patients with Localized Cerebral Lesions," *Brain* 101 (1978): 163–185.

S. J. Dimond, *Neuropsychology: A Textbook of Systems and Psychological Functions of the Human Brain* (London: Butterworths, 1980).

[7]N. Geschwind, "Disconnexion Syndromes in Animals and Man," *Brain* 88 (1965): 237–294.

N. Geschwind, "The Organization of Language and the Brain," *Science* 170 (1970): 940–944.

[8]Dimond, *Neuropsychology: A Textbook of Systems and Psychological Functions of the Human Brain.*

[9]Geschwind, "Disconnexion Syndromes in Animals and Man."

[10]J. C. Marshall, "On the Biology of Language Acquisition," in *Biological Studies of Mental Processes*, ed. D. Caplan (Cambridge, Mass.: MIT Press, 1980).

[11]J. W. Brown, *Mind, Brain, and Consciousness* (New York: Academic Press, 1977).

[12]P. MacLean, "Cerebral Evolution and Emotional Processes: New Findings on the Striatal Complex," *Annals of the New York Academy of Science* 193 (1972): 137–149.

G. Coghill, *Anatomy and the Problem of Behavior* (London and New York: Cambridge University Press, 1929).

[13]Dimond, *Neuropsychology: A Textbook of Systems and Psychological Functions of the Human Brain.*

[14]G. A. Ojemann, "Subcortical Language Mechanisms," in *Studies in Neurolinguistics*, Vol. 1, ed. H. Whitaker and H. A. Whitaker (New York: Academic Press, 1976).

G. A. Ojemann, "Asymmetric Function of the Thalamus in Man," *Annals of the New York Academy of Science* 299 (1977): 380–396.

[15]A. Smith, "Speech and Other Functions After Left (Dominant) Hemispherectomy," *Journal of Neurology, Neurosurgery and Psychiatry* 29 (1966): 467–471.

C. W. Burkland and A. Smith, "Language and the Cerebral Hemispheres," *Neurology* 27 (1977): 627–633.

[16]A. Smith, "Nondominant Hemispherectomy," *Neurology* 19 (1969): 442–445.

[17]Geschwind, "Disconnexion Syndromes in Animals and Man."

[18]M. Coltheart, "Deep Dyslexia: A Right-Hemisphere Hypothesis," in *Deep Dyslexia*, ed. M. Coltheart, K. Patterson, and J. C. Marshall (London: Routledge and Kegan Paul, 1980).

[19]D. Hines, "Differences in Tachistoscopic Recognition Between Abstract and Concrete Words as a Function of Visual Half-Field and Frequency," *Cortex* 13 (1977): 66–73.

[20]M. Danly and B. Shapiro, "Speech Prosody in Broca's Aphasia," *Brain and Language* 16 (1982): 171–190.

[21]K. M. Heilman, R. Scholes, and R. T. Watson, "Auditory Affective Agnosia: Disturbed Comprehension of Affective Speech," *Journal of Neurology, Neurosurgery and Psychiatry* 38 (1975): 69–72.

[22]E. D. Ross and M. M. Mesulam, "Dominant Language Functions of the Right Hemisphere?" *Archives of Neurology* 36 (1979): 144–148.

[23]M. L. Albert, R. W. Sparks, and N. A. Helm, "Melodic Intonation Therapy for Aphasia," *Archives of Neurology* 29 (1973): 130–131.

[24]E. Winner and H. Gardner, "The Comprehension of Metaphor in Brain-Damaged Patients," *Brain* 100 (1977): 717–729.

[25]N. S. Foldi, M. Cicone, and H. Gardner, "Pragmatic Aspects of Communication in Brain Damaged Patients," in *Language Functions and Brain Organization*, ed. S. J. Segalowitz (New York: Academic Press, 1983).

[26]W. R. Gowers, *A Manual of Diseases of the Nervous System* (London: J & A Churchill, 1893).

[27] M. Kinsbourne, "The Minor Cerebral Hemisphere as a Source of Aphasic Speech," *Archives of Neurology* 25 (1971): 302–306.

[28] J. L. Cummings, D. F. Benson, M. J. Walsh, and H. L. Levine, "Left-to-Right Transfer of Language Dominance: A Case Study," *Neurology* 29 (1979): 1547–1550.

[29] A. C. Papanicolaou, B. D. Moore, H. S. Levin, and H. M. Eisenberg, "Evoked Potential Correlates of Right Hemisphere Involvement in Language Recovery Following Stroke," *Archives of Neurology* 44 (1987): 521–524.

[30] G. Deutsch, A. C. Papanicolaou, and H. M. Eisenberg, "CBF During Tasks Intended to Differentially Activate the Cerebral Hemispheres: New Normative Data and Preliminary Applications in Recovering Stroke Patients," *Journal of Cerebral Blood Flow and Metabolism* 7, Suppl. (1987): S306.

[31] E. DeRenzi, P. Faglioni, and G. Scotti, "Hemispheric Contribution to Exploration of Space Through Visual and Tactile Modality," *Cortex* 6 (1970): 191–203.
D. J. Fontenot and A. L. Benton, "Tactile Perception of Direction in Relation to Hemispheric Locus of Lesion," *Neuropsychologia* 9 (1971): 83–88.

[32] B. Julesz, "Binocular Depth Perception without Familiarity Cues," *Science* 145 (1964): 356–363.

[33] A. Carmon and H. P. Bechtoldt, "Dominance of the Right Cerebral Hemisphere for Stereopsis," *Neuropsychologia* 7 (1969): 29–39.
A. L. Benton and Hecaen, "Stereoscopic Vision in Patients with Unilateral Cerebral Disease," *Neurology* 20 (1970): 1084–1088.

[34] A. L. Benton, "Visuoperceptive, Visuospatial and Visuoconstructive Disorders," in *Clinical Neuropsychology*, ed. K. M. Heilman and E. Valenstein (Oxford: Oxford University Press, 1979).
A. L. Benton, "The Neuropsychology of Facial Recognition," *American Psychologist* 35 (1980): 176–186.

[35] K. Heilman and S. Watson, "The Neglect Syndrome—A Unilateral Defect of the Orienting Response," in *Lateralization in the Nervous System*, ed. S. Harnad, R. Doty, L. Goldstein, J. Jaynes, and G. Krauthamer (New York: Academic Press, 1977).

[36] B. T. Volpe, J. E. LeDoux, and M. S. Gazzaniga, "Information Processing of Visual Stimuli in an 'Extinguished' Field," *Nature* 282 (1979): 122–124.

[37] G. Deutsch, J. Tweedy, and B. Lorinstein, "Some Temporal and Spatial Factors Affecting Visual Neglect" (paper presented at the Eighth Annual Meeting of the International Neuropsychological Society, San Francisco, 1980).

[38] E. K. Warrington, "Constructional Apraxia," in *Handbook of Clinical Neurology*, Vol. 4, ed. P. J. Vinken and G. W. Bruyn (Amsterdam: Elsevier/North-Holland Biomedical Press, 1969).

[39]Benton, "Visuoperceptive, Visuospatial, and Visuoconstructive Disorders."

[40]K. S. Lashley, "In Search of the Engram," in *Symposium of the Society for Experimental Biology*, No. 4 (London: Cambridge University Press, 1950).

[41]R. P. Kesner, "Mnemonic Functions of the Hippocampus: Correspondence Between Animals and Humans," in *Conditioning Representation of Neural Function*, ed. C. D. Woody (New York: Plenum Press, 1983).

B. Milner, "Hemispheric Specialization: Scope and Limits," in *The Neurosciences: Third Research Program*, ed. F. O. Schmitt and F. G. Warden (Cambridge, Mass.: MIT Press, 1974).

[42]C. B. Blakemore and M. A. Falconer, "Long Term Effects of Anterior Temporal Lobectomy on Certain Cognitive Functions," *Journal of Neurology, Neurosurgery and Psychiatry* 30 (1967): 364–367.

B. Milner and H. L. Teuber, "Alteration of Perception and Memory in Man: Reflections on Methods," in *Analysis of Behavioral Change*, ed. L. Wieskrantz (New York: Harper and Row, 1968).

[43]B. Milner, "Visual Recognition and Recall After Right Temporal-Lobe Excision in Man," *Neuropsychologia* 6 (1968): 191–209.

[44]B. Milner, "Visually Guided Maze Learning in Man: Effects of Bilateral Hippocampal, Bilateral Frontal, and Unilateral Cerebral Lesions," *Neuropsychologia* 3 (1965): 317–338.

[45]N. Geschwind, "The Organization of Language and the Brain," *Science* 170 (1970): 940–944.

M. S. Gazzaniga and J. E. LeDoux, *The Integrated Mind* (New York: Plenum Press, 1978).

[46]W. Penfield and P. Perot, "The Brain's Record of Auditory and Visual Experience. A Final Summary and Discussion," *Brain* 86 (1963): 595–696.

W. Penfield and L. Roberts, *Speech and Brain Mechanisms* (Princeton University Press, 1959).

[47]B. Milner, "Laterality Effects in Audition," in *Interhemispheric Relations and Cerebral Dominance*, ed. V. Mountcastle (Baltimore: Johns Hopkins University Press, 1962).

[48]J. E. Bogen and H. W. Gordon, "Musical Tests of Functional Lateralization with Intracarotid Amobarbital," *Nature* 230 (1971): 524–525.

[49]T. Alajouanine, "Aphasia and Artistic Realization," *Brain* 71 (1948): 229–241.

[50]A. Gates and J. Bradshaw, "The Role of the Cerebral Hemispheres in Music," *Brain and Language* 4 (1977): 403–431.

[51]T. Bever and R. Chiarello, "Cerebral Dominance in Musicians and Nonmusicians," *Science* 185 (1974): 137–139.

[52]G. Gainotti, "Reactions 'Catastrophiques' et Manifestations d'Indif-

ference au Cours des Atteintes Cerebrales," *Neuropsychologia* 7 (1969): 195–204.

[53]G. F. Rossi and G. Rosadini, "Experimental Analysis of Cerebral Dominance in Man," in *Brain Mechanisms Underlying Speech and Language*, ed. C. H. Milikan and F. L. Danley (New York: Grune & Stratton, 1967).

H. Terzian, "Behavioral and EEG Effects of Intracarotid Sodium Amytal Injection," *Acta Neurochirurgia (Wein)* 12 (1964): 230–239.

[54]Terzian, "Behavioral and EEG Effects of Intracarotid Sodium Amytal Injection."

[55]Ibid.

[56]B. Milner, "Comments of Rossi and Rosadini," in *Brain Mechanisms Underlying Speech and Language*, ed. C. H. Milikan and F. L. Danley (New York: Grune & Stratton, 1967).

T. Tsunoda and M. Oka 1976, "Lateralization for Emotion in the Human Brain and Auditory Cerebral Dominance," *Proceedings of the Japanese Academy* 52 (1976): 528–531.

[57]H. A. Sackheim, M. S. Greenberg, A. L. Weiman, R. C. Gur, J. P. Hungerbuhler, and N. Geschwind, "Hemispheric Asymmetry in the Expression of Positive and Negative Emotions: Neurological Evidence," *Archives of Neurology* 39 (1982): 210–218.

[58]K. M. Heilman, R. Scholes, and R. T. Watson, "Auditory Affective Agnosia: Disturbed Comprehension of Affective Speech," *Journal of Neurology, Neurosurgery and Psychiatry* 38 (1975): 69–72.

[59]D. M. Tucker, R. T. Watson, and K. M. Heilman, "Affective Discrimination and Evocation in Patients with Right Parietal Disease," *Neurology* 27 (1977): 947–950.

[60]H. A. Sackheim, R. C. Gur, and M. Saucy, "Emotions Are Expressed More Intensely on the Left Side of the Face," *Science* 202 (1978): 434–436.

[61]J. C. Borod and H. S. Caron, "Facedness and Emotion Related to Lateral Dominance, Sex, and Expression Type," *Neuropsychologia* 18 (1980): 237–242.

[62]J. Borod, E. Koff, and B. White, "Facial Asymmetry in Posed and Spontaneous Expressions of Emotion," *Brain and Cognition* 2 (1983): 165–175.

[63]F. L. King and D. Kimura, "Left Ear Superiority in Dichotic Perception of Vocal Nonverbal Sounds," *Canadian Journal of Psychology* 26 (1972): 111–116.

M. P. Haggard and A. M. Parkinson, "Stimulus and Task Factors as Determinants of Ear Advantages," *Quarterly Journal of Experimental Psychology* 23 (1971): 168–177.

[64]R. G. Ley and M. P. Bryden, "Hemispheric Differences in Recognizing Faces and Emotions," *Brain and Language* 7 (1979): 127–138.

## Chapter 7  Sex and Asymmetry

[1]M. Coltheart, E. Hull, and D. Slater, "Sex Differences in Imagery and Reading," *Nature* 253 (1975): 438–440.

[2]J. McGlone, "Sex Differences in Human Brain Asymmetry: A Critical Survey," *Behavioral and Brain Sciences* 3 (1980): 215–263.

[3]M. G. McGee, "Human Spatial Abilities: Psychometric Studies and Environmental, Genetic, Hormonal, and Neurological Influences," *Psychological Bulletin* 86 (1979): 889–918.

[4]H. Lansdell, "A Sex Difference in Effect of Temporal Lobe Neurosurgery on Design Preference," *Nature* 194 (1962): 852–854.

[5]J. McGlone, "Sex Differences in Functional Brain Asymmetry," *Cortex* 14 (1978): 122–128.

[6]J. Inglis and J. S. Lawson, "Sex Differences in the Effects of Unilateral Brain Damage on Intelligence," *Science* 212 (1981): 693–695.

[7]D. A. Lake and M. P. Bryden, "Handedness and Sex Differences in Hemispheric Asymmetry," *Brain and Language* 3 (1976): 266–282.

[8]D. M. Piazza, "The Influence of Sex and Handedness in the Hemispheric Specialization of Verbal and Nonverbal Tasks," *Neuropsychologia* 18 (1980): 163–176.

[9]M. P. Bryden, *Laterality: Functional Asymmetry in the Intact Brain* (New York: Academic Press, 1982).

[10]S. F. Witelson, "Sex and the Single Hemisphere: Specialization of the Right Hemisphere for Spatial Processing," *Science* 193 (1976): 425–427.

[11]J. A. Wada, R. Clark, and A. Hamm, "Cerebral Hemisphere Asymmetry in Humans," *Archives of Neurology* 32 (1975): 239–246.

[12]M. Diamond, "Age, Sex, and Environmental Influences on Anatomical Asymmetry in Rat Forebrain," in *Cerebral Dominance: The Biological Foundations*, ed. N. Geschwind and A. M. Galaburda (Cambridge, Mass.: Harvard University Press, 1984).

[13]D. M. Tucker, "Sex Differences in Hemispheric Specialization for Synthetic Visuospatial Functions," *Neuropsychologia* 14 (1976): 447–454.

[14]R. J. Davidson and G. E. Schwartz, "Patterns of Cerebral Lateralization During Cardiac Feedback versus the Self-Regulation of Emotion: Sex Differences," *Psychophysiology* 13 (1976): 62–68.

[15]R. C. Gur, R. E. Gur, W. D. Obrist, J. P. Hungerbuhler, D. Younkin, A. D. Rosen, B. E. Skolnick, and M. Reivich, "Sex and Handedness Differences in Cerebral Blood Flow During Rest and Cognitive Activity," *Science* 217 (1982): 659–661.

[16]D. Waber, "Sex Differences in Cognition: A Function of Maturation Rate?" *Science* 192 (1976): 572–573.

[17]J. Levy, "Lateral Differences in the Human Brain in Cognition and Behavioral Control," in *Cerebral Correlates of Conscious Experience,*

ed. P. Buser and A. Rougeul-Buser (New York: North Holland Publishing Co., 1978).

## Chapter 8  The Development of Asymmetry

[1] E. H. Lenneberg, *Biological Foundations of Language* (New York: Wiley, 1967).

[2] L. S. Basser, "Hemiplegia of Early Onset and the Faculty of Speech with Special Reference to the Effects of Hemispherectomy," *Brain* 85 (1962): 427–460.

[3] S. Krashen, "Lateralization, Language Learning, and the Critical Period: Some New Evidence," *Language Learning* 23 (1973): 63–74.

[4] M. Kinsbourne, "The Ontogeny of Cerebral Dominance," in *Developmental Psycholinguistics and Communication Disorders*, ed. D. Aaronson and R. W. Reiber (New York: New York Academy of Sciences, 1975).

[5] B. T. Woods and H. L. Teuber, "Changing Patterns of Childhood Aphasia," *Annals of Neurology* 3 (1978): 273–280.

[6] M. Nagafuchi, "Development of Dichotic and Monaural Hearing Abilities in Young Children," *Acta Otolaryngologica* 69 (1970): 409–414.

[7] A. K. Entus, "Hemispheric Asymmetry in Processing of Dichotically Presented Speech and Nonspeech Stimuli by Infants," in *Language Development and Neurological Theory*, ed. S. J. Segalowitz and F. Gruber (New York: Academic Press, 1977).

[8] F. Vargha-Khadem and M. C. Corballis, "Cerebral Asymmetry in Infants," *Brain and Language* 8 (1979): 1–9.

[9] C. Berlin, L. Hughes, S. Lowe-Bell, and H. Berlin, "Right Ear Advantage in Children 5 to 13," *Cortex* 9 (1973): 394–402.

P. Satz, D. J. Bakker, J. Tenunissen, R. Goebel, and H. Van der Vlugt, "Developmental Parameters of the Ear Asymmetry: A Multivariate Approach" *Brain and Language* 2 (1975): 171–185.

[10] D. L. Molfese, R. B. Freeman, Jr., and D. S. Palermo, "The Ontogeny of Brain Lateralization for Speech and Nonspeech Stimuli," *Brain and Language* 2 (1975): 356–368.

[11] J. A. Wada and A. Davis, "Fundamental Nature of Human Infants' Brain Asymmetry," *Canadian Journal of Neurological Sciences* 4 (1977): 203–207.

[12] G. Turkewitz and S. Creighton, "Changes in Lateral Differentiation of Head Posture in the Human Neonate," *Developmental Psychology* 8 (1974): 85–89.

J. Liederman and M. Kinsbourne, "The Mechanism of Neonatal Righward Turning Bias: A Sensory or Motor Asymmetry?" *Infant Behavior and Development* 5 (1980): 223–238.

[13] J. Viviani, G. Turkewitz, and E. Karp, "A Relationship Between Later-

ality of Functioning at 2 Days and at 7 Years of Age," *Bulletin of the Psychonomic Society* 12 (1978): 189–192.

[14]J. Chi, E. Dooling, and F. Giles, "Left-Right Asymmetries of the Temporal Speech Areas of the Human Fetus," *Archives of Neurology* 34 (1972): 346–348.

[15]J. A. Wada, R. Clark, and A. Hamm, "Cerebral Hemispheric Asymmetry in Humans," *Archives of Neurology* 32 (1975): 239–246.

[16]A. Galaburda, "Anatomical Asymmetries in the Human Brain," in *Biological Foundations of Cerebral Dominance,* ed. N. Geschwind and A. M. Galaburda (Cambridge, Mass.: Harvard University Press, 1984).

[17]C. Netley, "Cognitive Development, Cerebral Organization and the X Chromosome" (presented at NATO, Advanced Studies Institute, Neuropsychology and Cognition, Augusta, Georgia, September 1980).

[18]A. Smith, "Speech and Other Functions After Left (Dominant) Hemispherectomy," *Journal of Neurology, Neurosurgery, and Psychiatry* 29 (1966): 467–471.

A. Smith and C. W. Burkland, "Dominant Hemispherectomy," *Science* 153 (1966): 1280–1282.

[19]M. Dennis and W. Whitaker, "Language Acquisition Following Hemidecortication: Linguistic Superiority of the Left Over the Right Hemisphere," *Brain and Language* 3 (1976): 404–433.

[20]D. V. M. Bishop, "Linguistic Impairment After Left Hemidecortication for Infantile Hemiplegia? A Reappraisal," *Quarterly Journal of Experimental Psychology* 35 (1983): 199–207.

[21]C. Trevarthen, "Cerebral Embryology and the Split Brain," in *Hemispheric Disconnection and Cerebral Function,* ed. M. Kinsbourne and W. L. Smith (Springfield, Ill.: Charles C. Thomas, 1974).

[22]Berlin et al., "Right Ear Advantage in Children 5 to 13."

[23]Satz et al., "Developmental Parameters of the Ear Asymmetry: A Multivariate Approach."

[24]Ibid.

[25]Molfese et al., "The Ontogeny of Brain Lateralization for Speech and Nonspeech Stimuli."

[26]Wada et al., "Cerebral Hemispheric Asymmetry in Humans."

[27]S. Witelson, "Neurological Aspects of Language in Children," *Child Development* 58 (1987): 653–688.

[28]M. Morgan, "Embryology and Inheritance of Asymmetry," in *Lateralization in the Nervous System,* ed. S. Harnad, R. Doty, L. Goldstein, J. Jaynes, and G. Krauthamer (New York: Academic Press, 1977).

[29]M. P. Bryden, "Speech Lateralization in Families: A Preliminary Study Using Dichotic Listening," *Brain and Language* 2 (1975): 201–211.

[30]J. Liederman and M. Kinsbourne, "Rightward Motor Bias in Newborns Depends upon Parental Right Handedness," *Neuropsychologia* 18 (1980): 579–584.

[31]D. S. Geffner and I. Hochberg, "Ear Laterality Performance of Children from Low and Middle Socioeconomic Level on a Verbal Dichotic Listening Task," *Cortex* 7 (1971): 193–203.

[32]T. Borowy and R. Goebel, "Cerebral Lateralization of Speech: The Effects of Age, Sex, Race, and Socioeconomic Class," *Neuropsychologia* 14 (1976): 363–370.

[33]M. F. Dorman and D. Geffner, "Hemispheric Specialization for Speech Perception in Six Year Old Black and White Children from Low and Middle Socioeconomic Classes," *Cortex* 10 (1974): 171–176.

[34]S. Krashen, "Lateralization, Language Learning, and the Critical Period: Some New Evidence, *Language Learning* 23 (1973): 63–74.

[35]W. F. McKeever, H. Hoemann, V. Florian, and A. Van Deventer, "Evidence of Minimal Cerebral Asymmetries for the Processing of English Words and American Sign Language in the Congenitally Deaf," *Neuropsychologia* 14 (1976): 413–423.

[36]A. A. Manning, W. Goble, R. Markman, and T. LaBreche, "Lateral Cerebral Differences in the Deaf in Response to Linguistic and Nonlinguistic Stimuli," *Brain and Language* 4 (1977): 309–321.

H. Poizner and H. Lane, "Cerebral Asymmetry in the Perception of American Sign Language," *Brain and Language* 7 (1979): 210–226.

[37]McKeever et al., "Evidence of Minimal Cerebral Asymmetries for the Processing of English Words and American Sign Language in the Congenitally Deaf."

Poizner and Lane, "Cerebral Asymmetry in the Perception of American Sign Language."

[38]S. Virostek and J. E. Cutting, "Asymmetries for Ameslan Handshapes and Other Forms in Signers and Nonsigners," *Perception and Psychophysics* 26 (1979): 505–508.

[39]L. Obler, R. Zattore, L. Galloway, and J. Vaid, "Cerebral Lateralization in Bilinguals: Methodological Issues," *Brain and Language* 15 (1982): 40–54.

[40]J. Vaid and F. Genesee, "Neuropsychological Approaches to Bilingualism: A Critical Review," *Canadian Journal of Psychology* 34 (1980): 419–447.

[41]F. Genesee, J. Hamers, W. E. Lambert, M. Seitz, and R. Stark, "Language Processing in Bilinguals," *Brain and Language* 5 (1978): 1–12.

## Chapter 9  Asymmetries in Animals

[1]C. H. M. Beck and R. L. Barton, "Deviation and Laterality of Hand Preference in Monkeys," *Cortex* 8 (1972): 339–363.

R. L. Collins, "On the Inheritance of Handedness. I: Laterality in Inbred Mice," *Journal of Heredity* 59 (1968): 9–12.

J. M. Warren, J. M. Abplanalp, and H. B. Warren, "The Development of Handedness in Cats and Rhesus Monkeys," in *Early Behavior: Comparative and Developmental Approaches*, ed. H. W. Stevenson, E. H. Hess, and H. L. Reingold (New York: Wiley, 1967).

[2]R. L. Collins, "On the Inheritance of Handedness II: Selection for Sinistrality in Mice," *Journal of Heredity* 60 (1969): 117–119.

[3]G. Ettlinger and D. Gautrin, "Verbal Discrimination Performance in the Monkey: The Effect of Unilateral Removal of Temporal Cortex," *Cortex* 7 (1971): 315–331.

J. M. Warren and A. J. Nonneman, "The Search for Cerebral Dominance in Monkeys," in *Origins and Evolution of Language and Speech*, ed. S. Harnad, H. Steklis, and J. Lancaster (New York: New York Academy of Sciences, 1976).

[4]J. H. Dewson, A. Cowey, and L. Weiskrantz, "Disruptions of Auditory Sequence Discrimination by Unilateral and Bilateral Cortical Ablations of Superior Temporal Gyrus in the Monkey," *Experimental Neurology* 28 (1970): 529–548.

[5]J. H. Dewson, "Preliminary Evidence of Hemispheric Asymmetry of Auditory Function in Monkeys," in *Lateralization in the Nervous System,* ed. S. Harnad, R. Doty, L. Goldstein, J. Jaynes, and G. Krauthamer (New York: Academic Press, 1977).

[6]C. R. Hamilton, "An Assessment of Hemispheric Specialization in Monkeys," in *Evolution and Lateralization of the Brain*, ed. S. Dimond and D. Blizzard (New York: New York Academy of Sciences, 1977).

[7]F. F. Ebner and R. E. Myers, "The Corpus Callosum and Interhemispheric Transmission of Tactual Learning," *Journal of Neurophysiology* 25 (1962): 380–391.

[8]J. S. Stamm and R. W. Sperry, "Function of Corpus Callosum in Contralateral Transfer of Somesthetic Discrimination in Cats," *Journal of Comparative and Physiological Psychology* 50 (1957): 138–143.

H. Gulliksen and T. Voneida, "An Attempt to Obtain Replicate Learning Curves in the Split Brain Cat," *Physiological Psychology* 3 (1975): 77–85.

J. S. Robinson and T. J. Voneida, "Hemisphere Differences in Cognitive Capacity in the Split Brain Cat," *Experimental Neurology* 38 (1973): 123–134.

[9]Hamilton, "An Assessment of Hemispheric Specialization in Monkeys."

[10]G. H. Yeni-Komshian and D. Benson, "Anatomical Study of Cerebral Asymmetry in the Temporal Lobe of Humans, Chimpanzees, and Rhesus Monkeys," *Science* 192 (1976): 387–389.

[11]M. Lemay and N. Geschwind, "Hemispheric Differences in the Brains of Great Apes," *Brain, Behavior, and Evolution* 11 (1975): 48–52.

[12]C. P. Groves and N. K. Humphrey, "Asymmetry in Gorilla Skulls: Evidence of Lateralized Brain Function?" *Nature* 244 (1973): 53–54.

[13]M. Diamond, "Age, Sex, and Environmental Influences on Anatomical Asymmetry in Rat Forebrain," in *Cerebral Dominance: The Biological Foundations*, ed. N. Geschwind and A. M. Galaburda (Cambridge, Mass.: Harvard University Press, 1984).

[14]S. Glick and D. Ross, "Lateralization of Function in the Rat Brain. Basic Mechanism May Be Operative in Humans," *Trends in the Neurosciences* 12 (1981): 196–199.

[15]E. Mach (1885), cited in Glick and Ross, "Lateralization of Function in the Rat Brain. Basic Mechanism May Be Operative in Humans."

[16]M. R. Petersen, M. D. Beecher, S. R. Zoloth, D. B. Moody, and W. C. Stebbins, "Neural Lateralization of Species-Specific Vocalizations by Japanese Macaques," *Science* 202 (1978): 324–326.

[17]F. Nottebohm, "Asymmetries in Neural Control of Vocalization in the Canary," in *Lateralization in the Nervous System*, ed. S. Harnad et al. (New York: Academic Press, 1977).

[18]N. Geschwind, "Implications for Evolution, Genetics, and Clinical Syndromes" in *Cerebral Lateralization in Nonhuman Species*," ed. S. Glick (Orlando: Academic Press, 1985).

[19]Ibid., p. 273.

## Chapter 10  Role of Asymmetry in Developmental Disabilities and Psychiatric Illness

[1]S. T. Orton, *Reading, Writing, and Speech Problems in Children* (New York: Norton, 1937).

[2]E. B. Zurif and G. Carson, "Dyslexia in Relation to Cerebral Dominance and Temporal Analysis," *Neuropsychologia* 8 (1970): 351–361.

[3]M. P. Bryden, "Dichotic Listening—Relations with Handedness and Reading in Children," *Neuropsychologia* 8 (1970): 443–450.
M. E. Thomson, "Comparison of Laterality Effects in Dyslexics and Controls Using Verbal Dichotic Listening Tasks," *Neuropsychologia* 14 (1976): 243–246.
S. F. Witelson and M. Rabinovich, "Hemispheric Speech Lateralization in Children with Auditory-Linguistic Deficits," *Cortex* 8 (1972): 412–426.

[4]T. Marcel, L. Katz, and M. Smith, "Laterality and Reading Proficiency," *Neuropsychologia* 12 (1974): 131–139.

[5]S. F. Witelson, "Abnormal Right Hemispheric Specialization in Developmental Dyslexia," in *The Neuropsychology of Learning Disorders*, ed. R. Knights and D. Bakker (Baltimore: University Park Press, 1976).

[6]G. H. Yeni-Komshian, D. Isenberg, and H. Goldberg, "Cerebral Dominance and Reading Disability: Left Visual Field Deficit in Poor Readers," *Neuropsychologia* 13 (1975): 83–94.

[7]S. F. Witelson, "Developmental Dyslexia: Two Right Hemispheres and None Left," *Science* 195 (1977): 309–311.

[8]F. Pirozzolo and K. Rayner, "Cerebral Organization and Reading Disability," *Neuropsychologia* 17 (1979): 485–491.

[9]D. Hier, M. LeMay, P. Rosenberger, and V. Perlo, "Developmental Dyslexia," *Archives of Neurology* 35 (1978): 90–92.

[10]J. G. Sheenan, *Stuttering: Research and Therapy* (New York: Harper & Row, 1970).

[11]F. K. Curry and H. H. Gregory, "The Performance of Stutterers on Dichotic Listening Tasks Thought to Reflect Cerebral Dominance," *Journal of Speech and Hearing Research* 12 (1969): 73–82.

[12]P. Quinn, "Stuttering, Cerebral Dominance, and the Dichotic Word Test," *Medical Journal of Australia* 2 (1972): 639–643.
N. Slorach and B. Noehr, "Dichotic Listening in Stuttering and Dyslalic Children," *Cortex* 9 (1973): 295–300.

[13]R. K. Jones, "Observations on Stammering After Localized Cerebral Injury," *Journal of Neurology, Neurosurgery, and Psychiatry* 29 (1966): 192–195.

[14]G. Andrews, P. T. Quinn, and W. A. Sorby, "Stuttering: An Investigation into Verbal Dominance for Speech," *Journal of Neurology, Neurosurgery, and Psychiatry* 35 (1972): 414–418.

[15]H. Sussman and P. MacNeilage, "Studies of Hemispheric Specialization for Speech Production," *Brain and Language* 2 (1975): 131–151.

[16]H. Sussman and P. MacNeilage, "Hemispheric Specialization for Speech Production in Stutterers," *Neuropsychologia* 13 (1975): 19–26.

[17]R. Heltman, "Contradictory Evidence in Handedness and Stuttering," *Journal of Speech Disorders* 5 (1940): 327–331.

[18]L. Selfe, *Nadia: A Case of Extraordinary Drawing Ability in an Autistic Child* (New York: Academic Press, 1977).

[19]D. Fein, M. Humes, E. Kaplan, D. Lucci, and L. Waterhouse, "The Question of Left Hemisphere Dysfunction in Infantile Autism," *Psychological Bulletin* 95 (1984): 258–281.

[20]G. Dawson, S. Warrenburg, and P. Fuller, "Cerebral Lateralization in Individuals Diagnosed as Autistic in Early Childhood," *Brain and Language* 15 (1982): 353–368.

[21]Fein, Humes, Kaplan, Lucci and Waterhouse, "The Question of Left Hemisphere Dysfunction in Infantile Autism."

[22]M. R. Prior and J. L. Bradshaw, "Hemispheric Functioning in Autistic Children," *Cortex* 15 (1979): 73–81.

[23]P. Flor-Henry, "Schizophrenic-like Reactions and Affective Psychoses Associated with Temporal Lobe Epilepsy: Etiological Factors," *American Journal of Psychiatry* 26 (1969): 400–403.

[24]A. E. Qalker and S. Jablon, *A Follow-up Study of Head Wounds in World War II* (Washington, D.C.: U.S. Government Printing Office, 1961).

[25]D. Galin, "Implications for Psychiatry of Left and Right Cerebral Specialization," *Archives of General Psychiatry* 31 (1974): 572–583.

[26]J. Gruzelier and N. Hammond, "Schizophrenia—A Dominant Hemisphere Temporal Lobe Disorder?" *Research Communications in Psychology, Psychiatry, and Behavior* 1 (1976): 33–72.

[27]L. Schweitzer, E. Becker, and H. Welsh, "Abnormalities of Cerebral Lateralization in Schizophrenia Patients," *Archives of General Psychiatry* 35 (1978): 982–985.

[28]G. Beaumont and S. Dimond, "Brain Disconnection and Schizophrenia," *British Journal of Psychiatry* 123 (1972): 661–662.

[29]P. Flor-Henry, "Lateralized Temporal-Limbic Dysfunction and Psychopathology," in *Origins and Evolution of Language and Speech*, ed. S. Harnad, H. Steklis, and J. Lancaster (New York: New York Academy of Sciences, 1976).

## Chapter 11   Hemisphericity, Education, and Altered States

[1]Sri Aurobindo, quoted in J. E. Bogen, "The Other Side of the Brain. VII: Some Educational Aspects of Hemispheric Specialization," *UCLA Educator* 17 (1975): 24–32.

[2]R. Ornstein, *The Psychology of Consciousness* (New York: Harcourt Brace Jovanovich, 1977).

[3]R. Ornstein, "The Split and Whole Brain," *Human Nature* 1 (1978): 76–83.

[4]H. Gardner, "What We Know (and Don't Know) about the Two Halves of the Brain," *Harvard Magazine* 80 (1978): 24–27.

[5]J. A. Paredes and M. J. Hepburn, "The Split Brain and the Culture-and-Cognition Paradox," *Current Anthropology* 17 (1976): 121–127.

[6]J. E. Bogen, R. DeZare, W. D. TenHouten, and J. F. Marsh, "The Other Side of the Brain. IV: The A/P Ratio," *Bulletin of the Los Angeles Neurological Societies* 37 (1972): 49–61.

[7]J. A. Zook and J. H. Dwyer, "Cultural Differences in Hemisphericity: A Critique" *Bulletin of the Los Angeles Neurological Societies* 41 (1976): 87–90.

[8]S. Scott, G. Hynd, L. Hunt, and W. Weed, "Cerebral Speech Lateralization in the Native American Navajo," *Neuropsychologia* 17 (1979): 89–92.

[9]W. F. McKeever, "Evidence Against the Hypothesis of Right Hemisphere Language Dominance in the Native American Navajo," *Neuropsychologia* 19 (1981): 595–598.

[10]L. Rogers, W. TenHouten, C. Kaplan, and M. Gardiner, "Hemispheric Specialization of Language: An EEG Study of Bilingual Hopi Indian Children," *International Journal of Neuroscience* 8 (1977): 1–6.

[11]Ornstein, "The Split and Whole Brain."

[12]P. Bakan, "Hypnotizability, Laterality of Eye Movement, and Functional Brain Asymmetry," *Perceptual and Motor Skills* 28 (1969): 927–932.

[13]J. Dabbs, "Left–Right Differences in Cerebral Blood Flow and Cognition," *Psychophysiology* 17 (1980): 548–551.

[14]S. Arndt and D. Berger, "Cognitive Mode and Asymmetry in Cerebral Functioning," *Cortex* 14 (1978): 78–86.

[15]E. P. Torrance and C. Reynolds, "Norms—Technical Manual for 'Your Style of Learning and Thinking,'" (Athens, Ga.: Department of Educational Psychology, University of Georgia, 1980).

[16]M. E. Humphrey and O. L. Zangwill, "Cessation of Dreaming After Brain Injury," *Journal of Neurology, Neurosurgery, and Psychiatry* 14 (1951): 322–325.

[17]P. Greenwood, D. H. Wilson, and M. S. Gazzaniga, "Dream Report Following Commissurotomy," *Cortex* 13 (1977): 311–316.

[18]K. D. Hoppe, "Split Brains and Psychoanalysis," *The Psychoanalytic Quarterly* 46 (1977): 220–224.

[19]P. Bakan, "Hypnotizability, Laterality of Eye Movements, and Functional Brain Asymmetry," *Perceptual and Motor Skills* 28 (1969): 927–932.

[20]C. MacLeod and L. Lack, "Hemispheric Specificity: A Physiological Concomitant of Hypnotizability," *Psychophysiology* 19 (1982): 687–699.

[21]P. Bakan, "Handedness and Hypnotizability," *International Journal of Clinical and Experimental Hypnosis* 18 (1970): 99–104.

[22]L. Frumkin, H. Ripley, and G. Cox, "Changes in Cerebral Hemisphere Lateralization with Hypnosis," *Biological Psychiatry* 13 (1978): 741–750.

[23]J. E. Bogen, "The Other Side of the Brain. VII: Some Educational Aspects of Hemispheric Specialization," *UCLA Educator* 17 (1975): 24–32.

[24]G. Prince, "Putting the Other Half of the Brain to Work," *Training: The Magazine of Human Resources Development* 15 (1978): 57–61.

[25]Ibid.

[26]B. Edwards, *Drawing on the Right Side of the Brain* (Los Angeles, J. P. Tarcher, 1979).

[27]C. H. Delacato, *The Treatment and Prevention of Reading Problems (The Neuropsychological Approach)* (Springfield, Ill.: Charles C. Thomas, 1959).

[28]H. J. Cohen, H. G. Birch, and L. T. Taft, "Some Considerations for Evaluating the Doman–Delacato 'Patterning' Method," *Pediatrics* 45 (1970): 302–314.

[29]American Academy of Pediatrics, "The Doman–Delacato Treatment of Neurologically Handicapped Children," *Journal of Pediatrics* 72 (1968): 750.

[30]Cohen et al., "Some Considerations for Evaluating the Doman–Delacato 'Patterning' Method."

[31]C. Sagan, *The Dragons of Eden* (New York: Random House, 1977).

[32]Ibid.

[33]Ibid.

[34]Ibid.

## Chapter 12   Concluding Hypotheses and Speculations

[1]D. Kimura and Y. Archibald, "Motor Functions of the Left Hemisphere," *Brain* 97 (1974): 337–350.

[2]Ibid.

[3]M. Studdert-Kennedy and D. Shankweiler, "Hemispheric Specialization for Speech Perception, *Journal of the Acoustical Society of America* 48 (1970): 579–594.

[4]J. Schwartz and P. Tallal, "Rate of Acoustic Change May Underlie Hemispheric Specialization for Speech Perception," *Science* 207 (1980): 1380–1381.

[5]A. M. Liberman, F. S. Cooper, D. Shankweiler, and M. Studdert-Kennedy, "Perceptions of the Speech Code," *Psychological Review* 74 (1967): 431–461.

[6]E. Goldberg and L. D. Costa, "Hemispheric Differences in the Acquisition and Use of Descriptive Systems," *Brain and Language* 14 (1981): 144–173.

[7]E. Goldberg, H. G. Vaughan, Jr., and L. J. Gerstman, "Nonverbal Descriptive Systems and Hemispheric Asymmetry: Shape versus Texture Discrimination," *Brain and Language* 5 (1978): 249–257.

[8]D. Van Lancker and V. A. Fromkin, "Hemispheric Specialization for Pitch and 'Tone': Evidence from Thai," *Journal of Phonetics* 1 (1973): 101–109.

[9]T. G. Bever and K. Chiarello, "Cerebral Dominance in Musicians and Non-Musicians," *Science* 185 (1974): 537–539.

[10]C. J. Connoly, *External Morphology of the Primate Brain* (Springfield, Ill.: Thomas, 1950).

M. LeMay and A. Culebras, "Human Brain—Morphologic Differences in the Hemispheres Demonstrable by Carotid Arteriography," *New England Journal of Medicine* 287 (1972): 168–170.

A. M. Galaburda, M. LeMay, T. L. Kemper, and N. Geschwind, "Right–Left Asymmetries in the Brain," *Science* 199 (1978): 852–856.

[11]M. LeMay, "Morphological Cerebral Asymmetries of Modern Man, Fossil Man, and Nonhuman Primate," in *Origins and Evolution of Language and Speech*, ed. S. R. Harnad, H. D. Steklis, and J. Lancas-

ter. *Annals of the New York Academy of Sciences* 280 (1976): 349–366.

J. A. Wada, R. Clarke, and A. Hamm, "Cerebral Hemispheric Asymmetry in Humans," *Archives of Neurology* 32 (1975): 239–246.

[12]H. A. Whitaker and G. A. Ojemann, "Lateralization of the Higher Cortical Functions: A Critique," in *Evolution and Lateralization of the Brain*, ed. S. J. Dimond and D. A. Blizard. *Annals of the New York Academy of Sciences* 299 (1977): 459–473.

[13]R. C. Gur, I. K. Packer, J. P. Hungerbuhler, M. Reivich, W. D. Obrist, W. S. Amarnek, and H. A. Sackheim, "Differences in the Distribution of Gray and White Matter in Human Cerebral Hemispheres," *Science* 207 (1980): 1226–1228.

[14]J. Semmes, "Hemispheric Specialization: A Possible Clue to Mechanism," *Neuropsychologia* 6 (1968): 11–26.

[15]B. Kohn and M. Dennis, "Patterns of Hemisphere Specialization after Hemidecortication for Infantile Hemiplegia," in *Hemisphere Disconnection and Cerebral Function*, ed. M. Kinsbourne and W. L. Smith (Springfield, Ill.: Thomas, 1974).

[16]Goldberg and Costa, *"Hemispheric Differences in the Acquisition and Use of Descriptive Systems."*

[17]J. Levy, "Interhemispheric Collaboration: Single Mindedness in the Asymmetrical Brain," in *Hemispheric Function and Collaboration in the Child*, ed. C. T. Best (New York: Academic Press, 1985).

[18]N. D. Cook, "The Transmission of Information in Natural Systems," *Journal of Theoretical Biology* 108 (1984): 349–367.

N. D. Cook, "Callosal Inhibition: The Key to the Brain Code," *Behavioral Science* 29 (1984): 98–110.

[19]Ibid.

[20]S. H. Woodward, "An Anatomical Model of Hemispheric Asymmetry," *Journal of Clinical and Experimental Neuropsychology* 10 (1988): 68.

[21]G. Hinton, J. L.McClelland, and D. E. Rumelhart, "Distributed Representations," in *Parallel Distributed Processing: Explorations in the Microstructure of Cognition, Vol. 1: Foundations*, ed. D. E. Rumelhart, J. L. McClelland, and the PDP Research Group (Cambridge, Mass.: MIT Press, 1986).

[22]S. H. Woodward, "An Anatomical Model of Hemispheric Asymmetry."

[23]M. Dennis and H. Whittaker, "Hemispheric Equipotentiality and Language Acquisition," in *Language Development and Neurological Theory*, ed. S. J. Segalowitz and F. A. Gruber (New York: Academic Press, 1977).

[24]P. Somogyi and A. Cowey, "Double-Bouquet Cells," in *Cerebral Cortex: Vol. 1: Cellular Components of the Cerebral Cortex*, ed. A. Peters and E. G. Jones (Berlin: Springer, 1973).

[25]R. W. Sperry, "Brain Bisection and Consciousness," in *Brain and Conscious Experience*, ed. J. Eccles (New York: Springer-Verlag, 1966.)

[26]Eccles, *The Brain and Unity of Conscious Experience: The 19th Arthur Stanley Eddington Memorial Lecture* (Cambridge: Cambridge University Press, 1965).

[27]J. E. LeDoux, D. H. Wilson, and M. S. Gazzaniga, "A Divided Mind: Observation on the Conscious Properties of the Separated Hemispheres," *Annals of Neurology* 2 (1977): 417–421.

[28]Ibid.

[29]J. Jaynes, cited in S. Keen, "Reflections on the Dawn of Consciousness," *Psychology Today* 11 (1977): 58.

[30]Ibid.

[31]O. Loewi, *Perspectives in Biology and Medicine* 4 (Chicago: University of Chicago Press, 1960).

[32]A. Koestler, *The Act of Creation* (New York: Dell, 1964).

[33]Ibid.

[34]D. Galin, "Implications for Psychiatry of Left and Right Cerebral Specialization," *Archives of General Psychiatry* 31 (1974): 572–583.

[35]Ibid.

[36]Ibid.

[37]LeDoux et al., "A Divided Mind: Observations on the Conscious Properties of the Separated Hemispheres."

[38]M. S. Gazzaniga and J. E. LeDoux, *The Integrated Mind* (New York: Plenum Press, 1978).

[39]Ibid.

[40]R. Puccetti, "The Case for Mental Duality: Evidence from Split Brain Data and Other Considerations," *The Behavioral and Brain Sciences* 4 (1981): 93–123.

[41]Ibid.

[42]Ibid.

[43]Ibid.

[44]R. W. Sperry, E. Zaidel, and D. Zaidel, "Self Recognition and Social Awareness in the Disconnected Minor Hemisphere," *Neuropsychologia* 17 (1979): 153–166.

[45]Ibid.

[46]D. N. Robinson, "Cerebral Plurality and the Unity of Self," *American Psychologist* 37 (1982): 904–910.

[47]G. Sperling, "The Information Available in Brief Visual Presentations," *Psychological Monographs* 74 (1960): (11, Whole No. 498).

[48]D. H. Raab, "Backward Masking," *Psychological Bulletin* 60 (1963): 118–129.

[49]A. Binet, *Alterations of Personality* (H. Baldwin, trans.) (New York: Appleton, 1896).

[50]D. N. Robinson, "Cerebral Plurality and the Unity of Self."

[51]Ibid.

[52]R. Dubos, *Pasteur and Modern Science* (London: Heinemann, 1960).

[53]M. C. Corballis and I. L. Beale, *The Ambivalent Mind* (Chicago: Nelson-Hall, 1983).

[54]L. Wolpert, "Pattern Formation in Biological Development" *Scientific American* 239 (1978): 124–137.

[55]Corballis and Beale, *The Ambivalent Mind.*

[56]Ibid.

[57]B. Norden, "The Asymmetry of Life," *Journal of Molecular Evolution* 11 (1978): 313–332.

[58]E. M. Henley, "Parity and Time-Reversal Invariance in Nuclear Physics," *Annual Review of Nuclear Science* 19 (1969): 367–427.

[59]Corballis and Beale, *The Ambivalent Mind.*

# Index